PET/CT

Editor

YONG C. BRADLEY

RADIOLOGIC CLINICS
OF NORTH AMERICA

www.radiologic.theclinics.com

Consulting Editor
FRANK H. MILLER

September 2013 • Volume 51 • Number 5

ELSEVIER

1600 John F. Kennedy Boulevard • Suite 1800 • Philadelphia, Pennsylvania, 19103-2899

http://www.theclinics.com

RADIOLOGIC CLINICS OF NORTH AMERICA Volume 51, Number 5
September 2013 ISSN 0033-8389, ISBN 13: 978-1-4557-7610-8

Editor: Adrianne Brigido

Radiologic Clinics of North America (ISSN 0033-8389) is published bimonthly by Elsevier Inc., 360 Park Avenue South, New York, NY 10010-1710. Months of issue are January, March, May, July, September, and November. Periodicals postage paid at New York, NY and additional mailing offices. Subscription prices are USD 438 per year for US individuals, USD 685 per year for US institutions, USD 210 per year for US students and residents, USD 511 per year for Canadian individuals, USD 858 per year for Canadian institutions, USD 630 per year for international individuals, USD 858 per year for international institutions, and USD 302 per year for Canadian and foreign students/residents. To receive student and resident rate, orders must be accompanied by name of affiliated institution, date of term and the signature of program/residency coordinatior on institution letterhead. Orders will be billed at individual rate until proof of status is received. Foreign air speed delivery is included in all *Clinics* subscription prices. All prices are subject to change without notice. **POSTMASTER:** Send address changes to *Radiologic Clinics of North America*, Elsevier Health Sciences Division, Subscription Customer Service, 3251 Riverport Lane, Maryland Heights, MO63043. **Customer Service: Telephone: 1-800-654-2452** (U.S. and Canada); **1-314-447-8871** (outside U.S. and Canada). **Fax: 1-314-447-8029. E-mail: journalscustomerservice-usa@ elsevier.com** (for print support); **journalsonlinesupport-usa@elsevier.com** (for online support).

Reprints. For copies of 100 or more of articles in this publication, please contact the Commercial Reprints Department, Elsevier Inc., 360 Park Avenue South, New York, New York 10010-1710. Tel.: (+1) 212-633-3874; Fax: (+1) 212-633-3820; E-mail: reprints@elsevier.com.

Radiologic Clinics of North America also published in Greek Paschalidis Medical Publications, Athens, Greece.

Radiologic Clinics of North America is covered in *MEDLINE/PubMed (Index Medicus), EMBASE/Excerpta Medica, Current Contents/Life Sciences, Current Contents/Clinical Medicine, RSNA Index to Imaging Literature, BIOSIS, Science Citation Index,* and *ISI/BIOMED.*

Printed in the United States of America.

Contributors

CONSULTING EDITOR

FRANK H. MILLER, MD
Professor of Radiology; Chief, Body Imaging,
Section and Fellowship Program and GI
Radiology; Medical Director MRI, Department
of Radiology, Feinberg School of Medicine,
Northwestern University, Chicago, Illinois

EDITOR

YONG C. BRADLEY, MD
University of Tennessee Medical Center,
Knoxville, Tennessee

AUTHORS

MARTIN ALLEN-AUERBACH, MD
Ahmanson Translational Imaging Division/
Nuclear Medicine, Department of Molecular
and Medical Pharmacology, David Geffen
School of Medicine at UCLA, Los Angeles,
California

KEVIN P. BANKS, MD
Department of Radiology, Brooke Army
Medical Center, San Antonio Health Care
System; Department of Radiology, University
of Texas Health Science Center at San Antonio,
San Antonio, Texas; Department of Radiology,
Uniformed Services University of Health
Sciences, Bethesda, Maryland

AUSTIN C. BOURGEOIS, MD
University of Tennessee Medical Center,
Knoxville, Tennessee

YONG C. BRADLEY, MD
University of Tennessee Medical Center,
Knoxville, Tennessee

JACQUELINE BRUNETTI, MD
Director of Radiology, Department of
Radiology, Holy Name Medical Center,
Teaneck, New Jersey; Associate Clinical

Professor of Radiology, NewYork-Presbyterian
Hospital/Columbia University Medical Center,
New York, New York

TED T. CHANG, MD
University of Tennessee Medical Center,
Knoxville, Tennessee

JUNZO CHINO, MD
Assistant Professor, Department of Radiation
Oncology, Duke University Medical Center,
Durham, North Carolina

JOHANNES CZERNIN, MD
Ahmanson Translational Imaging Division/
Nuclear Medicine, Department of Molecular
and Medical Pharmacology, David Geffen
School of Medicine at UCLA, Los Angeles,
California

SHIVA DAS, PhD
Professor, Department of Radiation Oncology,
Duke University Medical Center, Durham,
North Carolina

SVEN DE VOS, MD, PhD
Division of Hematology/Oncology, Department
of Medicine, David Geffen School of Medicine
at UCLA, Los Angeles, California

SCOTT EMBRY, MD
University of Tennessee Medical Center,
Knoxville, Tennessee

EDWARD J. ESCOTT, MD
Associate Professor, Division of
Neuroradiology, Department of Radiology,
University of Kentucky Medical Center,
Lexington, Kentucky

TODD FAASSE, MPH, CNMT(PET), RT(N)(CT)
Radiologic Technologist, Nuclear Medicine
and Computed Tomography, Department of
Radiology, Spectrum Health Lemmen Holton
Cancer Pavillion, Grand Rapids, Michigan

LINDSAY M. FISH, MD
University of Tennessee Medical Center,
Knoxville, Tennessee

SIDNEY R. HINDS II, MD
Walter Reed National Military Medical Center,
Bethesda, Maryland

KATHLEEN HUDSON, MD
University of Tennessee Medical Center,
Knoxville, Tennessee

PATRICK J. PELLER, MD
Program Director, Nuclear Radiology;
Assistant Professor, Department of Radiology,
College of Medicine, Mayo Clinic, Rochester,
Minnesota

PAUL SHREVE, MD
Advanced Radiology Services, P.C., and
Medical Director of PET-CT, Spectrum Health,
Grand Rapids, Michigan

WON S. SONG, MD
Department of Radiology, Brooke Army
Medical Center, San Antonio Health Care
System, San Antonio, Texas

DEREK J. STOCKER, MD
Walter Reed National Military Medical Center,
Bethesda, Maryland

LANCE A. WARREN, MD
University of Tennessee Medical Center,
Knoxville, Tennessee

TERENCE WONG, MD, PhD
Associate Professor, Department of Radiology,
Duke University Medical Center, Durham,
North Carolina

Contents

Positron emission tomography (PET)–computed tomography (CT) has become a routine imaging modality in body oncology and is particularly well suited for the management of patients with lung cancer. Current clinical applications of PET-CT in patients with lung cancer include evaluation of indeterminate pulmonary nodules, initial staging of lung cancer, restaging of lung cancer following treatment, and radiation therapy planning. Contemporary PET-CT scanners allow comprehensive diagnostic PET and CT imaging in a single imaging session. Interpretation and reporting of PET-CT examinations of patients with lung cancer require a thorough and integrated approach taking advantage of the anatomic and metabolic information.

Although positron emission tomography (PET) imaging may not be used in the diagnosis of breast cancer, the use of PET/computed tomography is imperative in all aspects of breast cancer staging, treatment, and follow-up. PET will continue to be relevant in personalized medicine because accurate tumor status will be even more critical during and after the transition from a generic metabolic agent to receptor imaging. Positron emission mammography is an imaging proposition that may have benefits in lower doses, but its use is limited without new radiopharmaceuticals.

Positron emission tomography (PET) has proved itself to be valuable in the evaluation of patients with a wide array of gastrointestinal (GI) malignancies. Subsequent development of fusion imaging with PET and computed tomography (PET-CT) scanners has significantly advanced the capabilities of imaging by combining the functional data of the ^{18}F-labeled glucose analogue fluorodeoxyglucose (FDG) with the conventional anatomic data provided by CT. This article reviews the evolving role of FDG PET-CT imaging in the initial assessment and monitoring of GI tumors. Specific applications are discussed, and normal variants and benign findings frequently encountered during PET-CT of the GI tract are reviewed.

[^{18}F]Fluorodeoxyglucose (FDG) positron emission tomography (PET)/computed tomography (CT) scans provide patients and referring physicians with diagnostic

PET and CT information in a single imaging session. Because most lymphomas show high glucose metabolic activity and FDG avidity, they can be reliably assessed with FDG-PET/CT. PET/CT has emerged as the modality of choice for treatment strategy assessments in patients with lymphoma. Its ability to characterize masses as benign or malignant and its high sensitivity and specificity for staging, restaging, and treatment monitoring have led to widespread acceptance of PET imaging for managing patients with lymphoma.

This article presents an overview of positron emission tomography combined with computed tomography (PET/CT) imaging of bone tumors for the practicing radiologist. The clinical roles and utility of ^{18}F-labeled fluorodeoxyglucose PET/CT in patients with primary bone tumors, osseous metastases, and multiple myeloma are reviewed. The clinical and research data supporting the utility of PET/CT in the evaluation of skeletal malignancies continues to grow.

Fludeoxyglucose F 18 positron emission tomography/computed tomography (PET/CT) has been invaluable in the assessment of melanoma throughout the course of the disease. As with any modality, the studies are incomplete and more information will be gleaned as our experience progresses. Additionally, it is hoped that a newer PET agent in the pipeline will give us even greater success in the identification and subsequent treatment of melanoma. This article aims to examine the utilization of PET/CT in the staging, prognostication, and follow-up of melanoma while providing the physicians who order and interpret these studies practical guidelines and interpretive pitfalls.

Positron emission tomography/computed tomography (PET/CT) has an important role in the diagnosis and treatment of head and neck cancer. The technique can aid in the detection of an unknown primary tumor, assist in locoregional staging, evaluate for distant metastases or second primary tumors, and be a component of restaging and tumor surveillance. This article reviews the basic principles, pitfalls, and uses of PET/CT in head and neck cancer, as well as potential future applications.

Ovarian cancer and malignancies of the uterine cervix and corpus are the most commonly encountered gynecologic neoplasms in clinical practice. Although of little value in both diagnosis and early-stage gynecologic malignancy, fluorodeoxyglucose-PET and PET/computed tomography provide accurate detection of metastatic disease in advanced malignancy and better delineation of recurrent disease compared with conventional imaging.

PROGRAM OBJECTIVE:

The objective of the Radiologic Clinics of North America is to keep practicing radiologists and radiology residents up to date with current clinical practice in radiology by providing timely articles reviewing the state of the art in patient care.

TARGET AUDIENCE

Practicing radiologists, radiology residents, and other health care professionals who provide patient care utilizing radiologic findings.

LEARNING OBJECTIVES

Upon completion of this activity, participants will be able to:
1. Review the role of PET-CT in pulmonary neoplasms, head and neck cancer, gastrointestinal malignancies, lymphoma, bone malignancies, gynecologic malignancies, breast cancer, and dementia.
2. Discuss PET in radiation treatment planning.
3. Recognize the potential of metabolic imaging.

ACCREDITATION

The Elsevier Office of Continuing Medical Education (EOCME) is accredited by the Accreditation Council for Continuing Medical Education (ACCME) to provide continuing medical education for physicians.

The EOCME designates this enduring material for a maximum of 15 *AMA PRA Category 1 Credit*(s) ™. Physicians should claim only the credit commensurate with the extent of their participation in the activity.

All other health care professionals requesting continuing education credit for this enduring material will be issued a certificate of participation.

DISCLOSURE OF CONFLICTS OF INTEREST

The EOCME assesses conflict of interest with its instructors, faculty, planners, and other individuals who are in a position to control the content of CME activities. All relevant conflicts of interest that are identified are thoroughly vetted by EOCME for fair balance, scientific objectivity, and patient care recommendations. EOCME is committed to providing its learners with CME activities that promote improvements or quality in healthcare and not a specific proprietary business or a commercial interest.

The planning committee, staff, authors and editors listed below have identified no financial relationships or relationships to products or devices they or their spouse/life partner have with commercial interest related to the content of this CME activity:
Martin Allen-Auerbach, MD; Kevin P. Banks, MD; Austin C. Bourgeois, MD; Yong C. Bradley, MD; Adrianne Brigido; Jacqueline Brunetti, MD; Ted T. Chang, MD; Junzo Chino, MD; Nicole Congleton; Johannes Czernin, MD; Shiva Das, PhD; Sven de Vos, MD, PhD; Scott D. Embry; Todd Faasse, CNMT, MS; Lindsay M. Fish, MD; Sidney R. Hinds, MD; Kathleen Hudson, MD; Brynne Hunter; Sandy Lavery; Jill McNair; Frank H. Miller, MD; Paul Shreve, MD; Won S. Song, MD; Derek J. Stocker, MD; Karthikeyan Subramaniam; Lance A. Warren, MD.

The planning committee, staff, authors and editors listed below have identified financial relationships or relationships to products or devices they or their spouse/life partner have with commercial interest related to the content of this CME activity:
Edward J. Escott, MD has royalties/patents with Thieme Medical Publishers, Inc. and has a research grant from Athersys, Inc.
Patrick J. Peller, MD is on speakers bureau for Eli Lilly and Company.
Terence Wong, MD, PhD is a consultant/advisor for Eli Lilly and Company and Bayer AG.

UNAPPROVED/OFF-LABEL USE DISCLOSURE

The EOCME requires CME faculty to disclose to the participants:
1. When products or procedures being discussed are off-label, unlabelled, experimental, and/or investigational (not US Food and Drug Administration (FDA) approved); and
2. Any limitations on the information presented, such as data that are preliminary or that represent ongoing research, interim analyses, and/or unsupported opinions. Faculty may discuss information about pharmaceutical agents that is outside of FDA-approved labelling. This information is intended solely for CME and is not intended to promote off-label use of these medications. If you have any questions, contact the medical affairs department of the manufacturer for the most recent prescribing information.

TO ENROLL

To enroll in the *Radiologic Clinics of North America* Continuing Medical Education program, call customer service at 1-800-654-2452 or sign up online at http://www.theclinics.com/home/cme. The CME program is available to subscribers for an additional annual fee of USD 288.

METHOD OF PARTICIPATION

In order to claim credit, participants must complete the following:
1. Complete enrolment as indicated above.
2. Read the activity.
3. Complete the CME Test and Evaluation. Participants must achieve a score of 70% on the test. All CME Tests and Evaluations must be completed online.

CME INQUIRIES/SPECIAL NEEDS

For all CME inquiries or special needs, please contact elsevierCME@elsevier.com.

RADIOLOGIC CLINICS OF NORTH AMERICA

Dedication

I am dedicating this issue to my father, J. T. Bradley, who, after a prolonged battle, passed away on March 1, 2013 of pancreatic cancer; ironically, a cancer not well assessed using PET/CT. I love you, Dad, for you and Mom always provided strong and silent support throughout my life. I am also dedicating this issue to my family, who always supports me with unfailing and overflowing love.

Yong C. Bradley, MD
University of Tennessee Medical Center
1924 Alcoa Highway
Knoxville, TN 37920, USA

E-mail address:
YBradley@mc.utmck.edu

Radiol Clin N Am 51 (2013) xi
http://dx.doi.org/10.1016/j.rcl.2013.08.009
0033-8389/13/$ – see front matter © 2013 Published by Elsevier Inc.

Role of Positron Emission Tomography–Computed Tomography in Pulmonary Neoplasms

Paul Shreve, MD[a],*, Todd Faasse, MPH, CNMT(PET), RT(N)(CT)[b]

KEYWORDS

- FDG-PET • CT • PET-CT • Lung cancer • Diagnosis and staging

KEY POINTS

- Positron emission tomography (PET)–computed tomography (CT) is now a well-established imaging modality for the management of patients with lung cancer.
- Fully diagnostic anatomic and metabolic registered image sets can be rapidly obtained in a single examination session using contemporary PET-CT scanners.
- Interpretation and reporting of these imaging examinations can be demanding and time consuming, but provide indispensable information for initial diagnosis and staging, therapy response assessment, and radiation therapy planning.

INTRODUCTION

Computed tomography (CT) revolutionized the management of patients with cancer for diagnosis, staging, and assessing disease response to therapy. Continued improvements in the speed and spatial and contrast resolution of CT scanners has ushered in new eras of radiation therapy and image-guided therapies. Nonetheless, diagnosis and assessment by CT alone is limited to static anatomic features and any additional information contrast enhancement provides.

Imaging of tissue physiology using radiotracers was substantially bolstered by the development of positron emission tomography (PET) using the glucose analogue 2-[F-18]-fluoro-2-deoxy-D-glucose (FDG). In the late 1980s and early 1990s it became clear FDG imaging would depict the deranged glucose metabolism of a wide variety of malignant neoplasms. Among the first applications of body FDG-PET oncologic imaging was assessment of indeterminate pulmonary nodules and preoperative staging of non–small cell lung cancer.[1,2] FDG-PET body imaging was, to varying degrees, interpreted in conjunction with CT images performed on a separate CT scanner even though image registration was imperfect. In the 1990s, Townsend and Nutt developed an approach using a combined PET and CT scanner with a common gantry and rapid sequencing of the CT and PET image acquisitions permitting close imaging registration and explicitly merging anatomic and metabolic imaging diagnoses.[3] It soon became apparent that explicitly merging the two modalities resulted in improvements in diagnostic accuracy compared with FDG-PET and CT performed separately, and, specifically in the case of lung cancer, rigorous prospective studies showed that use of PET-CT could reduce unnecessary thoracotomies.[4]

[a] Advanced Radiology Services, P.C., Spectrum Health, 3264 North Evergreen Drive, Grand Rapids, MI 49525, USA; [b] Nuclear Medicine and Computed Tomography, Department of Radiology, Spectrum Health Lemmen Holton Cancer Pavillion, 145 Michigan Street, Suite 2100, Grand Rapids, MI 49503, USA
* Corresponding author.
E-mail address: pshreve@earthlink.net

Radiol Clin N Am 51 (2013) 767–779
http://dx.doi.org/10.1016/j.rcl.2013.05.001

PET-CT is now a routine body oncology imaging modality, and is particularly well suited for patients with lung cancer. Current clinical applications of FDG-PET-CT imaging in patients with lung cancer are listed in **Box 1**.

INDETERMINATE PULMONARY NODULE

Anatomic features such as size, spiculation, and contrast-enhancement features can give some indication of the likelihood that a nodule represents a primary lung cancer, and certain calcification patterns are considered diagnostic for a benign nodule. Unless a pulmonary nodule has a clear-cut benign calcification pattern or has been stable for at least 2 years,[5] malignancy cannot be reliably excluded. However, the presence of a PET-positive pulmonary nodule greatly increases the likelihood of malignancy and can significantly influence management decisions. It must be emphasized that a PET-positive or PET-negative nodule is not a perfect binary distinction with respect to a malignant or benign nature. The FDG-PET findings must be put in a broader context of anatomic findings and clinical information to arrive at the final patient management decision. **Table 1** shows some of the many clinical factors and imaging findings that contribute to the likelihood of a solitary pulmonary nodule being malignant.

Management of pulmonary nodules that are not clearly benign, such as a densely calcified granuloma, comes down to a decision to remove the nodule, biopsy the nodule by percutaneous or bronchoscopic means, or follow the nodule for growth by serial CT imaging. This management decision is typically made by the surgeon or pulmonologist in consultation with the patients and their families, and in some instances their primary care physician as well. Treatment alternatives to resection of a pulmonary nodule increasingly include stereotactic radiation therapy or percutaneous CT-guided radiotherapy ablation, although such methods almost always require tissue proof of malignancy and imaging-based staging studies.

Table 1 Malignancy likelihood ratios for a solitary pulmonary nodule	
Age 10–29 y	0.05
Age 60–89 y	2.6
Nonsmoker status	0.15
30–39 pack-years smoking	0.74
40 pack-years smoking	3.7
Hemoptysis	5.1
Nodule size 0–1 cm	0.52
Nodule size 1–2 cm	0.74
Nodule size 2–3 cm	3.7
Nodule size >3 m	5.2
Noncalcified nodule	2.2
Benign calcifications	0.01
Lobulated nodule	0.74
Spiculated nodule	5.5
Malignant growth rate	3.4
FDG-PET–positive nodule	4.3
FDG-PET–negative nodule	0.4

Data from Gurney JW. Determining the likelihood of malignancy in solitary pulmonary nodules with Bayesian analysis. Part I. Theory. Radiology 1993;186:405–13.

The practical indications of FDG-PET-CT in assessment of indeterminate pulmonary nodules in isolation are limited, because the indication often merges with the task of initial staging of lung cancer. A large spiculated noncalcified nodule or pulmonary mass (>3 cm maximum dimension) in a patient with a long smoking history is a malignancy until proved otherwise, and the imaging examination is treated as a staging study, even before histologic proof of malignancy is obtained. In contrast, small pulmonary nodules, generally less then 6 mm as measured on lung window images, are too small to be reliably detected on FDG-PET due to the reconstructed image resolution limitations of even contemporary PET tomographs,[6] necessitating serial CT assessment of the growth of FDG-PET–negative nodules, currently using at least the Fleischner Society criteria.[5] An FDG-PET–negative nodule may allow reduced CT follow-up frequency than is delineated in the Fleischner Society criteria, but consensus criteria for follow-up of pulmonary nodules negative on FDG-PET have not yet been reached.

Focal ground-glass opacities seen on CT imaging, raising the possibility of adenocarcinoma in situ, are formally referred to as bronchoalveolar carcinoma and are found on CT in routine practice (**Fig. 1**). These malignancies are characterized by slow growth but retain malignant potential.[7] Because of the typical low FDG avidity of

---

Box 1
Current clinical applications of PET-CT in the management of patients with lung cancer

- Indeterminate pulmonary nodule
- Pulmonary mass: suspected lung cancer
- Initial staging of lung cancer
- Restaging lung cancer following treatment
- Radiation therapy planning

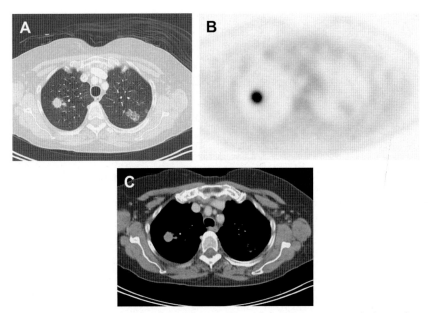

Fig. 1. PET-CT evaluation of pulmonary nodule. PET-CT was performed to assess an indeterminate pulmonary nodule in the right upper lobe. The CT image set (A, C) reveals a noncalcified pulmonary nodule in the right upper lobe, which on lung algorithm reconstruction/lung window images (B) is slightly lobulated with subtle spiculations. In the left upper lobe there is a 2.4 × 1.7 cm ground-glass opacity lacking a solid soft tissue component and a tiny satellite ground-glass opacity. The FDG-PET image set (B) shows intense FDG uptake in the right upper lobe nodule and only minimal FDG tracer activity, less than mediastinal background tracer activity, in the left upper lobe ground-glass opacity. Morphologic features as well as metabolic activity of pulmonary nodules should always be incorporated in PET-CT evaluation of pulmonary nodules.

these neoplasms and confounding false-positive potential of pulmonary inflammation, including in ground-glass pulmonary opacities, FDG-PET is only of limited additive value compared with CT alone.[8] The finding of a solid soft tissue component on CT imaging, growth on serial CT imaging, and possible biopsy, remain the mainstays for determining malignant potential of focal ground-glass opacities.

INITIAL STAGING OF LUNG CANCER

PET-CT can now be considered the standard of practice for staging non–small cell lung cancer, either suspected or histologically proven. There is a large body of accumulated peer-reviewed literature showing the improved sensitivity and specificity of FDG-PET compared with CT alone, and further improvement in diagnostic performance and effect on patient management of combined PET-CT compared with independently performed FDG-PET and CT.[9–11]

As locoregional spread of lung cancer is to hilar and mediastinal lymph nodes, adding FDG-PET to CT increases diagnostic accuracy by detecting metastatic involvement of nonenlarged nodes. Distant metastatic patterns for non–small cell lung cancer include chiefly liver, adrenal glands,

and bone, and here FDG-PET provides sensitivity for the small metastases easily overlooked on CT interpretation or occult on the CT images. Lung cancer also has a propensity for soft tissue metastases, especially in the setting of treated disease, and these are often depicted on FDG-PET and only identified on CT as easily overlooked or subtle findings. The metastases to the brain are not well detected on FDG-PET, and contrast-enhanced dedicated brain CT or magnetic resonance (MR) imaging is required to exclude brain metastases. Lung cancer staging is by the tumor-node-metastasis (TNM) classification and there have been recent updates to the TNM staging criteria for non–small cell and small cell lung cancer by the Joint Commission on Cancer.[12] PET-CT combines the advantages of CT for largely anatomically defined criteria such as T stage with the added sensitivity of FDG-PET metabolic assessment of small nodal or distant metastatic disease defining N and M stage (**Fig. 2**).

THERAPY RESPONSE ASSESSMENT

Therapy response assessment can be broadly thought of as both assessing response of malignant disease to therapy during the course of therapy, usually referred to as therapy monitoring, and

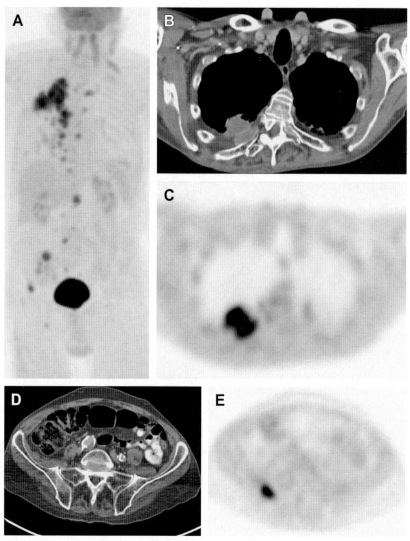

Fig. 2. PET-CT initial staging of lung cancer. PET-CT was performed for initial staging for a right upper lobe mass positive for non–small cell lung cancer on bronchoscopic biopsy. The maximum intensity projection FDG-PET image (A) shows a large hypermetabolic mass in the right hemithorax and multiple foci of abnormal FDG tracer activity in a distribution consistent with multiple osseous metastases. Transaxial CT and FDG-PET images (B, C) show the right upper lobe mass invading the posterior chest wall. The osseous metastases are readily shown on the FDG-PET images, but are seen on CT as only subtle sclerosis (D, E). The combined modality imaging combines the strengths of the precise anatomic delineation of CT with the sensitivity of the FDG metabolic assessment in a single imaging session generating registered and aligned CT and FDG-PET images sets.

restaging of extent of malignant disease following completion of a therapy regimen.[13] In either case, the imaging examination is performed for the purpose of guiding subsequent treatment, be it systemic or directed.

Restaging is becoming a more common indication for imaging of patients with lung cancer due to the continued improvements in treatment strategies with attendant increases in patient survival. The FDG-PET component of the PET-CT examination is particularly helpful in identifying recurrent malignancy in regions of postoperative or radiation therapy–induced soft tissue scarring, and, as with initial staging, identifying manifestations of locoregional or distant metastatic disease easily overlooked or occult on CT imaging alone (Fig. 3).

A developing application of FDG-PET imaging is therapy monitoring early in the course of chemotherapy or assessing neoadjunctive therapy before completion. FDG-PET has been shown to predict response of malignancy before anatomic changes of response are depicted on anatomic imaging in

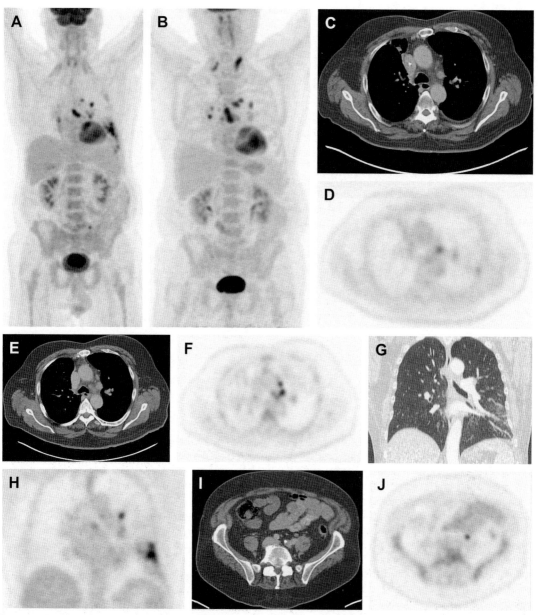

Fig. 3. PET-CT restaging of lung cancer. PET-CT was performed to assess disease status following chemoradiation therapy for recurrent lung cancer. Right upper lobe squamous cell carcinoma was treated by lobectomy but subsequently locoregional metastases to mediastinal, hilar, and supraclavicular lymph nodes developed. FDG-PET maximum intensity projection images after chemoradiation therapy (*A*) and before chemoradiation therapy (*B*) show resolution of the hypermetabolic supraclavicular nodes and improvement in the extent and intensity of the hypermetabolic mediastinal and hilar nodal metastases. Less intense FDG tracer activity is seen at the left lung base on the post treatment image, reflecting development of pneumonitis. A new tiny focus of increased FDG tracer activity is seen on the posttreatment image projecting adjacent to the medial left iliac crest. CT and FDG-PET images (*C, D*) show decrease in size and metabolism of aortopulmonary window lymph node metastases compared with the prechemoradiation study (*E, F*), but the persistent abnormal glucose metabolism in the remaining lymph node indicates a partial response. Radiation pneumonitis has developed at the left lung base (*G, H*); note the intensity of FDG uptake relative to the modest CT findings. The tiny focus of FDG tracer activity in the pelvis seen on the maximum intensity projection images corresponds with a 7-mm left common iliac lymph node, which is clearly hypermetabolic (*I, J*), and is a new finding compared with the prechemoradiation study (*K, L*), and indicates that a distant metastasis has developed outside the radiation-treated nodal basin volumes in the thorax. The loss of normal bone marrow FDG tracer activity throughout the thoracic spine on the posttreatment FDG-PET image compared with the pretreatment images (*M, N*) is expected following radiation therapy and reflects the extent of radiation treatment field in the thorax.

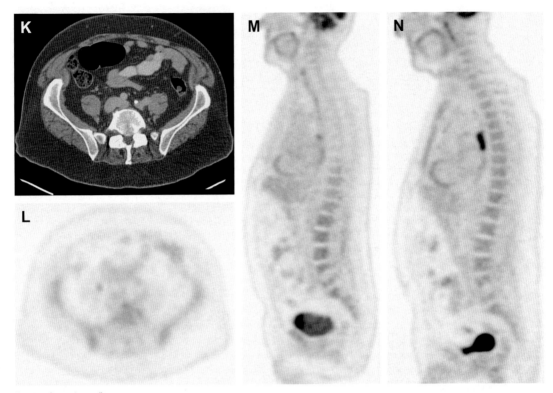

Fig. 3. (*continued*)

several cancers, particularly lymphoma.[14] There is emerging evidence that PET-CT can predict the benefit of neoadjunctive chemotherapy in patients with advanced-stage lung cancer[15]; however, presently such therapy monitoring cannot be considered a routine clinical indication for PET-CT in patients with lung cancer. In addition, although PET-CT is well suited for surveillance (imaging for recurrent disease when there are no clinical or laboratory findings to suggest disease recurrence), this is generally not an indication recognized by payors.

RADIATION THERAPY PLANNING

Cross-sectional imaging has revolutionized radiation therapy planning and treatment effectiveness by allowing for conformational focus of radiation using three-dimensional plans based on CT or MR imaging. The goal of radiation therapy is to control locoregional disease in the absence of distant metastatic disease. Here the value of adding FDG-PET to CT to detect unsuspected distant metastatic disease is a principal advantage of PET-CT in the evaluation of a patient under consideration for radiation therapy. To optimize conformational treatment plans, the radiation oncologist must know the precise delineation of

the primary malignant mass and the extent of locoregional nodal disease. Adding FDG-PET to the currently used CT imaging at simulation is becoming more widespread due to the improved delineation of tumor mass margins and assessment of locoregional tumor spread (**Fig. 4**).

PROTOCOLS FOR PET-CT FOR LUNG CANCER

Since the introduction of commercial PET-CT scanners in 2002, there has been continued evolution of the capability of the PET tomograph component and CT components as well as the operating systems and image reconstruction and archiving systems. Current PET-CT scanners can perform high-quality FDG-PET and CT scans of the torso (skull base to thighs) in as little as 10 minutes. With CT scanners of 16-detector, 64-detector, and up to 128-detector capability in contemporary PET-CT scanners, comprehensive diagnostic CT performed with PET imaging is now a routine capability.[16,17]

For staging or restaging lung cancer a torso scan is performed with axial coverage from the skull base to the thighs. Scans performed for evaluation of a pulmonary nodule can be more limited, covering the lungs only, or even a restricted portion of the lungs. In either case it is preferable

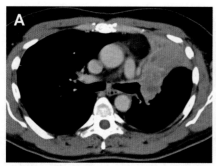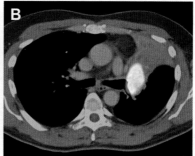

Fig. 4. PET-CT in radiation therapy planning. Patient with a non–small cell carcinoma of the left upper lobe with associated postobstructive left upper lobe atelectasis underwent PET-CT for radiation therapy planning. The CT images alone (*A*) show mass and atelectatic lung extending from the superior left hilum without clear distinction of soft tissue mass from consolidated lung, even on contrast-enhanced technique. The FDG-PET-CT fusion images (*B*) delineate the primary tumor mass from the postobstructive atelectasis, and depict the relationship between the primary tumor mass and atelectatic lung allowing for a treatment volume sparing the uninvolved lung parenchyma.

to have the patient's arms in a raised position, as this improves both FDG-PET and CT image quality and reduces artifacts from arm movement during the image acquisition.

With the first PET-CT scanners it was common practice to perform the CT portion of the examination at quiet breathing, rather than with breath hold, to avoid misregistration of the image sets, especially in the lower thorax and upper abdomen. This method resulted in poor-quality CT images and even reconstruction artifacts on the PET images. With multidetector CT of 16 slices or greater, the image degradation and artifacts associated with the respiratory movement are modest. It is also simple to incorporate a separate breath hold CT acquisition of the lungs in a routine imaging protocol (**Fig. 5**). This incorporation can be particularly important for characterizing lung nodules because the morphologic features are an important contribution to the overall assessment for likelihood of malignancy. Also, small pulmonary nodules, either primary malignancy or metastatic, can be missed on FDG-PET imaging, especially at the lung bases, and a full-inspiration breath hold CT acquisition can improve identification of such nodules compared with a free-breathing CT acquisition. As an alternative, a midexpiratory single breath hold on-the-fly CT acquisition can be performed with contemporary multidetector PET-CT scanners,[16,17] which can provide good image set registration and CT imaging quality in the lungs. A common practice of performing 2 CT acquisitions, one for attenuation correction and localization purposes and one diagnostic CT, is redundant and unnecessary, especially with contemporary PET-CT scanners.

In the initial treatment strategy of lung cancer, it is common to have a PET-CT examination ordered in response to the finding of a pulmonary nodule or

mass on a CT scan performed for chest pain or cough or a radiographic finding. In such cases a suitable diagnostic CT scan is available for interpretation with the FDG-PET examination and hence the diagnostic quality of the thoracic portion of the CT acquisition of the PET-CT examination can be simplified.

It is important for the imaging physician to work closely with the pulmonologists and surgeons in an effort to provide all the information possible for the care of patients with lung cancer. Continued improvements in bronchoscopic techniques have extended biopsy capabilities with the aid of CT image–generated virtual bronchoscopy (**Fig. 6**). These image reformats require thin overlapping transaxial reconstructed source image sets, which can easily be provided by contemporary PET-CT scanners with a breath hold acquisition.

PET-CT examinations to be used in radiation therapy planning require special considerations.[18] The scan may be used for staging and as an adjunct to the simulation process, or images from the examination, either the FDG-PET image sets or both PET and CT images sets, directly incorporated into the therapy planning software. As noted earlier, the radiation oncologist relies on the FDG-PET images to assist in delineating the extent of the primary tumor mass and to assess extent of locoregional nodal metastases. Radiation therapy planning software uses a simulation CT scan performed on a flat pallet with the patient in the therapy position with positioning devices in place. A PET-CT scan performed in the same manner can then be used as the simulation scan, and at some centers a PET-CT scanner is dedicated for such purposes. To be useful as an adjunct to a separately performed simulation CT, PET-CT should be performed on a flat pallet with

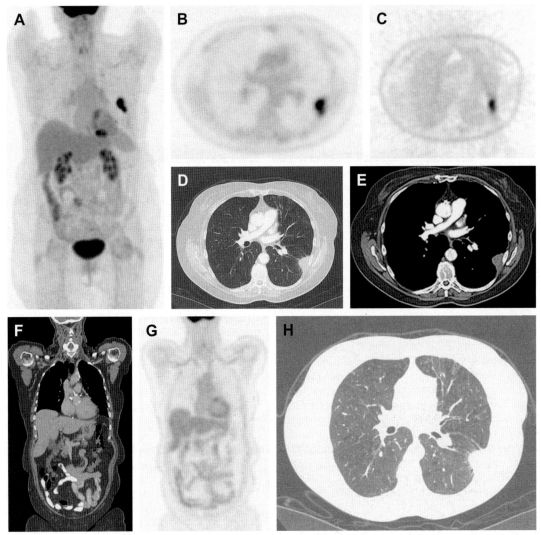

Fig. 5. Typical PET-CT protocol for lung cancer evaluation. Patient presented for initial staging of lung cancer. CT imaging included a full-inspiration breath hold scan through the lungs during the arterial phase of contrast enhancement and then scanning from the skull base to the thighs at the portal-venous phase of contrast enhancement. PET image acquisition was 1.5 minutes per bed position. The entire scanning session was performed in 10 minutes. Images sets generated include full maximum intensity FDG-PET projection image (*A*) and attenuation-corrected (*B*) and non–attenuation-corrected (*C*) PET transaxial image sets with sagittal and coronal reformats. CT image sets include lung algorithm reconstruction images of the lungs at full-inspiration breath hold (*D*) as well soft tissue algorithm reconstructed images of the full-inspiration thorax at arterial phase contrast enhancement (*E*). The whole-torso images at quiet breathing or near end-expiration breath hold to insure the CT images are properly aligned and registered with the PET images (*F, G*). CT images (and consequently PET images) are reconstructed typically at 2.5-mm or 3-mm slice thickness; however, with contemporary CT scanners, additional very thin section overlapping slice thickness image reconstruction, such as for virtual bronchoscopy, can routinely be derived from the raw (projection) data set (*H*).

the patient in the exact simulation position or a close approximation of it (**Fig. 7**).

INTERPRETATION AND REPORTING OF PET-CT IN LUNG CANCER

With the central role of PET-CT imaging in the care of patients with lung cancer, special attention to

interpretation and reporting of these examinations is required.[19,20]

As with all PET-CT examinations in body oncology patients, the interpretation and reporting is a process of integrating the metabolic information of the FDG-PET images with the morphologic diagnosis found in the CT images; the examination is not merely a PET scan with a

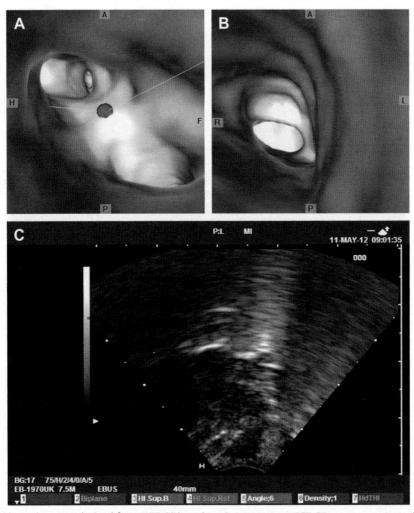

Fig. 6. Virtual bronchoscopy derived from PET-CT imaging. Contemporary PET-CT scanners can provide a comprehensive evaluation in a single imaging session. Image sets suitable for virtual bronchoscopy needed for such advanced endoscopic procedures such as virtual bronchoscopic navigation–assisted endobronchial ultrasound can routinely be generated (see **Fig. 5**). The virtual bronchoscopic images (*A*, *B*) are then used to provide virtual bronchoscopic navigation assistance for endobronchial ultrasound–guided biopsy (*C*). (*Courtesy of* Glen Van Otteren, MD, Spectrum Health Medical Group, Grand Rapids, MI.)

CT for localization purposes only. Also, as with all imaging examinations, the imaging findings must be integrated with the available clinical information and findings on prior imaging studies. Because of the large axial coverage and dual-modality nature of PET-CT body oncology scans, and in large part the complexity of the patients commonly encountered, oncologic PET-CT examinations are among the most complex and time-intensive interpretation and reporting imaging studies.

The principal tasks in the interpretation and reporting of PET-CT examinations are listed in **Box 2**. The T stage is determined largely by the

CT findings, and this is optimized by using thin-section image reconstruction and intravenous contrast. Locoregional nodal and distant metastatic disease are often obvious on CT alone; however, the addition of FDG-PET images significantly improves diagnostic sensitivity for detecting metastases involving nonenlarged lymph nodes and small or easily overlooked distant metastatic disease. Marrow-based osseous metastatic disease can be subtle or occult on CT (although easily seen on MR imaging), but, because most lung cancer is highly FDG avid, osseous metastases are readily depicted on FDG-PET images (see **Fig. 2**). Abnormally enlarged lymph nodes that

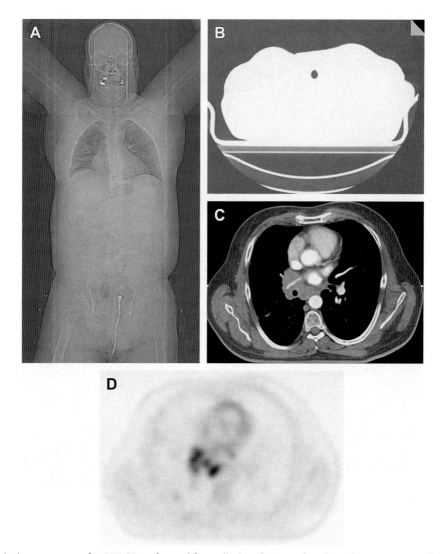

Fig. 7. Typical arrangement for PET-CT performed for radiation therapy planning when a separate simulation CT is performed. Patient is placed in a cradle on a flat radiation therapy pallet identical to that to be used at simulation and treatment and the patient is positioned in the same position as will be assumed during treatment (*A, B*). Fiducial markers, seen on the skin on the CT image (*C*), are used to define the isocenter for registration with the simulation CT images and positioning at each of the treatment fractions. Both the fully optimized CT and the PET image sets (*C, D*) can be imported into the radiation therapy planning software. The CT provides the precise delineation of the tumor margins for gross tumor volume determination, with the FDG-PET providing additional information when tumor margins are ill defined on the CT and providing improved sensitivity and specificity for locoregional nodal involvement.

are not FDG avid should not be dismissed as benign; mediastinal, and hilar lymph nodes with short axis diameter greater than 1.6 cm are considered suspicious, requiring biopsy at the time of mediastinoscopy or thorocotomy.[21] Hence reporting the size of abnormally enlarged lymph nodes remains important regardless of the FDG-PET findings (**Box 3**). Microscopic malignant disease does not reach the detection threshold of

FDG-PET; a tumor mass composed largely of malignant cells generally needs to be 5 to 6 mm in diameter to be detected on FDG-PET, and hence even nonenlarged lymph nodes in excess number in the mediastinum should be noted in the exam report.

Inflammation is the chief limitation of FDG-PET specificity, because inflammation can give rise to FDG tracer uptake in tissue in the range of FDG

Box 2

Principal tasks in interpretation of body oncology PET-CT examinations

For staging

- Primary mass size, metabolism, and adjacent organ or tissue involvement: T stage
- Distribution of abnormal lymph nodes and associated metabolism: N stage
- Distant metastases: M stage
- Incidental CT and FDG-PET findings unrelated to malignancy

For restaging and therapy monitoring

- Change in size and metabolism of primary and metastatic lesions
- Overall assessment of disease stability, response, or progression
- Incidental CT and FDG-PET findings unrelated to malignancy

For radiation therapy planning

- Identify margins of primary tumor mass
- Locoregional nodal basins node sizes, excess number, and metabolism
- Unexpected local and distant metastases
- Verify fiducial markers, if any

---

uptake caused by malignancy. Granulomatous infection can be especially FDG avid, showing levels of FDG activity as high as the highest levels caused by lung cancer. Inflammation is particularly

---

Box 3

Essential findings addressed in a PET-CT report of patients with lung cancer

- Primary lung nodule or mass size, morphologic features, metabolism
- Primary mass involvement of fissures, chest wall, mediastinum, hila
- Presence or absence of any additional pulmonary nodules
- Location of enlarged and/or hypermetabolic lymph nodes
- Presence or absence of distant metastases
- Presence or absence of pleural fluid collection
- Pulmonary abnormalities unrelated to malignancy
- Relevant unexpected findings (pneumothorax, pulmonary embolism)

---

confounding in the thorax, where 15% to 20% of FDG-PET–positive lymph nodes in the mediastinum and hila are caused by inflammation and not malignancy. Inflammation, principally granulomatous, similarly gives rise to the FDG-PET false-positive pulmonary nodules and the false-positive findings vary from 5% to 10% depending on the prevalence of granulomatous infection in a region.[22]

Most centers include standardized uptake values (SUVs) in PET-CT examination reports. SUVs are an attempt to provide a degree of quantification to the observed FDG tracer depiction of glucose metabolism on the PET images and have been a source of contention for nearly 2 decades.[23] One consensus effort concluded that SUVs should be reported with caution, if used at all, because they are not generally standardized, and values obtained at one center can differ significantly from those of another center due to several factors that influence the measured value.[24] There is also a great deal of overlap between the SUV of malignant tissue and inflammation; there is no discrete cutoff (such as 2.6). SUVs can be used to assess changes in tumor response to therapy, but comprehensive efforts must be made to ensure consistency within a given imaging center.[25]

Common pitfalls encountered when performing PET-CT on patients with known or suspected lung cancer are shown in **Box 4**. As noted earlier, inflammation can mimic malignant tissue on FDG-PET, and this must always be kept in mind. For example, small spiculated nodules can be caused by pneumonitis, and present a management dilemma as they are not generally suitable for biopsy. Radiation pneumonitis can be FDG-PET positive, making it difficult to assess possible residual or recurrent lung cancer after radiation treatment. A pulmonary abscess can be indistinguishable from a pulmonary abscess based on CT and FDG-PET findings. Not all malignant neoplasms are FDG avid, and, in the lungs, well-differentiated adenocarcinoma and carcinoid tumors can be minimal or essentially negative on FDG-PET images. Small foci of FDG tracer activity in the skeleton can be caused by degenerative joint changes or healing fractures, or even Schmorl's nodes at vertebral body endplates and mimic small metastatic deposits. Benign adrenal adenomas can present modest FDG uptake. In contrast, certain benign tumors such as Warthins tumor in the parotid gland or pituitary adenomas at the skull base can be very FDG avid and be mistaken for distant metastases based on the PET images alone.[26] Patients with lung cancer can have additional

---

Box 4
Some general pitfalls encountered in PET-CT examinations for lung cancer

- False-positive pulmonary nodules caused by inflammation
- Pneumonia and radiation pneumonitis
- Small pulmonary nodules (<5 mm) negative on PET images
- Non–FDG-avid neoplasm (well-differentiated adenocarcinoma, carcinoid)
- False-positive lymph nodes caused by inflammation
- Healing fractures, degenerative joint, Schmorl's node–related FDG uptake
- Hypermetabolic thyroid nodule (could be additional thyroid cancer)
- Small focal FDG uptake in colon (could be primary colon caner)
- Benign FDG-avid tumors (Warthin tumor, pituitary macroadenoma)
- Adrenal adenomas with modest FDG uptake
- Pneumothorax, pulmonary embolism, central vein thrombus

---

unrelated neoplasms, and incidental thyroid and early colon cancers are commonly seen on FDG-PET images.[27]

SUMMARY

PET-CT is now a well-established imaging modality for the management of patients with lung cancer. Fully diagnostic anatomic and metabolic registered image sets can be rapidly obtained in a single examination session using contemporary PET-CT scanners. Interpretation and reporting of these imaging examinations can be demanding and time consuming, but they provide indispensable information for initial diagnosis and staging, therapy response assessment, and radiation therapy planning.

REFERENCES

1. Gupta NC, Frank AR, Dewan NA, et al. Solitary pulmonary nodules: detection of malignancy with PET with 2-[F-18]-fluoro-2-deoxy-D-glucose. Radiology 1992;184:441–4.
2. Valk PE, Pounds TR, Hopkins DM, et al. Staging non-small-cell lung cancer by whole body positron emission tomographic imaging. Ann Thorac Surg 1995; 60:1573–81.
3. Beyer T, Townsend D, Brun T, et al. A combined PET/CT scanner for clinical oncology. J Nucl Med 2000; 41:1369–79.
4. Fischer B, Lassen U, Mortensen J, et al. Preoperative staging of lung cancer with combined PET-CT. N Engl J Med 2009;361:32–9.
5. MacMahon H, Austin J, Gamsu G. Guidelines for management of small pulmonary nodules detected on CT scans: a statement of the Fleischner Society. Radiology 2005;237:395–400.
6. Raylman RR, Kison PV, Wahl RL. Capabilities of two- and three-dimensional FDG-PET for detecting small lesions and lymph nodes in the upper torso: a dynamic phantom study. Eur J Nucl Med 1999; 26:39–45.
7. Travis WD, Brambilla E, Noguchi M, et al. International Association for the Study of Lung Cancer/American Thoracic Society/European Respiratory Society international multidisciplinary classification of lung adenocarcinoma. J Thorac Oncol 2011;6: 244–85.
8. Goudarzi B, Jacene HA, Wahl RL. Diagnosis and differentiation of bronchioloalveolar carcinoma from adenocarcinoma with bronchioloalveolar components with metabolic and anatomic characteristics using PET/CT. J Nucl Med 2008;49:1585–92.
9. Antoch G, Stattaus J, Nemat AT. Non-small cell lung cancer dual-modality PET/CT preoperative staging. Radiology 2003;229:526–33.
10. Shin SS, Lee KS, Kim B-T. Non-small cell lung cancer: prospective comparison of integrated FDG PET/CT and CT alone for preoperative staging. Radiology 2005;236:1011–9.
11. Keidar Z, Haim N, Guralnik L. PET/CT using 18F-FDG in suspected lung cancer recurrence: diagnostic value and impact on patient management. J Nucl Med 2004;45:1640–6.
12. Detterbeck FC, Boffa DJ, Tanoue LT. The new lung cancer staging system. Chest 2009;136: 260–71.
13. Segal GM. Therapy response evaluation with positron emission tomography-computed tomography. Semin Ultrasound CT MR 2010;31:490–5.
14. Wahl RL, Jacene H, Kasamon Y, et al. From RECIST to PERCIST: evolving considerations for PET response criteria in solid tumors. J Nucl Med 2009; 50(Suppl 1):122S–50S.
15. Eschmann SM, Friedel G, Paulsen F, et al. Impact of staging with 18F-FDG-PET on outcome of patients with stage III non-small cell lung cancer: PET identifies potential survivors. Eur J Nucl Med Mol Imag 2007;34:463–71.
16. Shyn PB. Protocol considerations for thoracic positron emission-tomography-computed tomography. Semin Ultrasound CT MRI 2008;29:242–50.
17. Shreve P, Agress H Jr. Performance and interpretation of PET-CT body oncology scans. In: Shreve P,

Townsend D, editors. Clinical PET-CT. Philadelphia: Springer; 2010. p. 285–97.

18. Shreve P, Swanston NM, Faasee T. Positron emission tomography-computed tomography protocols for radiation therapy planning and therapy response assessment. Semin Ultrasound CT MRI 2010;31: 468–79.

19. Agress H Jr, Wong TZ, Shreve P. Interpretation and reporting of positron emission tomography-computed tomography scans. Semin Ultrasound CT MRI 2008; 29:283–90.

20. Rohren EM. Positron emission tomography-computed tomography reporting in radiation therapy planning and response assessment. Semin Ultrasound CT MRI 2010;31:516–29.

21. de Langen AJ, Raijmakers P, Riphagen I, et al. The size of mediastinal lymph nodes and its relation with metastatic involvement: a meta-analysis. Eur J Cardiothorac Surg 2006;29:26–39.

22. Croft DR, Trapp J, Kernstinek K. FDG PET imaging and the diagnosis of non-small cell lung cancer in a region of high histoplasmosis prevalence. Lung Cancer 2002;36:297–301.

23. Keyes JW. SUV: standard uptake value or silly useless value? J Nucl Med 1995;36:1836–9.

24. Blodgett T. Best practices in PET/CT: consensus on performance of positron emission tomography-computed tomography. Semin Ultrasound CT MRI 2008;29:236–41.

25. Kinahan PE, Fletcher JW. Positron emission tomography-computed tomography standardized uptake values in clinical practice and assessing response to therapy. Semin Ultrasound CT MRI 2010;31:496–505.

26. Shreve P. Artifacts and normal variants in PET imaging. In: Wahl RL, Beanlands RSB, editors. Principles and practice of PET and PET/CT. Philadelphia: Lippincott; 2009. p. 139–68.

27. Agress H Jr, Cooper BZ. Detection of clinically unexpected malignant and premalignant tumors with whole-body FDG PET: histopathological comparison. Radiology 2004;23:417–23.

Role of Positron Emission Tomography/Computed Tomography in Breast Cancer

Austin C. Bourgeois, MD, Lance A. Warren, MD,
Ted T. Chang, MD, Scott Embry, MD, Kathleen Hudson, MD,
Yong C. Bradley, MD*

KEYWORDS

- Positron emission tomography • Computed tomography • Breast cancer
- Positron emission mammography

KEY POINTS

- Positron emission tomography (PET)/computed tomography is imperative in all aspects of breast cancer staging, treatment, and follow-up.
- PET will continue to be relevant in personalized medicine because the use of accurate tumor status will be even more critical during and after the transition from a generic metabolic agent to receptor imaging.
- Positron emission mammography is an imaging proposition that may have benefits in lower doses, but its use is limited without new radiopharmaceuticals.

INTRODUCTION

Epidemiology and Background

Breast cancer is the most common solid malignancy in women in the Western world, and a woman's lifetime risk of developing breast cancer exceeds 10%.[1] In 2012, an expected 226,870 patients will be diagnosed, accounting for 29% of all new cancer cases.[2] Although incidence of breast cancer increased in the 1970s and 1980s as a result of improved detection, its incidence has stabilized over the past 2 decades.[2]

Improved early detection, staging, and treatment methods have produced a steady decline in breast cancer–related mortality since 1991.[2] In spite of this, primary breast malignancies remain responsible for 15% of all female cancer-related deaths.[3] As with most malignancies, the presence of locoregional and distant metastasis at the time of diagnosis correlates with a poor prognosis. Multiple studies have shown that the presence and extent of locoregional nodal metastasis is the single most important prognostic factor in breast cancer.[4–6] This is reflected in 5-year survival rates of 99% in the absence of nodal metastasis, decreasing to 84% and 23% respectively for locoregional and distant metastatic disease.[4,5]

However, most patients diagnosed with breast cancer have neither locoregional nor distant metastatic disease at the time of diagnosis. Between 2001 and 2007, 60% of patients diagnosed with breast carcinoma had disease confined to the breast.[7] One-third of these patients had evidence of locoregional metastasis and only 5% had distant metastasis at the time of diagnosis.[7] The high proportion of patients with early-stage disease at diagnosis reflects intensive efforts at early detection and awareness.[8] Although a significant proportion of patients with local or locoregional-confined disease are cured, approximately 30% eventually relapse.[9,10] For this reason, patients with breast cancer commonly undergo close posttherapy follow-up over a period of 3 to 5 years, with emphasis on detecting treatable recurrence.[11]

University of Tennessee Medical Center, 1924 Alcoa Highway, Knoxville, TN 37920, USA
* Corresponding author.
E-mail address: ybradley@mc.utmck.edu

Radiol Clin N Am 51 (2013) 781–798
http://dx.doi.org/10.1016/j.rcl.2013.06.003
0033-8389/13/$ – see front matter © 2013 Elsevier Inc. All rights reserved.

Imaging plays a critical role in the initial evaluation of breast cancer and serves as an important adjunct to surgical, pathologic, and clinical staging. Mammography, ultrasound (US), physical examination, and tissue sampling are the mainstay of evaluating a suspicious breast mass. The current literature examines the role of metastatic work-up with computed tomography (CT), nuclear medicine bone scintigraphy (BS), and magnetic resonance (MR) imaging, as well as the role of lymphoscintigraphy (LS) in evaluating sentinel lymph node (SLN) status. Combined positron emission tomography (PET) and CT (PET/CT) plays an increasingly important role in breast cancer staging and restaging, although no consensus guidelines have set forth its proper use in this setting.

This article examines the use of PET/CT in the staging, prognostication, and follow-up of primary breast carcinoma and provides practical guidelines and interpretive pitfalls for the physicians who order and interpret these studies.

STAGING AND PROGNOSTIC CONSIDERATIONS

Primary breast carcinoma is a histologically and clinically heterogeneous disease.[12] Although the current model of staging based on tumor, node, metastasis (TNM) classification provides prognostic significance, it excludes important factors such as hormonal receptor typing and serum tumor markers. Breast cancer staging increasingly uses an integrated approach, incorporating clinical, pathologic, surgical, serologic, and radiologic factors.[13]

Carcinoma in Situ

With rare exceptions, primary breast carcinoma is an adenocarcinoma that develops in 2 primary sites: breast ducts or lobules.[13] Most breast cancers are of ductal origin.[13] Carcinoma in situ (CIN) refers to histologic evidence of breast tissue metaplasia without invasive characteristics, distinguishing it from malignancy. Although CIN does not represent a true malignancy, it does impart increased risk of developing breast cancer subsequently.[14] Therefore, both lobular and ductal CIN receive the tumor staging classification T0.

TNM Staging

The TNM system describes the extent of tumor burden in patients with breast cancer using a standardized approach. The presence of locoregional nodal disease has well-documented prognostic significance.[4–6] Therefore, evaluating the regional lymph node basin is a priority in clinical and surgical staging. Many other factors affect breast cancer prognosis such as nodal location and metastatic burden, primary tumor size, hormone receptor status, and site of distant metastasis. These factors form the basis of the current TNM classification criteria.

Large primary tumor size at the time of diagnosis implies a poor prognosis. In particular, patients with breast cancer with tumors greater than 5 cm (T3) carry a significantly increased risk of progressing to distant metastasis, which occurs in up to 15.1% of this subset.[15] Just as the presence of nodal metastasis is an important consideration, quantifying the degree of nodal metastatic burden is clinically significant. As the number of positive axillary lymph nodes increases, prognosis proportionally worsens irrespective of primary tumor characteristics.[4] Location of nodal metastasis is also of prognostic significance, because the presence of internal mammary (IM) nodal (IMN) or supraclavicular nodal involvement further decreases expected survival.[4]

The presence of distant metastasis is associated with markedly diminished long-term survival. The most common site of distant breast cancer metastasis is the skeleton, occurring in 69% of patients with advanced disease.[16] Other common sites include the lung, liver, and brain.[17] Although breast cancer metastases to the liver occur infrequently, their presence is associated with the worst prognosis (**Table 1**).[17]

Approach to Staging

Staging patients with breast cancer accurately is essential in directing appropriate treatment. In addition to a thorough history and physical examination, a complete blood count, liver function tests, and alkaline phosphatase value are recommended as part of the initial staging.[7] The results of clinical, laboratory, and pathologic factors guide imaging and further breast cancer work-up.

If cancer is detected at an early stage, surgical resection with curative intent is the mainstay of therapy.[18] Surgical resection is typically achieved using one of 2 techniques: (1) breast conservation therapy combined with total or partial breast irradiation, or (2) mastectomy. In contrast, disease that has spread beyond the locoregional lymph node basin is rarely curable via surgery alone.[17] In the setting of stage IV disease, surgical resection is replaced by chemotherapy, radiation, and/or hormonal therapy.[18] Detection of distant metastatic foci thus has the ability to profoundly alter both prognosis and clinical management.

Evaluation of nodal status is commonly performed using LS to identify the SLN for SLN biopsy

Table 1
TNM classification based on the American Joint Committee on Cancer's TNM staging

Stage	Primary Tumor (T)	Regional Lymph Node Status (N)	Distant Metastasis (M)
0	Carcinoma in situ	No evidence of nodal metastasis	No
I	Tumor ≤2 cm	No evidence of nodal metastasis	No
IIA	No evidence of primary tumor	Metastasis in 1–3 nodes	No
	Tumors ≤2 cm	Metastasis in 1–3 nodes	No
	Tumor ≥2 cm but ≤5 cm	No evidence of nodal metastasis	No
IIB	Tumor ≥2 cm but ≤5 cm	Metastasis in 1–3 nodes	No
	Tumor >5 cm	No evidence of nodal metastasis	No
IIIA	No evidence of primary tumor	Metastasis in 4–10 nodes	No
	Tumors ≤2 cm	Metastasis in 4–10 nodes	No
	Tumor ≥2 cm but ≤5 cm	Metastasis in 4–10 nodes	No
	Tumor >5 cm	Metastasis in 1–3 nodes	No
	Tumor >5 cm	Metastasis in 4–10 nodes	No
IIIB	Tumor of any size with direct extension to chest wall or skin	No evidence of nodal metastasis	No
	Tumor of any size with direct extension to chest wall or skin	Metastasis in 1–3 nodes	No
	Tumor of any size with direct extension to chest wall or skin	Metastasis in 4–10 nodes	No
IIIC	Any tumor designation	Metastasis in >10 nodes	No
IV	Any tumor designation	Any lymph node designation	Yes

Used with the permission of the American Joint Committee on Cancer (AJCC), Chicago, Illinois. The original source for this material is the AJCC Cancer Staging Manual, Seventh Edition (2010) published by Springer-Verlag New York, www.springer.com.

(LS-SLNB). This technique remains the standard of care for locoregional nodal evaluation, sparing patients with negative SLN status the potential morbidity related to unnecessary axillary lymph node dissection. This technique has high sensitivity of 88% for macrometastases and 72% for micrometastases (**Fig. 1**).[19]

Hormone Receptor Status

In addition to TNM factors, expression of hormonal receptors by tumor cells plays an important role in breast cancer prognostication and treatment. Estrogen receptor (ER) and progesterone receptor (PR) status predict both long-term survival and response to therapy.[8] Nearly 70% of breast cancers express ER, which is a favorable prognosticator and allows receptor-targeted endocrine therapy.[12] Even in the setting of incurable distant metastasis, endocrine therapy represents a low-toxicity option for disease control in those patients who are candidates.[12] Tumors positive for human epidermal growth factor 2 (HER2) with locoregional metastasis similarly have improved survival compared with HER2-negative tumors.[8] The triple-negative tumor subtype, which does not express ER, PR, or HER2, portends the worse prognosis of all hormone receptor subtypes.[10]

Heterogeneity of receptor status within cancer cells, nonfunctionality of receptors, and sampling error can result in an erroneous classification of the patient's receptor status.[12] These factors are likely to blame for the highly variable response

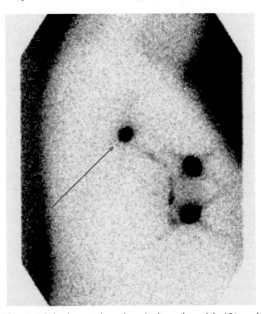

Fig. 1. Right breast lymphoscintigraphy with 12° and 6 o'clock technetium 99m SCOL injection identifying a single axillary lymph node (*arrow*).

rates to targeted therapy among ER-positive patients, which approach 30% to 40%.[12] For these reasons, research has recently turned to PET/CT for evaluating the efficacy of targeted therapy. In a pilot study of 22 patients, the degree of response to hormonal therapy by PET/CT correlated with progression-free survival.[20] Although limited evidence currently supports its widespread use in this manner, PET/CT may play an increasing role in hormonal treatment optimization and prognostication.

Tumor Markers

Current breast cancer guidelines regarding follow-up primarily emphasize sequential screening with mammogram and clinical examination, along with judicious integration of conventional imaging modalities.[9] In addition, tumor markers are often used to screen asymptomatic patients for evidence of recurrence. Markers that are commonly used for evaluating treatment response and monitoring for recurrent disease include cancer antigen 27.29 (CA 27.29), cancer antigen 15-3 (CA 15-3), and carcinoembryonic antigen (CEA). These tests represent serum values of proteins involved in cell adhesion.[21] Of these, CEA and CA 15-3 are most highly associated with recurrence in asymptomatic patients,[9] although their values lack specificity.

Other markers of cellular division and circulating tumor cells show potential benefit for evaluating recurrent and metastatic disease. Ki67 is a nuclear protein that serves as an indirect marker of tumor cellular proliferation by histopathologic analysis.[22] Expression of Ki67 is associated with aggressive primary tumor characteristics such as increased metabolic activity on PET/CT and increased rate of relapse after therapy.[23] Analysis by Keam and colleagues[6,22] suggests that Ki67 positivity carries a worse prognosis, particularly in the setting of triple-negative primary tumors.

A detailed discussion of serum tumor markers and their clinical application is outside of the scope of this article; however, they are likely to play an increasing role in the ordering and interpretation of imaging studies in the future.

INITIAL BREAST CANCER EVALUATION
Mammography and Ultrasound

Mammography and US imaging are the mainstays of evaluating suspicious breast masses. Although there has been recent controversy regarding the cost/benefit ratio of screening between the ages of 40 and 49 years, the American Cancer Society continues to recommend yearly mammogram screening beginning at the age of 40 years.[24,25]

Suspicious findings on diagnostic mammography or clinical examination are investigated further with US. Lesions meeting Breast Imaging-Reporting and Data System (BI-RADS) 4 or 5 criteria are generally referred for biopsy and histologic analysis.[26]

Although US provides known benefit in characterizing breast masses, its application elsewhere is limited. In particular, the accuracy of US in evaluating axillary lymph node status is controversial because of its strongly investigator-dependent and time-consuming nature.[3] Overall, sonographic evaluation of lymph node metastasis is suboptimal, with lesser sensitivity than both PET/CT and LS-SLNB. The role of US is thus generally confined to characterizing primary breast lesions, directing breast biopsy, and on rare occasion targeting suspected metastatic nodes for tissue sampling.

MR Imaging

Breast MR imaging is commonly used in screening high-risk patients, treatment planning, and monitoring neoadjuvant chemotherapy (NACT) response. The American Cancer Society recommends a yearly screening with MR imaging in conjunction with screening mammography for patients with a greater than 20% lifelong risk of breast cancer.[27] This patient subset includes those with BRCA1 or BRCA2 mutations, a personal history of radiation therapy to the chest, or a significant family history. The use of MR imaging outside of these limited indications is controversial, because it imparts high cost, increased burden of time, and may lead to increased false-positive rates.[28] For its indicated applications, the limited benefits of breast MR imaging include improved characterization of the primary tumor and detecting multicentric or multifocal malignancy.[27]

EVALUATING THE PRIMARY BREAST TUMOR WITH PET/CT

The role of PET/CT in staging, restaging, and prognostication continues to evolve as the extent of evidence regarding its impact in breast cancer management grows. Current literature describes the ability of PET/CT to accurately detect and characterize primary breast neoplasms as well as to detect locoregional and distant metastasis. Furthermore, PET/CT may also provide clinically relevant information in the setting of response to NACT and prognostication. In spite of these factors, PET/CT has yet to show improvement in disease-free survival or overall survival.[3]

In the setting of breast cancer, PET/CT is almost exclusively reserved as a staging tool for cases of pathology-proven disease. However, multiple studies have corroborated the high accuracy of PET/CT in detecting suspected primary breast malignancy.[6,29,30] In a study of 103 patients with newly diagnosed breast cancer, PET/CT identified 100 of 103 primary breast cancers (97%).[30] The 3 false-negatives comprised 2 cases of invasive ductal carcinoma, with tumors of 10 and 22 mm, as well as a single case of invasive lobular carcinoma.[30] These led the investigators to suggest a size threshold of approximately 2 cm for detection by PET/CT. A similar study by Garami and colleagues[31] noted a sensitivity of 93% in tumors less than 4 cm in size. In addition to its high sensitivity in detecting primary breast lesions, PET/CT has shown consistently high specificity and positive predictive value.[6] In spite of these reports, focally increased standardized uptake value (SUV) breast uptake can occur in the absence of malignancy.

False-positive Breast Lesions

Numerous physiologic and pathologic processes within the breast can produce focal fluorodeoxyglucose (FDG) avidity, mimicking breast malignancy or obscuring true disease. Fibroadenomata are a common false-positive finding on PET/CT, displaying increased FDG uptake as a result of their proliferation and growth.[32] Sterile chronic or acute inflammatory processes including fat necrosis and radiation necrosis may be indistinguishable from malignancy as well.[32] Gynecomastia, mastitis, silicone granulomas, postsurgical changes, and lactation are other known causes of false-positive results.[33] Thus, focally increased FDG avidity in the breast is not diagnostic for breast carcinoma. However, such findings should be regarded as highly suspicious for malignancy, warranting imaging with US, mammography, and tissue sampling.[34,35]

Correlation with Histopathology

Quantitative analysis of maximum SUV (SUV_{max}) values from PET/CT data provides information on a primary breast tumor's metabolic activity, potentially reflecting its histologic features and expected clinical course. In a study of 214 patients, Koolen and colleagues[36] showed that the presence of distant metastasis at the time of the staging examination was associated with significantly higher SUV_{max} values of the primary tumor. In this series, SUV_{max} levels correlated with aggressive histologic features, best shown by statistically significant increases in SUV_{max} in the triple-negative hormone receptor subtype. Several additional studies have corroborated that the more aggressive and prognostically poor invasive ductal carcinomas have increased average SUV_{max} relative to invasive lobular carcinomas.[36–38] Groheux and colleagues[38] summarized the relationship between SUV_{max} and histologic grade, noting a median SUV_{max} of 9.7 for grade III tumors, whereas all lower grade tumors displayed a median SUV_{max} of 4.8.

Incidentally Detected Breast Mass

Breast cancer can be discovered initially as an incidental finding on PET/CT performed for other indications, with an incidence of up to 0.82%.[34] In a study of 32,988 patients undergoing PET-CT for evaluation of nonbreast malignancy, focal breast hypermetabolic activity was identified in 131 (0.4%). Of these patients, 60 were subsequently found to have malignancy (32 benign and 28 malignant).[35] In this study, a SUV_{max} threshold of 2.3 yielded a specificity for malignancy detection of 76.3%.[35] A similar study found that incidentally detected focal hypermetabolic activity in the breast represented malignancy in up to 37.5% of cases. The incidentally detected breast mass should therefore be regarded as highly suspicious for malignancy, warranting, at minimum, further characterization with US and mammography.[34,39–41]

EVALUATING NODAL STATUS WITH PET/CT

SLNB remains the gold standard for nodal evaluation, offering high rates of sensitivity and specificity for detecting metastasis.[42–44] However, SLNB and axillary nodal dissection carry significant morbidity. The search for a noninvasive solution of evaluating nodal status has led to several studies examining the efficacy of both conventional imaging and PET/CT.

The accuracy of PET/CT for detecting axillary metastasis has primarily been studied in early-stage disease, in patients with low pretest probability for metastasis.[2] In this patient subset, sensitivity for detecting metastasis is suboptimal. A meta-analysis by Cooper and colleagues[45] examined 7 studies with a combined 862 patients who underwent PET/CT for breast cancer staging. The mean sensitivity for detecting nodal metastasis was only 56% (95% confidence interval, 44%–67%). However, additional studies regarding PET/CT sensitivity in this application are variable.[4,29,46] In an analysis of 311 patients, the sensitivity, specificity, positive predictive value (PPV), negative predictive value (NPV), and accuracy of PET/CT in evaluating axillary nodes were 82%, 92%, 98%, 53%, and 84% respectively.[4] Although overall sensitivity of nodal evaluation in early-stage breast cancer is low, PET/CT outperforms traditional imaging modalities[2] and may play a role in staging patients with certain histologic and clinical risk factors (**Fig. 2**).

The characteristics of a primary breast tumor and its metastases markedly affect its ability to be detected by PET/CT. A significantly higher proportion of metastases are detected in patients with aggressive histologic features including (1) N2 or N3 disease, (2) Ki67 positivity, (3) grade 3 tumors, and (4) triple-negative tumors.[4] Invasive ductal carcinoma is also more likely to be detected than invasive lobular carcinoma.[46] In contrast, those primary tumors with no or slightly increased FDG avidity are associated with a higher proportion of missed axillary metastasis.[4] The size of a nodal metastasis also affects its detection by PET/CT. Groheux and colleagues[38] described this relationship, noting a mean sensitivity of 11% in detecting micrometastases (<2 mm), compared with 57% in

detecting macrometastases (>2 mm). Understanding the correlation of PET/CT detection rates with these tumor characteristics provides an important understanding of the benefits and limitations of PET/CT on a patient-specific basis.

PET/CT IN PRETREATMENT EVALUATION

PET/CT serves as an adjunct to clinical and surgical staging, offering superior diagnostic accuracy for detecting metastases and the ability to guide optimal surgical management in a significant proportion of patients. In a prospective study of patients with primary breast tumors larger than 3 cm of all histologic types, 106 patients underwent staging with both PET/CT and conventional imaging. Conventional imaging included mammography, MR imaging, chest radiography, BS, and

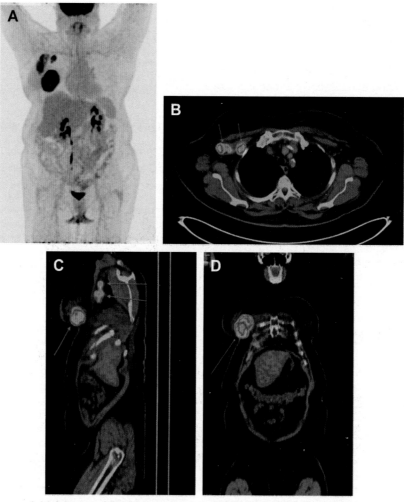

Fig. 2. Breast cancer initial staging. (*A*) Whole-body maximal intensity projection (MIP) showing a large primary lesion with local metastases. (*B*) Fused image reveals both axillary and subpectoral metastases (*arrows*). (*C*) Sagittal fused image showing the relationship of the primary tumor (*single arrow*) to axillary metastases (*double arrow*). (*D*) Coronal fused image exposes the central necrosis of the large primary lesion (*arrow*).

US of the breast, axilla, and liver.[30] PET/CT changed the initial staging in 42% of patients. In addition, 23 sites of extra-axillary malignancy in 15 (14%) patients were detected by PET/CT alone. Of these, treatment modification occurred in 8% based on PET/CT findings.[30] In a similar study of 106 patients, clinical management was changed in 14% of patients based on PET/CT findings alone, showing its clinical impact and superior diagnostic accuracy compared with conventional imaging.[3]

In low-risk patients, PET/CT may be useful for staging as well. A study of 115 patients with primary tumor less than 4 cm and no signs of distant metastasis showed a high rate of staging and treatment modification following PET/CT. In these patients, PET-CT led to changes in the TNM classification in 54 patients (47%) and altered treatment plans in 18 patients (15.6%).[31] Despite this high rate of altering clinical management, screening low-stage asymptomatic patients with PET/CT has not proved cost-effective.

PET/CT may provide clinically relevant information in evaluating nodal metastases, despite its overall suboptimal sensitivity.[47,48] In multiple studies, the specificity of PET/CT in nodal evaluation was high, often exceeding 90%.[2,4,29,30] This finding provides a rationale for omitting SLNB in favor of immediate axillary dissection in patients with FDG-avid axillary nodes.[2] PET/CT also plays an important role in evaluating nodal metastases that are often overlooked by LS and conventional imaging. The presence of metastases in IM chain and periclavicular chain nodes is of high prognostic significance and may be occult by conventional imaging modalities. In a study by Koolen and colleagues,[4] 311 patients were examined by PET/CT, and occult IM chain and periclavicular chain lymph nodes were detected in 26 and 32 patients respectively, which produced a change in regional radiation therapy in 50 of the initial 311 patients (16.1%).[4] Although PET/CT lacks sufficient sensitivity to routinely supplant SLNB, its high specificity and ability to detect occult IM and supraclavicular lymph nodes may serve as an adjunct in nodal evaluation (Fig. 3).

PET/CT in Evaluating Inflammatory Breast Cancer and Mastitis

Breast inflammation is an uncommon reason for patients to seek medical care, representing less than 1% of all office visits (22/3762).[49] Of these, infection is the most common cause, and is responsible for more than half of these clinical encounters.[49] Given the high incidence of infectious mastitis, breast inflammation is commonly treated with a 10-day antibiotic trial when such symptoms are accompanied by fever.[49] Nonresponders to antibiotic therapy at 15 days may be considered for malignancy work-up. Of all routine causes of breast inflammation, inflammatory breast cancer is the least common, with an incidence of 4.5% to 5.6%.[49]

Inflammatory breast cancer (IBC) is a form of breast cancer with aggressive clinical and imaging features. Although IBC is uncommon, its incidence is increasing in the United States. The clinical manifestations of IBC correlate with rapid growth, including edema, breast enlargement, warmth, tenderness, and peau de orange skin changes.[50] It also carries the worst prognosis among primary breast tumors and is associated with an expected 5-year survival of only 20% to 40%.[51] This poor prognosis is in part related to the approximately 30% of IBC patients who have metastatic disease at the time of presentation.[51] IBC is primarily a clinical diagnosis and is often confused with mastitis. Both PET/CT and breast MR imaging are of little usefulness in differentiating these causes.[49] However, PET/CT plays a critical role in metastatic work-up and planning systemic and locoregional therapy (Fig. 4).[51]

PET/CT shows high accuracy in diagnosing aggressive breast cancer histologic subtypes, and thus its benefit in staging IBC is intuitive. In a study of 41 patients with biopsy-proven IBC, PET/CT detected distant metastases in 49%.[50] Of these, 17% had no other clinical or radiologic manifestations of metastatic disease.[50] An additional prospective study of 59 patients showed a 100% sensitivity of PET/CT in detecting the primary IBC tumor.[51] Eighteen of these patients (31%) had distant metastases detected by PET/CT, only 6 of which were visible using conventional imaging techniques. PET/CT plays a critical role in evaluating IBC because of its aggressive nature and high pretest probability of metastasis.

EVALUATION OF DISTANT BREAST CANCER METASTASES WITH PET/CT

Most breast cancers are confined to the breast at the time of diagnosis. Approximately 30% of patients present with axillary lymph node metastases and 5% have distant metastatic disease at the time of diagnosis.[7] Although the current literature suggests a role for PET/CT in nodal evaluation (discussed earlier), it is effective in evaluating patients with high pretest probability of distant metastatic disease. This article discusses the role of PET/CT in evaluating distant metastases, with a focus on its limitations, alternative imaging modalities, proper use, and interpretive pitfalls.

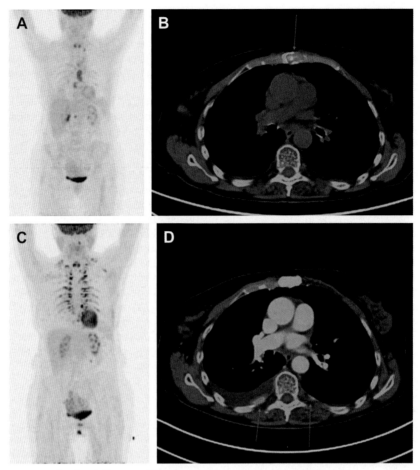

Fig. 3. Tumor response to chemotherapy. (*A*) Patient status post lumpectomy with bony metastases. (*B*) Fused axial image with a hypermetabolic lytic sternal metastasis (*arrow*). (*C*) Complete response to chemotherapy after chemotherapy. The multifocal supraclavicular and intercostal brown fat uptake can be a confounding factor. (*D*) Fused axial image shows the sclerotic sternum without significant FDG uptake consistent with a healed metastasis. Bilateral symmetric brown fat uptake between the ribs near the vertebral body (*arrows*) needs careful attention to rule out metastases.

Evaluation of Osseous Metastases

The skeletal system is the most common site of distant breast cancer metastases, which may be osteolytic and/or osteoblastic. Osseous metastases are present in 8% of patients with breast cancer and in 65% to 75% of all patients with stage IV disease.[16] BS has traditionally been used as a first-line evaluation for bone metastases, given its relative sensitivity and cost-effectiveness.[52] BS can also detect osseous metastases several months before plain radiography,[53] but has limited ability to characterize purely lytic metastases.[54] Suspicious findings on BS can be further evaluated with other imaging modalities, such as conventional radiographs, CT, or MR imaging, to increase the specificity of the examination. Comparative studies have shown that MR imaging can reveal significantly more metastases than BS; however, its widespread use is limited by increased time and cost, and by limited access.[53]

The high prevalence of bone metastases in patients with breast cancer has caused many clinicians to perform widespread screening of asymptomatic patients of all stages. Several investigations question the clinical usefulness and cost-effectiveness of this approach.[17] A large Italian clinical trial examined this relationship, in which 1243 women with breast cancer were randomized to only clinical screening or sequential screening with BS and chest radiography. The study showed no difference in survival between the two patient subsets.[17] Routine screening of patients for bone metastases is further refuted by evidence that early detection of bone metastases fails to reduce overall mortality.[17]

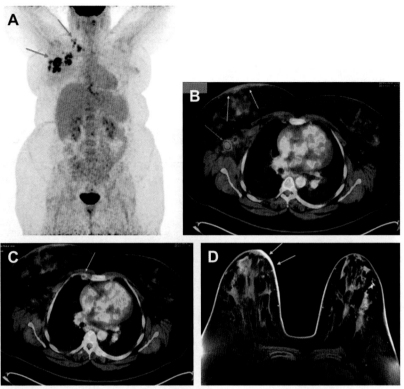

Fig. 4. IBC. (A) Whole-body MIP reveals right breast cancer with axillary and supraclavicular lymph nodes (arrows). (B) Fused image shows axillary nodes (red arrow) and thickened skin (yellow arrows) consistent with IBC. (C) IM lymph nodes (arrow) on fused image. (D) Contrast-enhanced MR imaging reveals thickened skin (arrows) consistent with inflammatory cancer.

The optimal modality for examining breast cancer metastases to bone has been the topic of extensive research. Studies evaluating the comparative efficacies of conventional BS, FDG-PET, PET/CT, and MR imaging suggest the superiority of PET/CT for this application.[15,54,55] Although BS remains a highly used modality, it is limited by its inability to evaluate purely lytic metastases.[54] Early studies of FDG-PET show its superiority compared with BS in characterizing lytic metastases, although this relationship has primarily derived from studies of non–small cell lung cancer in which purely lytic metastases are more common.[54] In comparative analysis including only patients with breast cancer, FDG-PET shows improved overall specificity in detecting bony metastases and no significant difference in detection rates.[56]

Combined PET with CT has emerged as a highly accurate method of characterizing breast cancer metastases, with superiority to both PET and CT alone.[57] In a study of 29 women with breast cancer, Hahn and colleagues[55] examined a total of 132 bone lesions evaluated with both PET/CT and BS. On a per-lesion basis, the sensitivity of PET/CT was 96%, whereas the sensitivity of conventional BS was 76%. The high relative accuracy of skeletal evaluation with PET/CT is corroborated by several additional studies,[15,54] leading many to consider it as the gold standard in the diagnosis of bone metastasis.[16] However, MR imaging allows similar diagnostic accuracy to PET/CT, offering a radiation-free alternative for following bone metastases.[16]

In addition, skeletal evaluation with PET/CT may provide relevant prognostic information. A study by Morris and colleagues[10] concluded that SUV_{max} levels of osseous lesions in patients with breast cancer were highly correlated with overall survival, after correcting for phenotype, grade, and the presence of visceral metastases. This finding suggests a role for quantitative PET/CT analysis in future prognostication models.[10] Anatomic and metabolic changes in sequential PET/CT imaging may serve a similar role in prognostication. In a study of 47 patients with bone metastases who underwent sequential PET/CT, both increased SUV_{max} and lytic change on coregistered CT images were associated with disease progression.[57] The presence of increased bone sclerosis was confounded by bisphosphonate therapy, and was not a reliable indicator of disease progression.[57]

PET/CT plays an important and increasing role in the detection of osseous metastases related to breast cancer. Its high diagnostic accuracy is attributable to its ability to characterize both anatomic and metabolic abnormalities, often occult by other modalities. Given the correlation between bone metastasis and prognostic significance, skeletal evaluation should be a primary goal of PET/CT in the patient with breast cancer, with close attention paid to morphologic and metabolic abnormalities (**Fig. 5**).

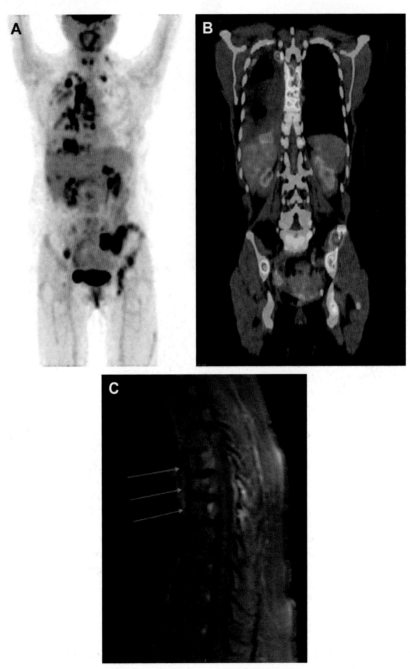

Fig. 5. Metastatic breast cancer with bony metastases. (*A*) A 42-year-old woman with diffuse bony metastases. (*B*) Fused coronal image confirms the extensive bony metastasis, typically a poor prognostic indicator. (*C*) Sagittal T1 FS with IV contrast showing T6 to T8 marrow enhancement (*arrows*) consistent with metastatic disease. Note that T7 has a pathologic fracture (breast cancer is the most common cause of pathologic fractures in women).

Evaluation of Thoracic Metastases

The presence of breast cancer metastasis to the lungs is associated with a bleak prognosis, with 5-year survival approaching 25%.[5] Early detection of pulmonary metastasis is important in both accurate staging and the likelihood of surgical cure. At present, no consensus criteria endorse screening of patients with asymptomatic, low-stage breast cancer. Those patients at higher risk of metastasis are commonly evaluated by means of thoracic CT or PET/CT. Because pulmonary nodules of both benign and malignant causes may be indistinguishable by CT, PET/CT may be used for further characterization. In a series of 29 patients with breast cancer with pulmonary nodules diagnosed by CT, less than half represented malignancy,[5] underscoring their nonspecificity, even in the patient with known primary malignancy.

PET-CT offers the additional benefit of assessing the metabolic activity of a lesion, increasing specificity. Nodules with focally increased FDG uptake should be considered as having high probability for malignancy. However, the diagnostic accuracy of PET imaging depends on pulmonary nodule size.[5] In one series, the sensitivity of PET in detecting pulmonary malignancy was 94% for nodules larger than 11 mm, decreasing to 78% in nodules 8 to 10 mm in diameter.[5] PET/CT is of low diagnostic usefulness in evaluating sub–8-mm lung nodules and should therefore not be used in the setting. This advice is secondary to the poor spatial resolution and increased motion artifacts, which are particularly problematic in the lung bases. PET/CT is beneficial in evaluating pulmonary nodules larger than 8 mm, with overall sensitivity and PPV of 77% and 89% respectively.[5]

A variety of infectious and inflammatory conditions may mimic thoracic metastasis. Radiation pneumonitis, pneumonia, and granulomatous disease are common reasons for false-positive PET/CT findings.[58] Metabolic activity of respiratory muscles and the diaphragmatic crura may also be mistaken for abnormalities and should be examined with caution.[58]

Evaluating Abdominal Visceral Metastases

The presence of hepatic disease portends the worst prognosis of all sites of distant breast cancer metastases.[17] Although PET/CT may detect liver metastasis, its accuracy is limited by background hepatic metabolic activity.[59] MR imaging has superiority in evaluating the liver, and thus may be a beneficial adjunct to PET/CT in cases of suspected isolated hepatic metastasis.

PET/CT has similarly limited usefulness in evaluating isolated adrenal metastases. In a study of 150 patients with suspicious adrenal nodules and known malignancy of various primary sources, the SUV_{max} values of malignant lesions were significantly higher than those of benign lesions.[60] However, because of the numerous physiologic and benign causes of increased FDG avidity, the investigators concluded that PET/CT has a limited role in the evaluation algorithm for adrenal nodules. Therefore, a suspicious adrenal nodule should be first characterized with contrast-enhanced CT or MR imaging, with attention paid to enhancement and washout characteristics. Indeterminate lesions may be considered for biopsy.[61]

Evaluating Brain Metastases

Screening for brain metastases is not recommended in patients with asymptomatic stage I breast cancer.[17] In patients with a high risk for brain metastases, accurate evaluation by PET/CT is hindered by background physiologic metabolic activity in the brain. FDG-PET has known poor accuracy in evaluating cerebral metastasis, with a reported sensitivity as low as 61%.[62] Evaluating brain metastasis with PET is also limited by poor spatial resolution, and its accuracy significantly decreases in proportion to decreasing lesion size.[62] For these reasons and because of its superior spatial resolution, brain MR imaging is the gold standard for evaluating cerebral, calvarial, and leptomeningeal metastases.[62] Therefore, PET/CT imaging protocols for breast cancer commonly exclude imaging the brain, in favor of dedicated brain MR imaging.

PET/CT in Evaluating Neoadjuvant Therapy

NACT consists of chemotherapy, targeted therapy, and/or endocrine therapy used in treating locally advanced breast cancer.[63] Neoadjuvant regimens are commonly used to shrink the tumor mass before breast conservation therapy,[63] and are increasingly used in large operable breast cancer.[4] However, up to 25% of patients treated in the neoadjuvant setting do not adequately respond to traditional NACT regimens.[63] Differentiating responders from the high proportion of nonresponders is of high clinical interest, sparing those nonresponders from side effects such as cardiotoxicity, neurotoxicity, alopecia, and nausea.[63] Because physical examination and other imaging modalities provide little benefit in evaluating response to NACT,[63] physiologic imaging with PET plays an important role.

Multiple studies have shown the success of PET/CT in differentiating responders and nonresponders to NACT.[6,63–65] Rousseau and colleagues[64] examined 52 patients undergoing NACT for locally advanced breast cancer who received PET/CT imaging at baseline and after the first, second, third, and sixth courses of chemotherapy. PET was able to accurately predict response to therapy after only 1 course of chemotherapy, using a threshold of a 50% decrease in SUV_{max}. PET imaging allowed identification of responders with sensitivity, specificity, NPV, and accuracy of 96%, 75%, 95%, and 84% respectively.[64] In an additional prospective evaluation of 78 patients with stage II and stage III breast cancer, PET/CT identified responders after 1 course of chemotherapy with high sensitivity and negative predictive values of 85.7% and 95.1%, respectively.[6] PET/CT provides a noninvasive means of predicting early response to NACT, directing nonresponders into modified chemotherapy regimens or early surgical intervention.

PET/CT in the neoadjuvant setting may also help determine nodal status and direct posttherapy clinical management. Nodal status remains an important prognosticator in patients undergoing NACT,[64] and is conventionally evaluated by SLNB and/or axillary lymph node dissection (ALND). Neoadjuvant therapy is known to alter the accuracy of the SLNB, resulting in false-negative rates as high as 19%.[4] In a study of 311 patients scheduled for NACT, the sensitivity of FDG-avid nodes for the detection of axillary metastases was 82%, which is similar to that of SLNB.[4] The investigators suggest that PET/CT may help monitor response to NACT and serve as an important adjunct to SLNB. In patients with FDG-avid axillary lymph nodes following NACT, ALND may be considered in the absence of nodal disease on SLNB.[4] Furthermore, PET/CT imaging resulted in a change of clinical management in a significant proportion of these patients. In 18% of these patients, occult IM or periclavicular chain lymph nodes were identified, changing regional radiation therapy in 16%.[4]

Physiologic response to NACT also carries prognostic significance. Metabolic alterations detected on PET or PET/CT commonly precede morphologic changes in a tumor, and often correlate with pathologic response to therapy.[37] Complete pathologic response is manifested by an absence of viable tumor cells on pathologic examination, and occurs in up to 25% of patients who undergo NACT.[64] This finding has an important clinical impact, because those patients with complete pathologic disease response to NACT carry a 96% expected 5-year survival.[37] By closely evaluating changes in SUV_{max}, clinicians and interpretive physicians gain important information that

may prevent unwarranted treatments, yield prognostic significance, and guide further clinical management.

Dual Time Point PET/CT

Breast tumors are associated with both increased glucose metabolism and increased angiogenesis relative to normal breast tissue. However, in breast cancer, these two factors are often mismatched.[23] High glucose metabolism relative to blood flow portends a worse prognosis, associated with decreased response to systemic therapy and earlier progression of disease.[23] Although this relationship was initially discovered using [15]O water, a study by Cochet and colleagues[23] suggests that similar information may be derived from dual time point PET/CT. In a prospective study of 59 patients with breast cancer, tumors were evaluated by both 2-minute dynamic imaging immediately following injection of FDG, as well as a static acquisition 90 minutes following FDG administration. In this small study, tumor blood flow on dynamic imaging was associated with immunohistochemical evidence of angiogenesis.[23] In contrast, increased tumor metabolism correlated with markers of proliferation such as Ki67.[23] Although its mainstream applicability has yet to be determined, dual time point PET/CT shows early potential in describing the phenotype profile of breast tumors.

Evaluation of Recurrent Breast Cancer and the Flare Phenomenon

PET-CT plays a prominent role in evaluating recurrent breast cancer, and provides an accurate means of assessing local and distant metastases.[66–70] Murakami and colleagues[70] examined the accuracy of PET/CT in 47 patients with suspected disease recurrence, concluding that its overall sensitivity and specificity were 96% and 91% respectively. Additional studies have corroborated this high sensitivity for characterizing breast cancer recurrence,[67] making it among the most accurate modalities for this application. Combined PET/CT provides more information than either PET or CT alone.[69] At present, debate surrounds the comparative benefit of PET/CT and MR imaging. Whole-body MR imaging shows promise in the evaluation of breast cancer, with similar accuracy and less acquisition time compared with PET/CT (average scan times at 1.5 T and 3.0 T were 51 and 43 minutes, respectively, compared with 103 minutes in PET/CT).[71,72] Focal hypermetabolic activity on PET/CT therefore indicates disease recurrence (with rare exceptions).

The tumor flare phenomenon (also known as the flare response) is characterized by an abrupt worsening of tumor-related symptoms following initiation of therapy, which may lead to the spurious diagnosis of disease progression. This syndrome may manifest with abruptly worsening clinical symptoms, which commonly include severe generalized pain and/or lymphadenopathy.[73] Imaging findings of disease progression may occur with or without these clinical manifestations, and are characterized by hypermetabolic lymphadenopathy that mimics metastasis. The flare phenomenon typically occurs within 7 to 10 days of beginning treatment,[12] but may present as late as 4 months following therapy cessation, which has led the European Organisation for Research and Treatment of Cancer (EORTC) PET group to suggest a minimum delay of 1 to 2 weeks following treatment cessation before PET imaging.[73] Although the flare phenomenon occurs infrequently,[12] it is an important cause of false-positive PET/CT examinations, so interpreting physicians should be aware of it.

Cost-Benefit Considerations

Ongoing efforts to reduce health care costs necessitate the close scrutiny of oncologic imaging, particularly in the setting of breast cancer because of its prevalence. The use of advanced imaging modalities in the work-up and management of breast cancer has significantly increased in recent years. Between 1992 and 2005, a 4-fold increase in PET/CT use was noted.[7] The average cost of imaging more than doubled over this time frame, and the average cost per patient has increased 4.1% annually.[7] In a review of 67,874 Medicare patients with stage II or stage III breast cancer, PET/CT imaging was often performed without clinical rationale and was commonly used in patients more than the 80 years of age, in whom its benefits are uncertain.[7] In spite of its high accuracy for breast cancer lesion detection, the mortality benefit and overall cost-effectiveness of PET/CT are unclear.

PET/CT provides improved detection of breast cancer metastases, changing clinical management in nearly 20% of patients. However, early detection does not always improve survival. An Italian clinical trial showed this phenomenon in 1243 patients who were randomized to either intensive imaging surveillance or clinical follow-up. In this study, breast cancer recurrence was detected an average of 1 month earlier in the group with intensive surveillance.[74] However, no significant difference in mortality in patients was shown between these two groups. In spite of this, surveys indicate that both patients and physicians prefer intensive imaging surveillance, even in asymptomatic patients.[17] However, these studies preceded the widespread use of PET/CT and breast MR imaging, and future research may help to delineate the role of each of these imaging modalities.

At present, no consensus guidelines advocate the use of PET/CT to evaluate for metastases in asymptomatic patients,[17] which is supported in research funded by the British National Institute for Health Research Health Technology Assessment program in which the investigators conclude that the routine use of PET/CT in all patients with breast cancer is not a cost-effective strategy.[45] PET/CT is likely best reserved for patients with breast cancer with high pretest probability for metastasis, such as T3 or greater lesions, stage III disease, or patients with early-stage disease and aggressive histopathologic features. Further research is needed to determine the proper cost-effective use of PET/CT and other advanced imaging modalities in the patient who has breast cancer.

Summary

The benefits of PET-CT in the initial evaluation of breast cancer include the high sensitivity for nodal and distant metastases as well as prognostic information based on the degree of FDG avidity. In addition, multiple studies have shown the benefit of PET-CT in the assessment of treatment response and recurrence in breast cancer. PET-CT should be used in concert with other imaging modalities in the initial and subsequent evaluation of patients with breast cancer. However, the cost-benefit considerations of PET-CT and other imaging needs to be considered, especially in patients at low risk for metastatic disease.

POSITRON EMISSION MAMMOGRAPHY

Anatomic imaging such as mammography, US, and MR imaging provide moderate specificity in determining the malignant potential of breast lesions. The desire to visualize and quantify primary breast tumors, as well as to follow treatment efficacy with functional/PET imaging, has driven the development of positron emission mammography (PEM). Traditional PET/CT imaging is limited in the detection of breast cancer, mainly because of its poor spatial resolution, but PEM may be a promising solution. It is a form of breast-specific functional imaging that combines the benefits of quantifying metabolic activity that comes with PET/CT and increased spatial resolution and anatomic imaging similar to traditional mammograms.

PEM uses high-resolution functional imaging in an immobilized breast. Initial protocols called for

10 mCi F18-FDG, but recent studies have shown that doses as low as 3 mCi may be adequate, and the *Journal of Nuclear Medicine* has approved a dose of 5 mCi for clinical use.[75] Patients are asked to fast before the study, which is similar to other forms of FDG imaging. After the injection of radiotracer, there is an approximate uptake time of 60 to 120 minutes. Following this wait time, the patient is positioned in the PEM scanner, which compresses the breast to obtain cranial-caudal (CC) and mediolatero-oblique (MLO) views, each scan taking approximately 7 to 10 minutes. Newer scanners are integrated into a traditional mammography unit, which allows accurate comparison of PEM and mammography images.[76] Although this is the most studied method, other techniques for dedicated functional breast imaging are being developed, particularly imaging a hanging breast with the patient prone instead of using compression.[77–80] This second technique is designed to improve on some of the drawbacks of PEM by allowing better visualization of posterior lesions near the pectoral muscle, reducing the patient discomfort that comes with compression, and allowing better comparison with MR imaging.[81]

Whole-body PET/CT has an important role in the initial work-up of stage II to III breast lesions, because it is useful in identifying metastatic disease and other primary tumors. However, traditional PET imaging is not particularly effective at visualizing/quantifying primary breast lesions, mainly because of its low spatial resolution. Current PET scanners provide spatial resolution of approximately 5 mm, making the detection of small or low-grade tumors difficult. PEM provides increased spatial resolution, down to 1.6 mm, and increased photon detection sensitivity as the detector is closer to the source. Another limitation of traditional PET imaging is patient positioning. Supine positioning does not allow the optimal visualization of tissue compared with compression, prone, or upright methods in MR imaging and mammography. A recent study showed PEM to have a significantly higher sensitivity for detecting primary breast tumors than PET/CT (95% vs 87%). This improvement was even greater in small lesions, with PEM maintaining a sensitivity of 60% to 70% in identifying lesions of less than 1 cm.[82]

PEM has shown comparable results with breast MR imaging in the detection of primary tumors, effectiveness in presurgical planning, and screening in the contralateral breast.[83–85] Unlike MR imaging, PEM is not affected by a patient's menopausal/hormonal status or breast density.[84] PEM is a possible alternative to MR imaging in patients with contraindications or claustrophobia, or in patients who have difficulty obtaining high-quality MR imaging because of motion. PEM is easy for breast imagers to learn because of the similarity in appearance of abnormalities. A recent study showed higher sensitivity and specificity for PEM (96% and 84%) compared with MR imaging (82% and 67%) in experienced breast imaging radiologists for the detection of breast lesions after a 2-hour didactic on PEM.[74]

Besides the detection and quantification of breast lesions, other uses for PEM are being developed. One promising use is PEM-guided breast biopsies. A multicenter study used a high-resolution PEM unit with biopsy guidance software to direct vacuum-assisted core biopsies, which resulted in successful sampling of all targeted lesions and no adverse events.[11] Not only does this provide another method of targeting lesions that may be difficult to see on other imaging modalities, it also allows the targeting of the most metabolically active portions of a lesion. Another potential use of PEM is to further characterize breast tumors. Studies have shown that there is a statistically significant higher mean lesion/background ratio on PEM imaging of ER-negative and PR-negative tumors, compared with the receptor-positive counterparts.[86] Tumors with higher histologic grade also had a significantly higher FDG uptake.[86] The use of other physiologic tracers, such as estradiol or thymidine, may also help further characterize or even better visualize certain lesions.[11]

PEM may in future be used for screening high-risk patients or those with other indications such as dense breasts, but its use as a general screening tool is currently limited by cost and radiation dose. A recent study compared the radiation exposure and radiation-induced cancer risk from screening mammography with screening PEM. Using the 10-mCi dose of F18-FDG, they calculated a 20 to 30 times higher cumulative cancer incidence and mortality for yearly screening of women aged 40 to 80 years with PEM versus conventional mammography. The benefit/risk ratio of annual digital mammography was estimated to be greater than 50:1, whereas the benefit/risk ratio for annual PEM screening of only women with dense breasts was estimated to be less than 10:1. The study concluded that, if the dose for PEM could be reduced to only 1 to 2 mCi, the benefit/risk ratio for yearly PEM screenings would approach that of annual mammography screening.[19]

SUMMARY

Although PET imaging may not be used in the diagnosis of breast cancer, the use of PET/CT is imperative in all aspects of breast cancer staging, treatment, and follow-up. PET will continue to be relevant in personalized medicine because accurate tumor status will be even more critical during and after the transition from a generic metabolic agent to receptor imaging. PEM is an imaging proposition that may have benefits in lower doses, but its use is limited without new radiopharmaceuticals.

REFERENCES

1. Robertson IJ, Hand F, Kell MR. FDG-PET/CT in the staging of local/regional metastases in breast cancer. Breast 2011;20(6):491–4.

2. Koolen BB, Vogel WV, Vrancken Peeters MJ, et al. Molecular imaging in breast cancer: from whole-body PET/CT to dedicated breast PET. J Oncol 2012;2012:438647.

3. Riegger C, Herrmann J, Nagarajah J, et al. Whole-body FDG PET/CT is more accurate than conventional imaging for staging primary breast cancer patients. Eur J Nucl Med Mol Imaging 2012;39(5):852–63.

4. Koolen BB, Olmos R, Elkhuizen P. Locoregional lymph node involvement on 18F-FDG PET/CT in breast cancer patients scheduled for neoadjuvant chemotherapy. Breast Cancer Res Treat 2012; 135(1):231–40.

5. Evangelista L, Panunzio A, Cervino AR, et al. Indeterminate pulmonary nodules on CT images in breast cancer patient: the additional value of 18F-FDG PET/CT. J Med Imaging Radiat Oncol 2012; 56(4):417–24.

6. Keam B, Im SA, Koh Y, et al. Predictive value of FDG PET/CT for pathologic axillary node involvement after neoadjuvant chemotherapy. Breast Cancer 2013;20(2):167–73.

7. Crivello ML, Ruth K, Sigurdson ER, et al. Advanced imaging modalities in early stage breast cancer: preoperative use in the United States Medicare population. Ann Surg Oncol 2013;20(1): 102–10.

8. Wang CL, MacDonald LR, Rogers JV, et al. Positron emission mammography: correlation of estrogen receptor, progesterone receptor, and human epidermal growth factor receptor 2 status and 18F-FDG. Am J Roentgenol 2011;197(2):W247–55.

9. Champion L, Brain E, Giraudet AL, et al. Breast cancer recurrence diagnosis suspected on tumor marker rising: value of whole-body 18FDG-PET/CT imaging and impact on patient management. Cancer 2011;117(8):1621–9.

10. Morris PG, Ulaner GA, Eaton A, et al. Standardized uptake value by positron emission tomography/computed tomography as a prognostic variable in metastatic breast cancer. Cancer 2012;118(22): 5454–62.

11. Auguste P, Barton P, Hyde C, et al. An economic evaluation of positron emission tomography (PET) and positron emission tomography/computed tomography (PET/CT) for the diagnosis of breast cancer recurrence. Health Technol Assess 2011; 15(18):iii–iiv, 1–54.

12. Evangelista L, Rubello D, Saladini G. Can FDG PET/CT monitor the response to hormonal therapy in breast cancer patients? Eur J Nucl Med Mol Imaging 2012;39(3):446–9.

13. Malhotra GK, Zhao X, Band H, et al. Histological, molecular and functional subtypes of breast cancers. Cancer Biol Ther 2010;10(10):955–60.

14. Bodian CA, Perzin KH, Lattes R. Lobular neoplasia. Long term risk of breast cancer and relation to other factors. Cancer 1996;78(5):1024–34.

15. Niikura N, Costelloe CM, Madewell JE, et al. FDG-PET/CT compared with conventional imaging in the detection of distant metastases of primary breast cancer. Oncologist 2011;16(8):1111–9.

16. Grankvist J, Fisker R, Iyer V, et al. MRI and PET/CT of patients with bone metastases from breast carcinoma. Eur J Radiol 2012;81(1):e13–8.

17. Huynh PT, Lemeshko SV, Mahoney MC, et al. ACR Appropriateness Criteria® stage I breast carcinoma. J Am Coll Radiol 2012;9:463–7.

18. Buck AK, Herrmann K, Stargardt T, et al. Economic evaluation of PET and PET/CT in oncology: evidence and methodologic approaches. J Nucl Med 2010;51(3):401–12.

19. Shiller SM, Weir R, Pippen J, et al. The sensitivity and specificity of sentinel lymph node biopsy for breast cancer at Baylor University Medical Center at Dallas: a retrospective review of 488 cases. Proc (Bayl Univ Med Cent) 2011;24(2):81–5.

20. Mortazavi-Jehanno N, Giraudet AL, Champion L, et al. Assessment of response to endocrine therapy using FDG PET/CT in metastatic breast cancer: a pilot study. Eur J Nucl Med Mol Imaging 2012;39(3):450–60.

21. Bidard FC, Hajage D, Bachelot T, et al. Assessment of circulating tumor cells and serum markers for progression-free survival prediction in metastatic breast cancer: a prospective observational study. Breast Cancer 2012;14(1):R29.

22. Keam B, Im SA, Lee KH, et al. Ki-67 can be used for further classification of triple negative breast cancer into two subtypes with different response and prognosis. Breast Cancer 2011;13(2):R22.

23. Cochet A, Pigeonnat S, Khoury B, et al. Evaluation of breast tumor blood flow with dynamic first-pass 18F-FDG PET/CT: comparison with angiogenesis markers and prognostic factors. J Nucl Med 2012;53(4):512–20.

24. Karimi P, Shahrokni A, Moradi S. Evidence for US Preventive Services Task Force (USPSTF) recommendations against routine mammography for females between 40–49 years of age. Asian Pac J Cancer Prev 2013;14(3):2137–9.

25. Smith RA, Saslow D, Sawyer KA. American Cancer Society guidelines for breast cancer screening: update 2003. CA Cancer J Clin 2003; 53(3):141–69.

26. Eberl MM, Fox CH, Edge SB, et al. BI-RADS classification for management of abnormal mammograms. J Am Board Fam Med 2006;19(2):161–4.

27. Saslow D, Boetes C, Burke W, et al. American Cancer Society guidelines for breast screening with MRI as an adjunct to mammography. CA Cancer J Clin 2007;57(2):75–89.

28. Agrawal G, Su MY, Nalcioglu O, et al. Significance of breast lesion descriptors in the ACR BI-RADS MRI lexicon. Cancer 2009;115(7):1363–80.

29. Sanli Y, Kuyumcu S, Ozkan ZG, et al. Increased FDG uptake in breast cancer is associated with prognostic factors. Ann Nucl Med 2012;26(4): 345–50.

30. Bernsdorf M, Berthelsen AK, Wielenga VT. Preoperative PET/CT in early-stage breast cancer. Ann Oncol 2012;23(9):2277–82.

31. Garami Z, Hascsi Z, Varga J, et al. The value of 18-FDG PET/CT in early-stage breast cancer compared to traditional diagnostic modalities with an emphasis on changes in disease stage designation and treatment plan. Eur J Surg Oncol 2012;38(1):31–7.

32. Adejolu M, Huo L, Rohren E, et al. False-positive lesions mimicking breast cancer on FDG PET and PET/CT. Am J Roentgenol 2012;198(3):W304–14.

33. Grubstein A, Cohen M, Steinmetz A, et al. Siliconomas mimicking cancer. Clin Imaging 2011;35(3): 228–31.

34. Kang BJ, Lee JH, Yoo IR, et al. Clinical significance of incidental finding of focal activity in the breast at 18F-FDG PET/CT. AJR Am J Roentgenol 2011; 197(2):341–7.

35. Chae EY, Cha JH, Kim HH, et al. Analysis of incidental focal hypermetabolic uptake in the breast as detected by 18F-FDG PET/CT: clinical significance and differential diagnosis. Acta Radiol 2012;53(5):530–5.

36. Koolen BB, Vrancken Peeters MJ, Wesseling J, et al. Association of primary tumour FDG uptake with clinical, histopathological and molecular characteristics in breast cancer patients scheduled for neoadjuvant chemotherapy. Eur J Nucl Med Mol Imaging 2012;39(12):1830–8.

37. Tateishi U, Miyake M, Nagaoka T, et al. Neoadjuvant chemotherapy in breast cancer: prediction of pathologic response with PET/CT and dynamic contrast-enhanced MR imaging–prospective assessment. Radiology 2012;263(1):53–63.

38. Groheux D, Giacchetti S, Moretti JL, et al. Correlation of high 18F-FDG uptake to clinical, pathological and biological prognostic factors in breast cancer. Eur J Nucl Med Mol Imaging 2011;38(3):426–35.

39. McEachen JC, Kuo PH. Male primary breast cancer found on FDG-PET/CT. Clin Nucl Med 2008; 33(9):630–2.

40. Beatty JS, Williams HT, Gucwa AL, et al. The predictive value of incidental PET/CT findings suspicious for breast cancer in women with non-breast malignancies. Am J Surg 2009;198(4):495–9.

41. Litmanovich D, Gourevich K, Israel O, et al. Unexpected foci of 18F-FDG uptake in the breast detected by PET/CT: incidence and clinical significance. Eur J Nucl Med Mol Imaging 2009; 36(10):1558–64.

42. Lyman GH, Giuliano AE, Somerfield MR, et al. American Society of Clinical Oncology guideline recommendations for sentinel lymph node biopsy in early-stage breast cancer. J Clin Oncol 2005; 23:7703–20.

43. Mabry H, Giuliano AE. Sentinel node mapping for breast cancer: progress to date and prospects for the future. Surg Oncol Clin N Am 2007;16(1): 55–70.

44. Straver ME, Meijnen P, van Tienhoven G, et al. Sentinel node identification rate and nodal involvement in the EORTC 10981-22023 AMAROS trial. Ann Surg Oncol 2010;17(7):1854–61.

45. Cooper KL, Meng Y, Harnan S, et al. Positron emission tomography (PET) and magnetic resonance imaging (MRI) for the assessment of axillary lymph node metastases in early breast cancer: systematic review and economic evaluation. Health Technol Assess 2011;15(4):iii–iiv, 1–134.

46. Groves AM, Shastry M, Ben-Haim S, et al. Defining the role of PET-CT in staging early breast cancer. Oncologist 2012;17(5):613–9.

47. Heusner TA, Kuemmel S, Hahn S, et al. Diagnostic value of full-dose FDG PET/CT for axillary lymph node staging in breast cancer patients. Eur J Nucl Med Mol Imaging 2009;36(10):1543–50.

48. Groheux D, Hindié E, Rubello D, et al. Should FDG PET/CT be used for the initial staging of breast cancer? Eur J Nucl Med Mol Imaging 2009;36(10): 1539–42.

49. De Bazelaire C, Groheux D, Chapellier M, et al. Breast inflammation: indications for MRI and PET-CT. Diagn Interv Imaging 2012;93(2):104–15.

50. Carkaci S, Macapinlac HA, Cristofanilli M, et al. Retrospective study of 18F-FDG PET/CT in the diagnosis of inflammatory breast cancer: preliminary data. J Nucl Med 2009;50(2):231–8.

51. Alberini JL, Lerebours F, Wartski M, et al. 18F-fluorodeoxyglucose positron emission tomography/computed tomography (FDG-PET/CT) imaging in the staging and prognosis of inflammatory breast cancer. Cancer 2009;115(21):5038–47.

52. Hamaoka T, Madewell JE, Podoloff DA, et al. Bone imaging in metastatic breast cancer. J Clin Oncol 2004;22(14):2942–53.

53. Piccardo A, Altrinetti V, Bacigalupo L, et al. Detection of metastatic bone lesions in breast cancer patients: fused (18)F-fluoride-PET/MDCT has higher accuracy than MDCT. Preliminary experience. Eur J Radiol 2012;81(10):2632–8.

54. Koolen BB, Vrancken Peeters MJ, Aukema TS, et al. 18F-FDG PET/CT as a staging procedure in primary stage II and III breast cancer: comparison with conventional imaging techniques. Breast Cancer Res Treat 2012;131(1):117–26.

55. Hahn S, Heusner T, Kümmel S, et al. Comparison of FDG-PET/CT and bone scintigraphy for detection of bone metastases in breast cancer. Acta Radiol 2011;52(9):1009–14.

56. Koolen BB, Vegt E, Rutgers EJ, et al. FDG-avid sclerotic bone metastases in breast cancer patients: a PET/CT case series. Ann Nucl Med 2012; 26(1):86–91.

57. Katayama T, Kubota K, Machida Y, et al. Evaluation of sequential FDG-PET/CT for monitoring bone metastasis of breast cancer during therapy: correlation between morphological and metabolic changes with tumor markers. Ann Nucl Med 2012. [Epub ahead of print].

58. Gorospe L, Raman S, Echeveste J, et al. Whole-body PET/CT: spectrum of physiological variants, artifacts and interpretative pitfalls in cancer patients. Nucl Med Commun 2005; 26(8):671–87.

59. Tatsumi M, Cohade C, Mourtzikos KA, et al. Initial experience with FDG-PET/CT in the evaluation of breast cancer. Eur J Nucl Med Mol Imaging 2006; 33(3):254–62.

60. Boland GW, Blake MA, Holalkere NS, et al. PET/CT for the characterization of adrenal masses in patients with cancer: qualitative versus quantitative accuracy in 150 consecutive patients. Am J Roentgenol 2009;192(4):956–62.

61. Berland LL, Silverman SG, Gore RM, et al. Managing incidental findings on abdominal CT: white paper of the ACR incidental findings committee. J Am Coll Radiol 2010;7(10):754–73.

62. Rohren EM, Provenzale JM, Barboriak DP, et al. Screening for cerebral metastases with FDG PET in patients undergoing whole-body staging of non–central nervous system malignancy1. Radiology 2003;226(1):181–7.

63. Buchbender C, Kuemmel S, Hoffmann O, et al. FDG-PET/CT for the early prediction of histopathological complete response to neoadjuvant chemotherapy in breast cancer patients: initial results. Acta Radiol 2012;53(6):628–36.

64. Rousseau C, Devillers A, Campone M, et al. FDG PET evaluation of early axillary lymph node response to neoadjuvant chemotherapy in stage II and III breast cancer patients. Eur J Nucl Med Mol Imaging 2011;38(6):1029–36.

65. Groheux D, Hindié E, Giacchetti S, et al. Triple-negative breast cancer: early assessment with 18F-FDG PET/CT during neoadjuvant chemotherapy identifies patients who are unlikely to achieve a pathologic complete response and are at a high risk of early relapse. J Nucl Med 2012; 53(2):249–54.

66. Constantinidou A, Martin A, Sharma B, et al. Positron emission tomography/computed tomography in the management of recurrent/metastatic breast cancer: a large retrospective study from the Royal Marsden Hospital. Ann Oncol 2011;22(2): 307–14.

67. Aukema TS, Rutgers EJ, Vogel WV, et al. The role of FDG PET/CT in patients with locoregional breast cancer recurrence: a comparison to conventional imaging techniques. Eur J Surg Oncol 2010; 36(4):387–92.

68. Pennant M, Takwoingi Y, Pennant L, et al. A systematic review of positron emission tomography (PET) and positron emission tomography/computed tomography (PET/CT) for the diagnosis of breast cancer recurrence. Health Technol Assess 2010;14(50):1–103.

69. Dirisamer A, Halpern BS, Flöry D, et al. Integrated contrast-enhanced diagnostic whole-body PET/CT as a first-line restaging modality in patients with suspected metastatic recurrence of breast cancer. Eur J Radiol 2010;73(2):294–9.

70. Murakami R, Kumita SI, Yoshida T, et al. FDG-PET/CT in the diagnosis of recurrent breast cancer. Acta Radiol 2012;53(1):12–6.

71. Schmidt GP, Baur-Melnyk A, Haug A, et al. Comprehensive imaging of tumor recurrence in breast cancer patients using whole-body MRI at 1.5 and 3 T compared to FDG-PET-CT. Eur J Radiol 2008;65(1):47–58.

72. Schmidt G, Dinter D, Reiser MF, et al. The uses and limitations of whole-body magnetic resonance imaging. Dtsch Arztebl Int 2010;107(22): 383–9.

73. Tu DG, Yao WJ, Chang TW, et al. Flare phenomenon in positron emission tomography in a case of breast cancer–a pitfall of positron emission tomography imaging interpretation. Clin Imaging 2009; 33(6):468–70.

74. Palli D, Russo A, Saieva C, et al. Intensive vs clinical follow-up after treatment of primary breast cancer: 10-year update of a randomized trial. National Research Council Project on Breast Cancer Follow-up. JAMA 1999;281(17):1586.

75. MacDonald L, Luo W, Lu X. Low dose lesion contrast on the PEM Flex Solo II [slides 1-9]. 2010. Retrieved from AAPM website: http://www.aapm.org/meetings/amos2/pdf/49-13625-50296-366.pdf.

76. MacDonald L, Edwards J, Lewellen T, et al. Clinical imaging characteristics of the positron emission

mammography camera: PEM Flex Solo II. J Nucl Med 2009;50(10):1666–75.

77. Raylman RR, Abraham J, Hazard H, et al. Initial clinical test of a breast-PET scanner. J Med Imaging Radiat Oncol 2011;55(1):58–64.

78. Wu Y, Bowen SL, Yang K, et al. PET characteristics of a dedicated breast PET/CT scanner prototype. Phys Med Biol 2009;54(13):4273–87.

79. Bowen SL, Wu Y, Chaudhari AJ, et al. Initial characterization of a dedicated breast PET/CT scanner during human imaging. J Nucl Med 2009;50(9): 1401–8.

80. Soriano A, González A, Orero A, et al. Attenuation correction without transmission scan for the MAMMI breast PET. Nucl Instrum Methods Phys Res A 2011;648:S75–8.

81. Murthy K, Aznar M, Thompson CJ, et al. Results of preliminary clinical trials of the positron emission mammography system PEM-I: a dedicated breast imaging system producing glucose metabolic images using FDG. J Nucl Med 2000;41(11):1851–8.

82. Eo JS, Chun IK, Paeng JC, et al. Imaging sensitivity of dedicated positron emission mammography in relation to tumor size. Breast 2012;21(1):66–71.

83. Berg WA, Madsen KS, Schilling K, et al. Breast cancer: comparative effectiveness of positron emission mammography and MR imaging in presurgical planning for the ipsilateral breast. Radiology 2011;258(1):59–72.

84. Schilling K, Narayanan D, Kalinyak JE, et al. Positron emission mammography in breast cancer presurgical planning: comparisons with magnetic resonance imaging. Eur J Nucl Med Mol Imaging 2011;38(1):23–36.

85. Berg WA, Madsen KS, Schilling K. Comparative effectiveness of positron emission mammography and MRI in the contralateral breast of women with newly diagnosed breast cancer. AJR Am J Roentgenol 2012;198(1):219–32.

86. Sloka JS, Hollett PD, Mathews M. Cost-effectiveness of positron emission tomography in breast cancer. Mol Imaging Biol 2005;7(5):351–60.

Role of Positron Emission Tomography–Computed Tomography in Gastrointestinal Malignancies

Kevin P. Banks, MD[a,b,c],*, Won S. Song, MD[a]

KEYWORDS

- Positron emission tomography–computed tomography • ^{18}F-Fluorodeoxyglucose
- Gastrointestinal malignancies • Neoadjuvant therapy

KEY POINTS

- Positron emission tomography (PET) combined with computed tomography (CT) has become the standard of care for staging and/or monitoring of many gastrointestinal (GI) malignancies.
- The physiologic information of PET provides a functional map of abnormal versus normal tissue metabolism while CT provides complementary anatomic data to include accurate localization of PET findings. Together, these two modalities are synergistic and provide valuable information not available from other imaging tests.
- PET-CT is becoming the first-line imaging tool at many institutions for assessing patients with suspected recurrent GI malignancies, as it is able to detect recurrent lesions earlier and with greater accuracy which, in turn, improves management decisions.
- Its value when added to conventional imaging evaluations is clear, with the metabolic information obtained from PET-CT resulting in a change in treatment for a large percentage of patients with GI cancers.
- The addition of a dedicated contrast-enhanced CT to the PET-CT protocol has been demonstrated to further improve its accuracy, and will likely become the standard of care for the majority of PET-CT examinations in the near future.

INTRODUCTION

Colorectal, stomach, and esophageal cancer rank third, fourth, and eighth, respectively, in terms of incidence worldwide, with nearly 3 million new cases of gastrointestinal (GI) malignancy diagnosed each year.[1] Many of these GI neoplasms are not only prevalent, but, in the cases of stomach and esophageal cancer, have some of the highest mortality-to-incidence ratios amongst all tumors.[2] As such, cancers of the GI tract are a serious health concern, with intense efforts focusing on improving both the diagnosis and management of these diseases. As part of this effort, positron emission tomography–computed tomography (PET-CT) using the ^{18}F-labeled glucose analogue fluorodeoxyglucose (FDG) has emerged as a valuable imaging

[a] Department of Radiology, Brooke Army Medical Center, San Antonio Health Care System, 3851 Roger Brooke Drive, San Antonio, TX 78234, USA; [b] Department of Radiology, Uniformed Services University of Health Sciences, 4301 Jones Bridge Rd, Bethesda, MD 20814, USA; [c] Department of Radiology, University of Texas Health Science Center at San Antonio, 7703 Floyd Curl Drive, San Antonio, TX 78229, USA
* Corresponding author. Department of Radiology, Brooke Army Medical Center, 3851 Roger Brooke Drive, San Antonio, TX 78234.
E-mail address: kevin.banks@amedd.army.mil

Radiol Clin N Am 51 (2013) 799–831
http://dx.doi.org/10.1016/j.rcl.2013.05.003
0033-8389/13/$ – see front matter Published by Elsevier Inc.

tool for the diagnosis, staging, and monitoring of these entities. First entering clinical use in 2001, combined PET-CT imaging has quickly become ubiquitous in oncologic imaging. The physiologic information of FDG PET provides a functional map of abnormal versus normal tissue metabolism while CT provides complementary anatomic data to include accurate localization of PET findings. Together, the two modalities have proved to be synergistic, with the images from PET-CT systems routinely outperforming PET alone as well as PET and CT examinations acquired separately but viewed together.[3]

Long known for its utility in imaging lymphoma, FDG PET-CT has likewise become the standard of care for staging and/or monitoring of many GI malignancies such as esophageal cancer, gastrointestinal stromal tumors (GIST), and colorectal carcinoma. The diagnostic information it provides has proved extremely valuable, with referring physicians reporting that the information supplied by FDG PET-CT changes management in 20% to 140% of patients.[4,5] Meanwhile, its role in imaging less common entities such as cholangiocarcinoma and cystic pancreatic neoplasms shows great promise, and will undoubtedly continue to grow as more research provides clearer guidance regarding the best utilization in the care of these patients.

METHODOLOGY

FDG PET provides information on tissue function while CT provides morphologic characterization as well as accurate localization of organs and lesions. Combined, the two modalities allow for maximal identification and localization of pathologic processes. Before the advent of integrated systems, attenuation correction was accomplished by rotating a positron-emitting material such as germanium-68 (^{68}Ge) around the patient. This step accounted for 40% or more of the scan time.[6] With the development of PET-CT scanners and subsequent use of CT for attenuation correction, examination times for patients have decreased significantly. Initially these CT examinations were acquired using a low-dose protocol that only provides attenuation correction and gross anatomic localization of abnormalities identified on PET. Thus the CT examinations were not considered diagnostic, and many oncologic patients were required to obtain a separate normal/full-dose CT using intravenous and oral contrast as clinically indicated. Nowadays PET-CT scans routinely come with 8-, 16-, or even 64-slice capability, providing the same anatomic imaging capabilities of stand-alone CT scanners. In recent

years, research has shown the value of contrast-enhanced diagnostic CT examinations as part of PET-CT protocols as well as important information that can be obtained from diligent review of such scans.[5,7] Given these promising results, more and more facilities are performing diagnostic-quality CT examinations with contrast as part of the PET-CT study (Box 1).

Early on during this transition to diagnostic quality CT, there was concern that the presence of intravenous iodinated contrast could induce significant artifacts on the attenuation-corrected PET images. Because of the significant photoelectric

---

Box 1
Generic GI tumor PET-CT protocol with diagnostic CT

- Measure of serum blood glucose following 4 to 6 hours' fast (consider rescheduling if exceeds 200 mg/dL)
- Administer 1 L of dilute oral contrast starting 1 hour before scan (consider H_2O immediately before scanning for gastric and pancreatic cancers)
- Inject 8 to 12 mCi of FDG 60 to 90 minutes before scan
- Have patient void urinary bladder immediately before scan
- Administer an additional 50 to 100 mL of oral contrast immediately before patient positioning (except for gastric and pancreatic cancers)
- Head fixation with arms up beside head
- CT and PET both acquired during shallow respiration
- Diagnostic CT settings of approximately 120 kV and 160 mA (adjusted per clinical indications and institutional preferences)
- Administer 100 mL of low-osmolar iodinated intravenous contrast
- Obtain CT scan in cranial-caudal direction following injection of intravenous contrast
  - Typically acquired in portal-venous phase occurring 60 to 70 seconds after injection
  - Preceding arterial phase obtained 30 to 40 seconds after injection may be helpful with certain GI tumors such as pancreatic and cholangiocarcinoma
- Immediately perform PET scan in caudal-cranial direction using 3-dimensional acquisition (scan direction limits time for filling of bladder with excreted FDG and potential for obscuring pelvic lesions)

effect at lower photon energies, contrast-enhanced blood absorbs 40% of the photons used in CT imaging ($\sim$80 kEv), but only 2% of the higher-energy photons (511 kEv) inherent to PET imaging.[3] Despite this difference, a decade of experience has proved that intravenous contrast rarely induces a diagnostically significant artifact.[8] With enteric contrast, there is a similar concern related to the difference in photon absorption secondary to positive contrast agents. Although some significant artifacts have been reported, this appears to be limited to the use of high-density contrast material, particularly in the right colon where contrast desiccation is thought to result in barium concentration.[9] Studies using orally administered iodine-based agents or dilute barium-based compounds showed a paucity of clinically relevant PET artifacts while often providing diagnostically useful information in the CT portion of the examination, particularly in the assessment of GI malignancies.[10,11]

The undergoing evolution from low-dose noncontrast CT to standard-dose contrast-enhanced CT (CECT) appears to be beneficial. Initial studies show a change in clinical management in almost one-fifth of all patients with cancer, while more than three-quarters of those with tumors of the GI tract receive additional benefit, predominantly related to improved localization of PET-avid lesions and more accurate staging of local tumors.[7,12]

ESOPHAGEAL CANCER

Esophageal cancer is the third most frequent GI malignancy, comprising a mix of squamous cell carcinoma and adenocarcinoma.[13] Squamous cell carcinoma is the most common histology, typically found in the upper two-thirds of the esophagus, and is associated with smoking and alcohol consumption. Adenocarcinoma is less frequent but is rapidly increasing in incidence. It is most likely to arise in the distal esophagus and at the gastroesophageal junction. Obesity and reflux are the major risk factors, with smoking and alcohol appearing to have no significant roles.[14]

Despite advancements in treatment, esophageal cancer continues to carry a poor long-term prognosis, with a 5-year survival rate of 38% for those presenting with isolated esophageal disease, 20% for patients with regional spread, and only 3% for those diagnosed initially with distant disease.[15] From 20% to 30% of patients will present with distant metastases, precluding any surgical cure.[16] For those without metastatic disease, treatment options are far from benign, with esophagectomy with or without neoadjuvant chemotherapy or chemoradiotherapy currently providing the only hope for cure. Even with aggressive curative surgical attempts, most patients will have recurrence within 2 years following initial therapy. In an effort to improve outcomes and reduce futile surgeries, FDG PET-CT is being used increasingly in an attempt to more accurately stage and monitor these patients.

[^{18}F]Fluorodeoxyglucose PET-CT for the Diagnosis and Staging of Esophageal Cancer

To date there is little evidence supporting the use of PET-CT for differentiating benign from malignant esophageal disease in either symptomatic or asymptomatic individuals, owing to unacceptable sensitivity and specificity (Box 2).[3] Although overall detection of primary lesions using FDG PET and PET-CT exceeds 90% in patients with esophageal carcinoma, results vary significantly by stage and size of the primary tumor.[17] In a

---

Box 2
FDG PET-CT pitfalls in evaluation of primary or recurrent esophageal cancer

False Negatives

T1 lesions: 57% of lesions are not detected

T2 lesions: 17% of lesions are not detected

Locoregional lymph node metastases: up to 64% of malignant nodes are not detected

Small volume of residual disease following chemotherapy/chemoradiotherapy: can be indistinguishable from complete pathologic response (defined as less than 10% viable tumor cells)

False Positives

Gastroesophageal sphincter uptake (typically circumferential, uniform, and without mass/soft tissue irregularity)

Hiatal hernia

Biopsy site

Anastomosis/suture line

Esophagitis (linear in distribution: can be secondary to reflux, radiation therapy, or infection). The abnormal FDG uptake associated with radiation therapy–induced esophagitis usually does not present until 2 weeks after treatment and may last several months

Reactive hilar/mediastinal lymph nodes (increased FDG uptake due to chronic inflammation is often seen in heavy smokers and patients with chronic respiratory diseases)

Focal liver necrosis (secondary to radiation therapy for tumors of gastroesophageal junction)

PET study of 149 patients, T1 lesions (carcinoma confined to the mucosa or submucosa) were detected only 43% of the time, and T2 lesions (carcinoma invading the muscularis propria) 83% of the time.[18,19] Other investigators have had similar findings using PET, demonstrating that only 51% to 53% of superficial esophageal cancers will have increased FDG avidity.[20] More recently, PET-CT has shown more promise than PET alone. Evaluating 81 patients with biopsy-proven adenocarcinoma or squamous cell carcinoma, PET-CT identified the primary tumor in 91.4% of cases.[21]

Conversely, false-positive findings are also a problem. Physiologic FDG accumulation at the gastroesophageal (GE) sphincter can impersonate a GE-junction tumor, and inflammatory FDG accumulation at sites of recent biopsy, ulcers, and esophagitis may be mistaken for malignancy (Fig. 1).[22] Following radiation therapy, focal liver necrosis secondary to radiation therapy for lower esophageal/GE junction tumors has also be reported as a potential mimic of liver metastasis.[23]

Once the diagnosis of esophageal malignancy is established, accurate staging of esophageal

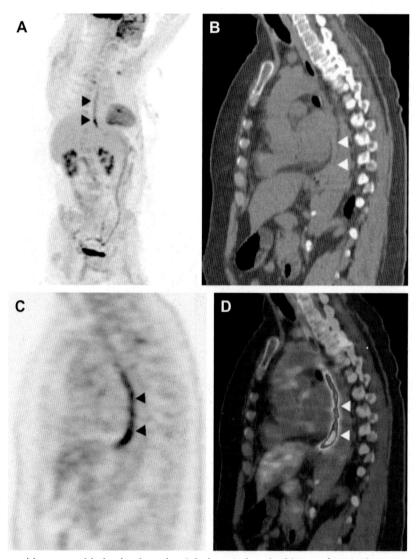

Fig. 1. A 71-year-old woman with dysphagia and weight loss, and a prior history of stage I breast cancer. (A) Right anterior oblique view from maximum-intensity projection (MIP) from FDG PET-CT shows a long segment of moderately intense linear FDG uptake in the mid to distal esophagus (arrowheads). Additional degenerative FDG uptake is present in spine as well as left sternoclavicular joint. (B–D) Sagittal noncontrast CT, PET, and fused PET-CT confirms the activity to be localized to a normal-appearing esophagus (arrowheads). Findings were consistent with esophagitis, and confirmed at endoscopy.

cancer becomes critical in determining appropriate therapy. Staging is performed using the standardized American Joint Committee on Cancer (AJCC) Tumor-Node-Metastasis (TNM) classification (**Box 3**). PET-CT generally offers little information regarding the depth of mural invasion, with the exception of invasion into adjacent organs (T4) that can sometimes be detected with confidence. Its inability to differentiate between T1, T2, and T3 lesions is likely due to limitations of spatial resolution on PET as well as the inability of CT to distinguish the separate layers of the esophagus. In a study by Lowe and colleagues[24] looking at the combined capabilities of FDG PET and CT to accurately assess the tumor (T) stage found it was correct in only 42% of patients, compared with 71% of cases evaluated by endoscopic ultrasonography (EUS). Similarly, Bar-Shalom and colleagues[25] found that PET-CT offered no additional value for the assessment of primary tumors over PET alone. As of now, EUS remains the best means for T-staging in the majority of cases.

Box 3
AJCC TNM staging for esophageal carcinoma

T1: carcinoma confined to mucosa or submucosa

T2: carcinoma invades muscularis propria

T3: carcinoma invades the adventitia

T4: carcinoma invades adjacent structures

N0: no locoregional lymph node metastases

N1: locoregional lymph node metastases

M0: no distant metastases

M1a: metastases to celiac or cervical lymph nodes (for distal and upper carcinomas, respectively)

M1b: nonregional lymph node or organ metastases

Stage 0: Tis N0 M0

Stage I: T1 N0 M0

Stage IIA: T2 N0 M0 or T3 N0 M0

Stage IIB: T1 N1 M0 or T2 N1 M0

Stage III: T3 N1 M0, T4 N0 M0, or T4 N1 M0

Stage IVA: Any T, Any N, M1a

Stage IVB: Any T, Any N, M1b

Used with the permission of the American Joint Committee on Cancer (AJCC), Chicago, Illinois. The original source for this material is the AJCC Cancer Staging Manual, Seventh Edition (2010) published by Springer-Verlag, New York, www.springer.com.

Paraesophageal nodal metastases and abdominal nodes cephalad to the celiac axis when the primary lesion is located in the distal esophagus are considered N1 disease, and do not preclude surgical resection. CT has suboptimal performance in the noninvasive determination of N1 disease, having sensitivity of 84% and specificity of 67%.[24] FDG PET as a stand-alone modality has better specificity but poorer sensitivity, with a meta-analysis of 12 PET studies showing pooled sensitivity of 51% and specificity of 84%.[26] Because of its limited spatial resolution, the performance of PET is particularly poor in assessing lymph nodes located near the primary tumor, a common manifestation of esophageal cancer.[27] The use of combined PET-CT may potentially overcome shortcomings of both modalities (**Fig. 2**). In a preoperative study of 45 patients with esophageal cancer, PET-CT had sensitivity, specificity, and accuracy of 94%, 92%, and 92%, respectively.[28] In a separate study specifically evaluating the benefit of PET-CT over PET, investigators found that PET-CT improved the definition of locoregional nodal disease in 7 of 11 (64%) areas of concern.[25] Unfortunately, other researchers have not had such promising results. A study of 81 patients by Walker and colleagues[21] found PET-CT to have a sensitivity of only 34% for locoregional adenopathy while Shimizu and colleagues[29] found a sensitivity of 14% for mediastinal nodal disease in a study of 20 patients. Both of these studies used a noncontrast CT technique, and it is possible that improved accuracy could be obtained with the use of such a method. Until more studies are performed to determine the accuracy of PET-CT with diagnostic-quality CT with intravenous contrast, EUS remains the first choice for the evaluation of locoregional lymph nodes.

Metastatic disease precludes surgery in patients with esophageal cancer and, thus, preoperative detection of such is critical in avoiding the morbidity and mortality associated with esophagectomy in patients who will not see a survival benefit. Conventional imaging consists of diagnostic CT of the chest, abdomen, and pelvis, in combination with EUS. The shortcomings of these modalities may be related to the high percentage of patients who historically experience recurrent disease soon after radical resection. Similar to its utility in other malignancies, FDG PET has shown usefulness in this aspect of staging.[30–32] This fact is of particular importance given that 20% to 30% of patients with esophageal carcinoma present with metastatic disease, to either nonregional lymph nodes or other organs.[16] The most common sites of visceral metastases are the liver, lungs,

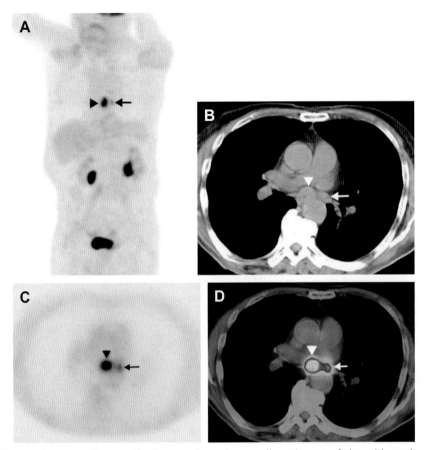

Fig. 2. An 81-year-old man with recently diagnosed squamous cell carcinoma of the mid esophagus. (*A*) Left anterior oblique view of an MIP from FDG PET-CT shows a hypermetabolic lesion in region of mid esophagus (*arrowhead*) and adjacent small focus (*arrow*) of additional abnormal FDG accumulation. (*B–D*) Axial noncontrast CT, PET, and fused PET-CT shows irregular hypermetabolic esophageal thickening (*arrowhead*). Immediately adjacent is a subcentimeter lymph node, occult by CT, with FDG avidity (*arrow*) consistent with regional metastatic disease.

bones, and adrenal glands.[33] In an evaluation of 97 patients, investigators found that CT and EUS missed surgically proven metastatic disease in 47% of cases, whereas the addition of PET reduced underdiagnosis of metastases to 11%.[26] Similarly, in 76 patients with curable disease as assessed by CT and EUS, Gananadha and colleagues[34] found that 25% were excluded from surgery because of metastatic disease identified on PET, as well as 1 patient with a synchronous primary lung cancer. Bar-Shalom and colleagues[25] specifically looked at the additional value of noncontrast PET-CT over PET, and found that the combined modalities further improved accuracy, changing interpretation in 22% of patients, in part by identifying 2 of 18 surgical candidates with metastatic disease missed by PET and excluding distal metastases in 4 patients with physiologic bowel activity that was concerning on PET. The results of Walker and colleagues[21]

were similarly impressive, with PET-CT detecting metastatic disease in 25% of patients and appropriately redirecting care to either chemoradiation or palliative therapy.

[^{18}F]Fluorodeoxyglucose PET-CT for Evaluating the Response of Esophageal Cancer to Neoadjuvant Therapy

Neoadjuvant therapy has become a standard part of the treatment regimen for patients with locally advanced disease. The addition of preoperative chemotherapy and radiation therapy to esophagectomy in this subset of patients has been shown to have a higher chance of complete resection and decreased likelihood of local recurrence, resulting in an improved 3-year survival.[23,35,36] Unfortunately, only 40% to 50% of patients respond to neoadjuvant therapy.[14] Early identification of this select group of patients is critical, as several studies have demonstrated that individuals who receive neoadjuvant chemotherapy and do not respond have a worse outcome than if they had undergone esophagectomy alone.[37,38] The most likely explanation of this deleterious result is a combination of the toxic side effects of chemotherapy/chemoradiotherapy as well as surgical delay, during which up to 1 in 6 patients will develop metastatic disease.[23]

Assessment of therapeutic response has traditionally made use of a combination of EUS and CT. These morphologic modalities are hindered by chemoradiation-related necrosis and fibrosis that distort pretreatment anatomy, but do not accurately reflect a corresponding tumor response. By contrast, the metabolic information inherent to FDG PET-CT provides a means of assessing tumor response that is not dependent on structural changes. Despite false-positive findings related to esophagitis or ulceration (see **Box 2**), PET has proved to be far superior to CT or EUS. In a literature review, Westerterp and colleagues[39] assessed response to neoadjuvant therapy, finding the sensitivity and specificity of PET to be 71% to 100% and 55% to 100%, in comparison with 33% to 55% and 50% to 71% for CT, and 50% to 100% and 36% to 100% for EUS. For the reasons stated earlier, it is beneficial to identify a response to neoadjuvant therapy early in its course so that nonresponders may have their chemotherapy altered or proceed to surgery without further delay. PET-CT was used to evaluate patients after 14 days of neoadjuvant chemoradiotherapy for both squamous cell carcinoma and adenocarcinoma of the esophagus. In patients with squamous cell carcinoma, a decrease in FDG uptake of 30% from baseline was found to accurately differentiate patients who went on to have a histologic response (<10% viable tumor cells) from nonresponders, with sensitivity and specificity of 93% and 88%.[40] In patients with adenocarcinoma, a decrease in FDG uptake of 33% from baseline was found to accurately differentiate responders from nonresponders, with sensitivity and specificity of 100% and 63%.[41] These findings were prospectively investigated in the MUNICON trial, where PET was used to modify treatment in patients with adenocarcinoma of the esophagus. Using a tumor standardized uptake value (SUV) decrease of 35% from baseline after 2 weeks on induction chemotherapy, patients were identified as responders or nonresponders. Responders completed neoadjuvant chemoradiotherapy before surgery, whereas nonresponders went on immediately to surgery. With a median follow-up of 2.3 years, overall survival was 25.8 months in nonresponders, but had not been

reached in responders. Event-free survival was 14.1 months in nonresponders and 29.7 months in responders.[42] This study was the first to prospectively demonstrate the feasibility of using early metabolic assessment with PET to guide neoadjuvant treatment algorithms in esophageal cancer.

[¹⁸F]Fluorodeoxyglucose PET-CT for the Diagnosis of Recurrent Esophageal Cancer

Recurrent disease is frequent after surgery. Historically, two-thirds of recurrences occur within the first year following treatment, with the remainder presenting by 2 years.[43] Patients who develop recurrent disease are incurable, but may benefit from additional therapy that can improve symptoms and increase survival time.[44] FDG PET-CT has shown definite utility in this role. In a study of 56 patients who had undergone curative therapy and presented with possible recurrence by symptoms or equivocal results on conventional imaging, PET-CT identified recurrence in 45 cases.[45] Overall, PET-CT had sensitivity of 93% and accuracy of 87% for identifying recurrent esophageal cancer. There were 9 false-positive results in the study, with 5 being due to increased uptake at the esophagogastric anastomosis. Other researchers have encountered a similar limitation, with Flamen and colleagues[46] finding PET to have a specificity of only 57% for recurrence at the site of anastomosis. Additional promising results for the use of PET-CT in detecting recurrent esophageal cancer were reported by Bar-Shalom and colleagues.[25] In a study of a mixed patient population comprising 23 individuals following resection of the primary tumor and 18 patients before surgery, they demonstrated increased accuracy of PET-CT versus PET interpreted side by side with CT, with sensitivity of 96%, specificity of 81% (vs 59% for side by side), and accuracy of 90% (vs 83% for side by side).

Summary

FDG PET-CT is useful in the initial staging of patients who have esophageal cancer and, as such, is included in the National Comprehensive Cancer Network (NCCN) 2012 guidelines for staging workup. Although its role in the evaluation of the primary tumor is limited, it shows promise in the assessment of locoregional nodal disease and is clearly a valuable tool for the identification of distal metastases. In this regard, PET-CT can help avoid unnecessary surgeries in patients who are failed by conventional imaging in accurately diagnosing M1 disease. In patients receiving neoadjuvant chemotherapy and/or radiation therapy, PET-CT has likewise shown usefulness, accurately identifying responders and nonresponders both following therapy and early in therapy when changes to treatment may benefit nonresponders. After esophagectomy, recurrent disease is frequent. In this setting, PET-CT is more sensitive and specific than conventional imaging assessment, although it is somewhat limited by its high rate of false-positive results at the site of anastomosis.

GASTRIC CANCER

Gastric cancer is relatively infrequent in the United States and Europe, but worldwide it is the fourth most frequent type of cancer.[47] It is an adenocarcinoma and has 2 major subtypes, the intestinal type and the nonintestinal or diffuse type. *Helicobacter pylori* is the main risk factor in 65% to 80% of cases, yet gastric cancer only develops in 2% of infected individuals.[48] Increased risk is also seen in individuals with chronic atrophic gastritis as well as in those with diets high in salted fish or meats, smoked foods, and pickled vegetables, possibly because of increased levels of nitrates and nitrites.

At present, the only cure is complete resection of the tumor and any involved regional lymph nodes. Many patients unfortunately present with advanced disease, with only 25% of European and United States patients in 2 studies, and only 5% of patients in a high-risk population from South America, presenting with Stage I or Stage II disease.[49–51] Treatment options for those with advanced disease are limited to palliative chemotherapy or neoadjuvant therapy with the goal of downstaging the carcinoma. Recurrence rates following radical gastrectomy are as high as 48%, recurrence being most frequently seen as peritoneal metastases or at distant sites, with locoregional recurrence the exception.[52] Five-year survival following gastrectomy remains only moderate, with 63% of patients succumbing to their disease.[52] In comparison with conventional diagnostic techniques, PET with FDG has been reported to provide increased accuracy and, thus, PET-CT is being applied more regularly in patients with gastric cancer.

[¹⁸F]Fluorodeoxyglucose PET-CT for the Diagnosis and Staging of Gastric Cancer

FDG PET is not considered an appropriate first-line diagnostic tool for the diagnosis of gastric cancer, which in part is likely due to the highly variable, but normal, uptake of FDG in the stomach, making detection of early gastric cancer difficult with PET. In a study by Stahl and colleagues,[53] PET identified only 60% of locally advanced gastric carcinomas. A challenge of early detection is also related to the poor FDG avidity of the nonintestinal subtypes including signet-ring cell and mucinous carcinomas. This group of gastric carcinomas is known to have low tumor-cell density and a high percentage of metabolically inert mucus, which explains why they were detected in only 41% of cases whereas the intestinal subtype was detected in 83% of cases.[53] Other researchers have obtained better results in detecting locally advanced gastric cancers (90%), but still could only identify 40% of patients with early-stage gastric cancer (**Fig. 3**).[54] A recent study specifically examined PET-CT in 71 patients with surgically proven advanced gastric cancer and found its sensitivity to be similar to CECT: 93% versus 90%.[55] False positives remain a challenge with both PET and PET-CT, owing to physiologic uptake and various inflammatory processes such as gastritis and ulcers (**Box 4, Fig. 4**).

The role of PET and PET-CT in the staging of gastric cancer is evolving, but the 2012 NCCN guidelines recommend PET-CT when conventional imaging fails to identify metastatic disease (with the exception of T1 patients). Similar to that for esophageal cancer, staging is based on the AJCC TNM classification (**Box 5**). As with many malignancies, tumor stage is poorly assessed with PET-CT because of the limited spatial resolution of PET and the inability of CT to reliably differentiate the layers of the gastric wall. This task is best performed preoperatively with EUS, which has a diagnostic accuracy of 78% to 93%.[56,57]

The limitations of using CT for the N-staging of regional lymph node metastases are related to its inability to differentiate reactive hyperplasia from metastatic disease as well as the frequent presence of malignant lymph nodes that are normal in morphology. Even so, CT appears to be better than PET and at least as good as PET-CT (performed using low-dose, noncontrast CT) for this task, and remains the mainstay for preoperative staging with or without EUS. In a study of 85 patients, Mochiki and colleagues[54] found FDG PET to have excellent specificity (100%) but only 23% sensitivity. Using a long-axis diameter of greater than 1 cm for the diagnosis of malignant lymph nodes, CT had specificity of 77% but sensitivity of 65%. In a similar study of 78 patients with gastric cancer, with postoperative abnormality as the gold standard, PET-CT had an accuracy of sensitivity of 31% versus 61% for diagnostic CT.[58] Specificity of PET-CT was again seen to be excellent, at 97%. Part of the shortcomings of PET appears to be related to perigastric lymph nodes that are often indistinguishable from the

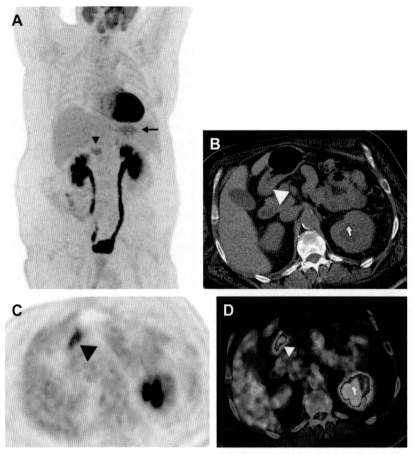

Fig. 3. A 63-year-old man with nonhealing gastric ulcer proven to be early-stage gastric carcinoma by endoscopic biopsy. (*A*) Right anterior oblique view of an MIP from FDG PET-CT shows a mild focus of abnormal FDG accumulation in region of gastric antrum (*arrowhead*). Physiologic uptake is present in the fundus (*arrow*). (*B–D*) Axial noncontrast CT, PET, and fused PET-CT show mild FDG avid mural thickening (*arrowhead*) correlating with the tumor and surrounding inflammation. Histology was diffuse signet-ring cell type, which typically demonstrates low FDG avidity as seen in this example. Focal gastritis could have a similar appearance, making prospective diagnosis of early gastric carcinoma difficult.

immediately adjacent tumor or physiologic FDG uptake in the stomach. The clinical impact of this may be negligible in patients with advanced gastric cancer because these nodes are part of standard dissection.[59] When PET-CT was compared with CECT in 71 patients who underwent gastrectomy, CECT showed a better, though suboptimal, sensitivity of 75% versus 41% for PET-CT, and accuracy of 77% versus 51% for PET-CT.[55] PET-CT had a slightly better specificity of 100% in comparison with CECT's 92%. This study, as with many evaluating the utility of PET-CT, used a low-dose, noncontrast CT as part of the PET-CT examination. Thus, it is foreseeable that PET-CT performed with diagnostic-quality CECT would yield accuracy better than either of the modalities investigated in this study.

Mixed results have been demonstrated with regard to accuracy of PET-CT in comparison with conventional imaging for the assessment of metastatic disease. In a study by Kim and colleagues,[55] 11 patients had distant metastatic disease. Whereas PET-CT identified all 4 cases of distant lymph node metastases in comparison with CECT, which missed one owing to its small size, PET-CT correctly identified 2 of the 10 patients with surgically proven peritoneal seeding (20%) while CECT suggested the presence of such in 5 of the 10 cases (50%). Sim and colleagues obtained similar results when looking at the detection of peritoneal spread of disease in 15 patients. Their study showed CECT to have a sensitivity of 87% versus 47% for PET-CT. Other metastatic lesions often not identified by PET-CT include subcentimeter lung nodules and sclerotic bone

Box 4
FDG PET-CT pitfalls in evaluation of primary or recurrent gastric cancer

False Negatives

Signet cell and mucinous subtypes: 59% of lesions are not detected

Early gastric cancer: 60% of lesions are not detected

Locoregional lymph node metastases: up to 69% of malignant nodes are not detected

False Positives

Gastroesophageal sphincter uptake (typically circumferential, uniform, and without mass/soft tissue irregularity)

Hiatal hernia

Physiologic uptake (often diffuse or regional, most typically involving proximal stomach; if more intense distally, focal, or with associated CT abnormality, further evaluation should be considered). Physiologic uptake is decreased with gastric distention by H_2O or oral contrast

Gastritis (diffuse or regional, typically without associated abnormality on CT)

Peptic ulcer disease

Biopsy site

lesions.[60] Combining the findings of diagnostic CT and PET-CT has been shown to provide a sensitivity of 78%.[61] Given these results, it is logical to assume that PET-CT using diagnostic-quality CECT will provide the most optimal means for detection of metastatic gastric cancer (**Fig. 5**).

Of note, in a study specifically looking at the ability of PET-CT to predict surgical success in patients with locally advanced gastric cancer, researchers found that valuable information could be gained. Looking at 142 patients, they found that a combination of high SUV for the primary tumor (>5.0) and concurrent presence of FDG-avid lymph nodes was specific for noncurable operations (91%).[62] However, sensitivity was low at 35%, with an overall accuracy of 77%.

[^{18}F]Fluorodeoxyglucose PET-CT for Evaluating the Response of Gastric Cancer to Neoadjuvant Therapy

Several studies have looked at the prospective capability of PET to assess response in patients undergoing neoadjuvant chemotherapy for gastric cancer. Results are promising, and strongly suggest that the metabolic changes measured by PET/PET-CT can predict a histologic response to therapy. In 71 patients undergoing cisplatin-based chemotherapy, FDG PET was performed at baseline and 14 days after the start of treatment. Using a decrease in SUV of 35% from baseline studies, 65% of the 17 patients with a metabolic response also showed a histologic response, whereas only 17% of the 32 patients who did not have a metabolic response demonstrated a histologic response.[63] This same study showed that non–FDG-avid tumors (comprising 22 of 71 of the cases) at baseline had a histologic response (24%) and prognosis similar to FDG-avid tumors that were metabolic nonresponders, suggesting that therapy modification in this subgroup of patients may be beneficial despite an inability to assess them for a metabolic response. In a second study using PET-CT, 42 patients with locally advanced gastric cancer were evaluated at baseline. Thirty-one had FDG-avid disease, and underwent repeat PET-CT at day 35 following neoadjuvant therapy with irinotecan and cisplatin. The investigators found that a 45% decrease in SUV best distinguished pathologic responders (<50% residual tumor) from nonresponders.[64] Metabolic response was also found to have prognostic implications, with nonresponders having a median time of 14.4 months until recurrence while responders' median disease-free survival was not reached by the time of the study's conclusion at 23.3 months. This study did not incorporate CT findings in the assessment and, as seen with GIST, it is plausible that accuracy may benefit from incorporation of these additional data.

[^{18}F]Fluorodeoxyglucose PET-CT for the Diagnosis of Recurrent Gastric Cancer

To date, there are no published studies evaluating the accuracy of PET-CT for gastric cancer recurrence using diagnostic-quality CT (standard dose with intravenous and oral contrast). PET-CT using a low-dose, noncontrast CT technique is less effective than conventional CT in the follow-up of patients with gastric cancer, and is considered optional by the 2012 NCCN guidelines. Park and colleagues[65] prospectively studied 105 patients with clinical or radiologic suspicion of recurrence of gastric cancer, of whom 75 were subsequently confirmed to have recurrence. PET-CT had sensitivity, specificity, and accuracy of 75%, 77%, and 75%, respectively. These values are better than those seen with PET alone, but the researchers noted that recurrence from low–FDG-avid tumor subtypes such as signet-ring cell and mucinous carcinoma was still commonly occult on PET-CT. Comparing CECT with PET-CT in 38 patients with recurrent gastric

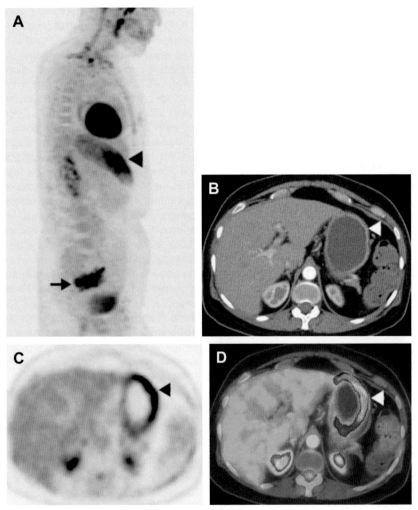

Fig. 4. A 59-year-old man undergoing PET-CT for staging of colon cancer. (*A*) Lateral view of an MIP from FDG PET-CT shows a segment of intense FDG uptake in the sigmoid colon (*arrow*) corresponding with the patient's primary lesion. Diffuse uptake is seen in the stomach with an area of superimposed intense uptake in the body (*arrowhead*). (*B–D*) Axial contrast-enhanced CT, PET, and fused PET-CT show normal gastric wall thickness, but abnormal mucosal enhancement corresponding to site of intense FDG avidity (*arrowhead*). Given the intense, but nonfocal nature of the uptake and lack of a mass, this was not thought to be physiologic or malignant, and gastritis was suggested. Subsequent endoscopy revealed active chronic gastritis.

cancer, Sim and colleagues[66] found PET-CT to be less sensitive (68%) than CECT (89%), but slightly more specific (71% vs 64%, respectively). The difference was most significant in patients with recurrent disease presenting as peritoneal seeding. When these 15 cases were excluded, the sensitivity and specificity of the two modalities were similar. The investigators found no increase in diagnostic accuracy on comparing PET-CT with CECT.

Summary

PET-CT has a limited role in detecting and evaluating the local extent of gastric cancer, mainly attributable to its poor sensitivity for early gastric cancer and nonintestinal subtypes. It shows good specificity and positive predictive value in identifying regional lymph node and distant metastasis, but sensitivity remains suboptimal, primarily in the setting of malignant perigastric lymph nodes and peritoneal spread of disease. Metabolic assessment of gastric cancer during neoadjuvant chemotherapy has been shown to be feasible and provides an early noninvasive means of stratifying patients' response to therapy, providing the future opportunity to customize treatment. In the diagnosis of recurrent gastric cancer, PET-CT enjoys moderate success. In the future, as

Box 5
AJCC TNM staging for gastric carcinoma

T1: carcinoma invades lamina propria/muscularis mucosa (T1a) or submucosa (T1b)

T2: carcinoma invades muscularis propria

T3: carcinoma penetrates subserosal connective tissue

T4: carcinoma invades serosa (visceral peritoneum) (T4a) or adjacent structures (T4b)

N0: no locoregional lymph node metastases

N1: metastases in 1 to 2 regional lymph nodes

N2: metastases in 3 to 6 regional lymph nodes

N3: metastases in 7 to 15 (N3a) or 16+ (N3b) regional lymph nodes

M0: no distant metastases

M1: distant metastases

Stage 0: Tis N0 M0

Stage IA: T1 N0 M0

Stage IB: T2 N0 M0 or T1 N1 M0

Stage IIA: T3 N0 M0 or T2 N1 M0 or T1 N2 M0

Stage IIB: T4a N0 M0 or T3 N1 M0 or T2 N2 M0 or T1 N3 M0

Stage IIIA: T4a N1 M0 or T3 N2 M0 or T2 N3 M0

Stage IIIB: T4b N0/1 M0 or T4a N2 M0 or T3 N3 M0

Stage IIIC: T4b N2/3 M0 or T4a N3 M0

Stage IV: Any T, Any N, M1

Used with the permission of the American Joint Committee on Cancer (AJCC), Chicago, Illinois. The original source for this material is the AJCC Cancer Staging Manual, Seventh Edition (2010) published by Springer-Verlag, New York, www.springer.com.

research assesses the accuracy of PET-CT using diagnostic-quality CT acquisition, it will undoubtedly see greater success in its role in the evaluation of recurrent disease as well as the N- and M-staging of gastric cancer.

GASTROINTESTINAL STROMAL TUMORS

GIST is a rare subset of mesenchymal tumors found in the GI tract. GIST are the most common mesenchymal lesion of the alimentary tract, yet only account for 0.1% to 3% of all GI malignancies.[67] Historically misclassified as leiomyomas, leiomyoblastomas, and leiomyosarcomas, it was subsequently discovered that the GIST cell of origin is the intestinal cell of Cajal rather than smooth muscle cells.[68] Ninety-five percent of

GIST express c-kit, a tyrosine kinase receptor (CD117).[69] Mutation of this receptor is present in nearly all patients with GIST and is thought to be the main cause of malignant transformation, providing growth and survival signals to tumor cells. GIST most frequently occur in middle-aged or older patients and are often asymptomatic until their size exceeds 5 cm[70] Once symptoms develop, patients most commonly present with abdominal pain, GI bleeding, and/or anemia. A GIST is typically a solitary circumscribed mass at the time of diagnosis, with the majority arising from the stomach and one-quarter of them developing in the small bowel. The rectum, colon, appendix, and esophagus are all rare sites of primary GIST. Fortunately, the majority of patients (50%–90%) are diagnosed before metastases have developed.[71,72] Of interest, when metastases do occur they are most commonly seen in the liver and peritoneum, with nodal, pulmonary, and osseous metastases being rare.[73] Surgery is the initial treatment for eligible patients. Despite apparent complete resection, many patients experience recurrence, with a similar distribution of disease as seen in patients who initially present with metastases.[74]

GIST are known to be chemoresistant and insensitive to radiation therapy, leaving few options for treating patients with unresectable or metastatic/recurrent disease.[75] In 2001, a clinical trial showed that a tyrosine kinase inhibitor, imatinib mesylate (Gleevac; Novartis, Basel, Switzerland), was successful in treating GIST.[76] Since then this agent has proved to be extremely effective, with most patients experiencing clinical benefits and long-term disease stability. This revolution in treatment was soon paralleled by a revolution in imaging assessment, with PET-CT now the current standard of care for evaluating response to therapy in these patients.

[18F]Fluorodeoxyglucose PET-CT for the Diagnosis and Staging of Gastrointestinal Stromal Tumors

Several studies have shown that most untreated GIST demonstrate high FDG avidity and thus can be readily detected with PET/PET-CT.[77,78] However, given that they typically present as a large mass and do not often metastasize to lymph nodes, PET-CT is not used for the diagnosis of GIST, nor is it generally recommended for their T- and N-staging (**Box 6**). One exception may be in the targeting of diagnostic biopsies. PET can best identify the metabolically active cellular areas of the tumor, which can improve the accuracy of histologic assessment while avoiding sampling

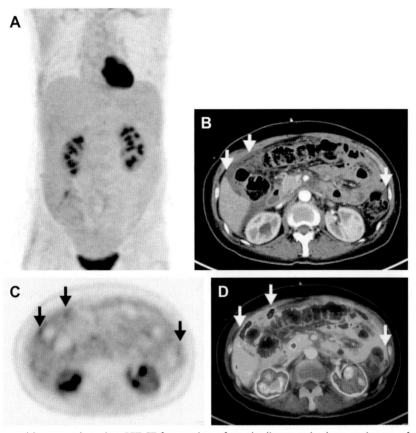

Fig. 5. A 53-year-old man undergoing PET-CT for staging of newly diagnosed adenocarcinoma of the stomach. (A) Frontal view of an MIP from FDG PET-CT shows diffuse increased FDG uptake throughout the entire abdomen, obscuring the normal outlines of physiologic hepatic and splenic FDG avidity. (B–D) Axial contrast-enhanced CT, PET, and fused PET-CT show FDG-avid ascites and nodular peritoneal/omental thickening (arrows). Peritoneal carcinomatosis was suggested, and subsequently proved by exploratory laparotomy.

error related to regions of tumor necrosis or cystic change.

Although PET-CT is not recognized as a standard means for diagnosing metastatic disease, research has shown it to be extremely accurate for such diagnoses. In a study of 20 patients with GIST using PET-CT with a diagnostic CECT technique, Antoch and colleagues[79] found that PET-CT identified more metastatic lesions (282) compared with PET (135) and CT (249). Even when PET and CT were read side by side, 3 lesions were missed that were properly diagnosed on fused PET-CT.

A separate study evaluated the potential role of PET-CT for the detection of occult metastatic disease following clinically complete resection, given that abdominal spread of disease may be missed in a large number of patients at the time of surgery. In 48 consecutive patients, PET-CT detected only 2 cases of occult metastatic disease and overdiagnosed metastatic disease in 6 patients, resulting in sensitivity and specificity of 25% and 88%,

respectively.[80] The investigators concluded that PET-CT performed immediately after R0 resection (removal of all visible and microscopic tumor) was not a sufficient tool for detecting clinically occult disease.

[18F]Fluorodeoxyglucose PET-CT for Evaluating the Response of Gastrointestinal Stromal Tumors to Therapy

The benefit of monitoring the treatment of GIST with protein kinase inhibitors stems from the fact that administration of these drugs (imatinib and, more recently, sunitinib) quickly switches off metabolic activity in the tumor.[81] This change can be seen with PET imaging as soon as 24 hours following initiation of therapy. By contrast, morphologic changes may take weeks to months to become apparent on CT and magnetic resonance (MR) imaging. A further confounding factor in CT and MR imaging assessment is that some liver lesions undergoing treatment with tyrosine kinase inhibitors have been shown to increase in size as they become more cystic while occult isodense hepatic metastases may liquefy and become hypodense, suggesting the presence of new metastatic lesions.[79,82,83] Capitalizing on these discordant findings, Goerres and colleagues[84] compared PET-CT with CECT in 34 patients with GIST who were undergoing therapy with imatinib mesylate. Posttreatment PET scans were able to predict overall survival and time to progression, whereas CECT provided insufficient prognostic power. Numerous other studies have likewise shown PET to be superior to CT for the identification of tumor response from imatinib treatment.[78,85–87] The value of metabolic assessment can be seen very early after initiation of treatment. In a study of patients with metastatic or unresectable primaries, patients underwent a baseline PET and again at 1 week after therapy with imatinib mesylate. Changes in SUV (mean decrease of 65% for PET responders and 16% for PET

nonresponders) matched treatment response in 14 of 15 cases.[88] PET-CT further increases the diagnostic accuracy over PET and/or CECT alone. Antoch and colleagues[79] examined 20 patients before and at 1, 3, and 6 months after initiating imatinib treatment. Response was determined using the metabolic response criteria recommended by the European Organization for Research and Treatment of Cancer (EORTC) and the anatomic response criteria according to the Response Evaluation Criteria in Solid Tumors (RECIST), with the additional stipulation that a response was considered to be present if attenuation decreased by 25%. Using these criteria and comparing results over a mean follow-up of 381 days, 95% of responders were correctly identified with PET-CT (performed with standard-dose, CECT) versus 85% with PET alone and 44% with CECT. At 3 months, PET-CT accurately identified 100% of responders. The study also pointed out the potential value gained from the CECT portion of the PET-CT examination. Twelve of 14 responders were correctly identified by a decrease in lesion density of 25%, further adding to the accuracy of the PET-CT.

[^{18}F]Fluorodeoxyglucose PET-CT for the Diagnosis of Recurrent Gastrointestinal Stromal Tumors

Although no reports of PET-CT for the detection of recurrent disease have been published, results from studies evaluating FDG PET in comparison with CECT imply its success in this role (Fig. 6). Gayed and colleagues[89] used both modalities to assess 54 patients with recurrent GIST. These investigators found CT to have a sensitivity and positive predictive value of 93% and 100% for CT, whereas PET had a sensitivity and positive predictive value of 86% and 98%. Of interest, the 5 false-positive findings on PET were related to osseous degenerative/stress changes and physiologic bowel activity that PET-CT would likely correctly assess as benign. Likewise, two-thirds of the false-negative findings were small lesions in the lungs, liver, and peritoneum, which would likely be detected with PET-CT using a diagnostic CT technique.

Summary

PET-CT currently does not have a significant role in the diagnosis or T- and N-staging of GIST. For M-staging it appears to be more accurate than PET or diagnostic CT, and will likely soon become a standard part of the evaluation of such tumors. In addition, some researchers have shown that preoperative PET-CT can help predict curability in

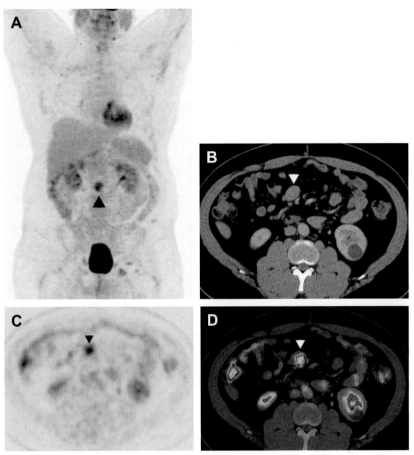

Fig. 6. A 52-year-old man with history of small bowel GIST, status post resection and 12 months of therapy with Gleevac, presented with new abdominal pain. (*A*) Frontal view of an MIP from FDG PET-CT shows a focal area of abnormal FDG avidity in the central abdomen (*arrowhead*). (*B–D*) Axial contrast-enhanced CT, PET, and fused PET-CT show a solid FDG-avid mesenteric mass (*arrowhead*) consistent with recurrent GIST.

surgery for locally advanced gastric carcinoma. The current value of PET-CT is in the assessment of tumor response to tyrosine kinase inhibitors. Metabolic findings precede morphologic changes by months, and numerous investigators have proved the accuracy of PET in assessing the early metabolic changes. Use of dedicated PET-CT further improves identification of patients responding to treatment, making it an essential part of monitoring therapy.

PANCREATIC CANCER

Adenocarcinoma of the pancreas is the fifth leading cause of cancer-related mortality in the United States, accounting for 5% of all cancer-related deaths.[90] It is most commonly seen in the seventh and eighth decade of life, and the most significant risk factor is smoking, with obesity and chronic pancreatitis also associated with an increased incidence.[91] Tumors arise from the pancreatic

ducts and are most frequently found in the head of the gland. Given their location, patients classically present with a triad of obstruction of the common bile duct, jaundice, and pain. Surgery remains the only potential hope for long-term survival but, because of the aggressive biology of these tumors, most patients are unresectable at the time of initial diagnosis, and overall 5-year survival rate remains poor at 20% with a median survival of less than 2 years.[92] Extension of disease is common, and typically involves direct invasion into adjacent structures and spread to regional lymph nodes or the liver. In patients who are deemed resectable and undergo surgery, recurrence is common, occurring within 6 to 12 months, thus suggesting the presence of surgically occult extrapancreatic spread of disease at the time of presentation.[93] Given the high rate of relapse, surveillance is critical, traditionally accomplished by monitoring of carbohydrate antigen 19-9 (CA 19-9) and the use of various imaging modalities.

Recent research adding PET-CT to the initial assessment and subsequent follow-up examinations shows improved accuracy, although improved clinical outcomes remain to be proved.

[¹⁸F]Fluorodeoxyglucose PET-CT for the Diagnosis and Staging of Pancreatic Adenocarcinoma

The use of PET for diagnosing pancreatic adenocarcinoma has been well researched, with a summary of the literature published in 2001 reporting an average sensitivity of 94% and specificity of 90%.[94] More recently evaluations of PET-CT have been performed, and results generally support the idea that it improves assessment of primary lesion when compared with conventional noninvasive imaging in the setting of an indeterminate solid pancreatic mass. Kauhanen and colleagues[95] evaluated 37 patients with PET-CT, CECT, and MR imaging, and found the diagnostic accuracy of PET-CT to be 89% in comparison with 79% for MR imaging and 76% for CECT. Farma and colleagues[96] obtained similar results on investigating 82 patients using PET-CT and standard diagnostic CT. PET-CT had sensitivity of 89% and specificity of 88% for the diagnosis of pancreatic cancer (with a limited negative predictive value of only 68%). In a different study,[97] investigators evaluated 19 patients with pancreatic masses that conventional imaging had been unable to differentiate between neoplasm and focal chronic pancreatitis. PET-CT was found to be very valuable, correctly identifying all 10 benign cases and all 9 malignant cases. Despite this, most providers prefer tissue confirmation of all suspect solid lesions to avoid inappropriately denying a patient potentially curative surgery. Given the excellent sensitivity of EUS in detecting pancreatic lesions (98% in a study of 80 patients with cancer) and the ability to perform fine-needle aspiration, it is understandable why PET-CT remains an adjunct in the assessment of indeterminate solid pancreatic lesions.[98] It has been suggested that PET-CT be primarily used for diagnosis in patients who cannot undergo EUS or have had nondiagnostic biopsy results.

Of note, FDG PET has shown only moderate sensitivity of 70% to 80% for the detection of periampullary carcinomas,[99] which is thought to result from adjacent physiologic bowel FDG uptake and the small size of these lesions at detection.

As with many tumors, there is no current role for PET-CT in the T-staging of pancreatic carcinoma (**Box 7**). However, this could change as more facilities incorporate the use of diagnostic CECT into their PET-CT protocols, with possible inclusion of

---

> **Box 7**
> **AJCC TNM staging for pancreatic adenocarcinoma**
>
> T1: cancer smaller than 2 cm and has not spread beyond the pancreas
> T2: cancer larger than 2 cm and has not spread beyond the pancreas
> T3: cancer has spread beyond the pancreas but not to major blood vessels/nerves
> T4: cancer has spread beyond the pancreas and involves major blood vessels/nerves
> N0: no regional lymph node metastases
> N1: metastases to regional lymph nodes
> M0: no distant metastases
> M1: distant metastases
>
> | | | |
> |---|---|---|
> | Stage IA: | T1 N0 M0 | Resectable |
> | Stage IB: | T2 N0 M0 | |
> | Stage IIA: | T3 N0 M0 | Typically resectable |
> | Stage IIB: | T1-3 N1 M0 | |
> | Stage III: | T4 Any N M0 | Unresectable |
> | Stage IV: | Any T, Any N, M1 | |
>
> Used with the permission of the American Joint Committee on Cancer (AJCC), Chicago, Illinois. The original source for this material is the AJCC Cancer Staging Manual, Seventh Edition (2010) published by Springer-Verlag, New York, www.springer.com.

---

dual-phase techniques. Strobel and colleagues[100] examined the ability of PET-CT with a dual-phase CECT to accurately determine the resectability of pancreatic cancer. Fifty patients were evaluated, and operative findings, histology, and follow-up imaging were used as the reference standard. Dual-phase contrast-enhanced PET-CT (obtained during arterial and portal-venous phases of intravenous contrast administration) showed sensitivity, specificity, and accuracy of 96%, 82%, and 88%, respectively. By comparison, routine PET-CT with low-dose noncontrast CT acquisition had an accuracy of only 76%. Of particular interest was the ability of dual-phase contrast-enhanced PET-CT to correctly identify all 5 patients with arterial infiltration, whereas unenhanced PET-CT missed all 5 (**Fig. 7**). Similarly, dual-phase contrast-enhanced PET-CT identified 4 of 5 patients with peritoneal carcinomatosis, whereas unenhanced PET-CT identified 3 of 5 cases. Both modalities missed 5 instances of surgically unresectable disease: 2 with liver metastases, 2 with infiltration of the mesenteric root, and 1 with peritoneal carcinomatosis. Of particular interest was that PET-CT detected 2 patients with other primary malignancies; a stage T1 non–small cell lung cancer and a stage T1 uterine cancer.

For N-staging, PET-CT has not proved itself to be superior to CECT, yet does appear to offer

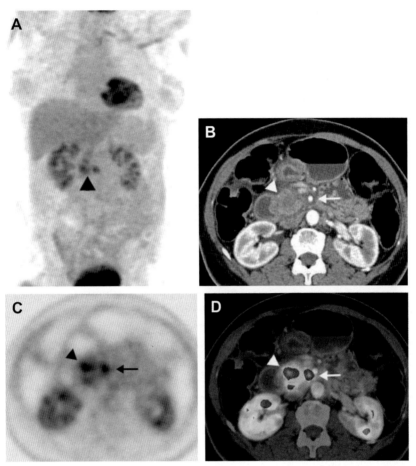

Fig. 7. A 63-year-old woman with pancreatic adenocarcinoma. (*A*) Frontal view of an MIP from FDG PET-CT shows a focal area of abnormal FDG avidity (*arrowhead*) in the medial to right kidney. (*B–D*) Axial contrast-enhanced CT, PET, and fused PET-CT show a hypermetabolic mass in the head of the pancreas (*arrowhead*), consistent with pancreatic adenocarcinoma. There is loss of the normal fat plane around the superior mesenteric artery (SMA) caused by extension of FDG-avid tissue (*arrow*), consistent with SMA involvement.

complementary information (**Box 8**). In the previously discussed study by Farma and colleagues,[96] adenopathy was best assessed using a combination of CECT, EUS, and PET-CT, yet remained suboptimal at 53%. PET-CT by itself was found to be limited in identifying malignant lymph nodes, being less sensitive than either CECT or EUS. The poor sensitivity of PET-CT for N-staging was further confirmed in a different study of 17 patients with pancreatic adenocarcinoma. Only 30% of surgically proven cases were prospectively identified, without improvement in the sensitivity when compared with CT and MR imaging.[95] In the future, the use of PET-CT with diagnostic-quality CT in combination with EUS will likely result in the most accurate means of preoperative assessment.

PET-CT is most helpful, and superior to CECT, for the identification of unsuspected distal metastases. Numerous studies have proved that FDG PET identifies more metastatic lesions than does CT, and is also helpful in characterizing indeterminate lesions seen on CT. In the previously cited study by Kauhanen and colleagues,[95] the sensitivity of PET-CT was compared with that of CECT and MR imaging for M-staging. Both CECT and MR imaging had a sensitivity of 38%, whereas PET-CT had a sensitivity of 88% (**Fig. 8**). In the study by Farma and colleagues,[96] CECT was compared with PET-CT as well as the combination of both in 82 patients. Detection of distant metastases rose from 57% for diagnostic CT to 61% for PET-CT and to 87% when both modalities were combined. This study supports the ongoing shift of using diagnostic-quality CT instead of noncontrast low-dose CT when performing PET-CT, obviating a separate dedicated CT examination. Of note, in both the Kauhanen

---

Box 8
FDG PET-CT pitfalls in evaluation of primary or recurrent pancreatic cancer

False Negatives

Elevated serum glucose levels (high incidence of hyperglycemia in patients with pancreatic pathology): elevated glucose can cause decreased FDG uptake by tumor owing to competitive inhibition, although not all researchers have found hyperglycemia to have a significant impact on accuracy

Mucinous tumors

Well-differentiated neuroendocrine tumors (best assessed with In-111 Octreoscan or I-123 metaiodo-benzylguanidine [MIBG]); of note, almost all neuroendocrine tumors that are negative on Octreoscan or MIBG are positive by FDG PET and such a finding carries a worse prognosis

Periampullary carcinoma: 70% to 80% sensitivity, likely due to small size at presentation and adjacent physiologic bowel activity

Locoregional lymph node metastases: up to 70% of malignant nodes are not detected

False Positives

Acute pancreatitis

Chronic active pancreatitis

Biliary stent: approximately 50% of patients will demonstrate FDG avidity along stent tract, likely due to combination of procedural inflammation and attenuation artifact

Recent endoscopic retrograde cholangiopancreatography

Radiation therapy: most intense during first 4 to 6 weeks following treatment

Serous cystadenoma

Retroperitoneal fibrosis

---

and Farma studies the detection of additional metastases not seen on conventional imaging led to a change in management in up to 26%.

[¹⁸F]Fluorodeoxyglucose PET-CT for Evaluating the Response of Pancreatic Adenocarcinoma to Neoadjuvant Therapy

Research is showing that the metabolic changes assessed by FDG PET can be useful for the evaluation of pancreatic tumor response to neoadjuvant therapy. An early study looked at 9 patients with potentially resectable pancreatic cancer who received chemoradiation therapy. Using a reduction in SUV of 50% in comparison with a baseline scan, 4 responders who all went on to successful resection were identified by PET, which demonstrated histologic evidence of tumor necrosis.[101] Despite a clear response to therapy, none of these same 4 patients showed a decrease in tumor size by CT evaluation. More recent research looking at PET-CT has confirmed these findings. Heinrich and colleagues[102] assessed PET-CT in 28 patients who underwent neoadjuvant therapy, and found that a metabolic response correlated with a histologic response. Similarly, in a retrospective review of 12 patients with borderline resectable pancreatic cancer who underwent neoadjuvant chemoradiation therapy, researchers found that a decrease

in SUV of 35% was 83% sensitive for predicting a histopathologic response.[103]

[¹⁸F]Fluorodeoxyglucose PET-CT for the Diagnosis of Recurrent Pancreatic Adenocarcinoma

CA 19-9 is a useful marker in the surveillance of patients with a history of pancreatic carcinoma. Unfortunately, it can only indicate the presence of recurrent disease but cannot localize it. Although recurrence can be difficult to detect and localize by conventional imaging, PET-CT has been shown to provide an effective alternative imaging modality. As with other tumors of the GI tract, PET-CT has been proved to be effective in early detection and assessment of disease relapse after initial definitive treatment. In a study of 72 patients with suspected recurrent pancreatic adenocarcinoma, PET-CT was found to be markedly superior to diagnostic CT, identifying 61 of 63 patients with proven recurrence, whereas CT only diagnosed 35 of 63 cases.[104] PET-CT findings influenced treatment strategies in almost half of the study's patients, mainly by identifying who would be the best candidates for surgical exploration. Kitajima and colleagues[93] obtained comparable results. These investigators looked at 45 patients with suspected recurrence and found

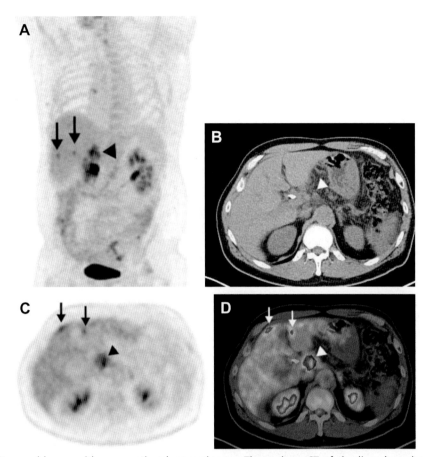

Fig. 8. A 63-year-old man with pancreatic adenocarcinoma. Three-phase CT of the liver (not shown) showed malignant local lymph nodes without evidence of visceral metastases. (*A*) Left anterior oblique view of an MIP from FDG PET-CT shows a focal area of abnormal FDG avidity (*arrowhead*) projecting over the right renal hilum, representing the patient's primary pancreatic adenocarcinoma. In addition, two small foci of abnormal FDG avidity are seen in the liver (*arrows*). (*B–D*) Noncontrast CT, PET, and fused PET-CT show hypermetabolic adenopathy in the porta hepatis (*arrowhead*) representing regional lymph node metastases. In addition, PET confirms 2 abnormal foci (*arrows*) of FDG uptake in the anatomically normal appearing liver, representing occult metastases; these were confirmed as hepatic metastases on follow-up examination.

contrast-enhanced PET-CT to have overall sensitivity, specificity, and accuracy of 92%, 95%, and 93%, respectively, versus 83%, 91%, and 87% for noncontrast low-dose PET-CT and 67%, 86%, and 76% for standard diagnostic CECT. In conclusion, PET-CT is a highly accurate method for assessing recurrent pancreatic cancer, particularly when performed with standard-dose CECT. With continued research, it will likely be the optimal first-line imaging tool in patients with elevation of CA 19-9 or other features suspicious for recurrent disease.

[18F]Fluorodeoxyglucose PET-CT for the Assessment of Pancreatic Intraductal Papillary Mucinous Neoplasm

Pancreatic intraductal papillary mucinous neoplasm (IPMN) develops from the epithelium of the pancreatic main duct or a major side branch. Often discovered incidentally in geriatric patients, the lesions can be premalignant or malignant. Unfortunately these tumors cannot be sufficiently characterized by CT or MR imaging, thus presenting a diagnostic dilemma because prognosis and treatment varies significantly. Premalignant lesions may undergo limited surgical resection or even imaging surveillance, whereas malignant IPMN are treated with radical resection. Current research using PET-CT shows excellent promise. Sperti and colleagues[105] evaluated 64 patients with suspected IPMN who were prospectively investigated using FDG PET as well as CECT and MR cholangiopancreatography (MRCP). Using focal increased metabolic activity as positive criteria, they found that PET correctly identified 4 of 5 (80%) cases of carcinoma in situ and 20 of 21 (95%) cases of invasive cancer. This finding is in contrast to those of conventional imaging, which only diagnosed 2 of 5 (40%) cases of carcinoma in situ and 13 of 21 (62%) cases of invasive cancer. Furthermore, FDG uptake was absent in all 13 cases of adenomas and in 7 of 8 cases of borderline IPMN, outperforming conventional imaging in both cases (**Fig. 9**). Baiocchi and colleagues[106] found FDG PET to be of comparable utility, with the presence of focal FDG avidity correctly identifying 5 benign and 2 malignant IPMN, whereas MRCP failed to correctly diagnose 3 of the 7 patients. Given the limitations of CT and MR imaging, it appears that the main diagnostic utility of PET-CT is derived from the PET portion of the examination, and it is thus unlikely that the addition of diagnostic-quality CT to the examination protocol will add much value in this scenario.

Summary

Despite its relatively high accuracy, FDG PET-CT is not typically used for the preoperative diagnosis of pancreatic adenocarcinoma. One particular exception is its excellent utility in patients who do not have a discrete mass on CT and/or non-diagnostic EUS fine-needle aspiration. By confirming malignancy in these individuals, surgery may be confidently undertaken with curative intent while avoiding the morbidity associated with a re-operative pancreaticoduodenectomy. For staging, contrast-enhanced PET-CT has recently shown increased sensitivity for the detection of regional lymph node extension of disease, and is clearly more sensitive and accurate for M-staging. Its integration of anatomic and metabolic information improves detection, characterization, and localization of lesions. Researchers have found the metabolic data of FDG PET to be helpful for assessing response to neoadjuvant therapy, and PET-CT shows a clear benefit in the detection of recurrence, being particularly helpful in differentiating between local recurrence and benign changes in postsurgical/radiation therapy.

In patients with IPMN seen on conventional imaging, FDG PET appears to have excellent utility, improving risk stratification of these heterogeneous lesions and better identifying those who should progress to surgery rather than conservative management.

CHOLANGIOCARCINOMA

Cholangiocarcinoma is a tumor originating from the bile duct epithelium, and is the second most common primary tumor of the liver after

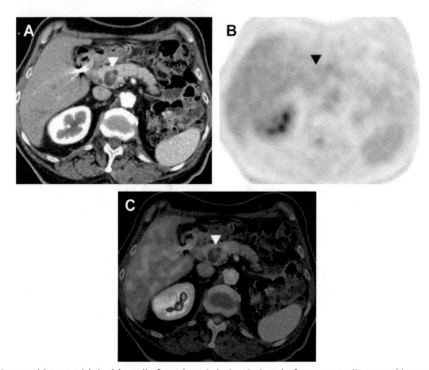

Fig. 9. A 76-year-old man with incidentally found cystic lesion in head of pancreas, diagnosed by magnetic resonance imaging (not shown) as intraductal papillary mucinous neoplasm of indeterminate malignant potential. (A–C) Contrast-enhanced CT, PET, and fused PET-CT show a cystic lesion without associated focal FDG avidity (*arrowhead*). Given the findings, the patient chose to undergo conservative management by means of imaging surveillance. Lesion was stable at follow-up PET-CT 1 year later.

hepatocellular carcinoma. The disease is encountered in the elderly, with several risk factors including primary sclerosing cholangitis, choledochal cyst(s), familial polyposis, hepatolithiasis, and clonorchiasis.[107] Although it is typically of an adenocarcinomatous origin (95% of cases), it can present with highly variable growth patterns and clinical manifestations, which make early diagnosis extremely difficult.[108,109]

Cholangiocarcinoma can arise in 3 locations: intrahepatic/peripheral (5%–10% of cases), extrahepatic (10%–20% of cases), and perihilar (60%–70% of cases).[110] It can also demonstrate 4 growth patterns: mass forming (exophytic), periductal (infiltrating), intraductal (polypoid), or mixed.[107] As with many other GI tumors, surgery

is the only curative treatment. Complete resection of hilar cholangiocarcinomas usually requires a partial hepatectomy. Unfortunately, many patients present with extension of disease that precludes surgery, to include invasion of local structures, malignant adenopathy (50% of patients), or distant metastases (10%–20% of cases at presentation).[111] Prognosis remains dismal, with a 5-year survival rate of only 5%.[112]

[¹⁸F]Fluorodeoxyglucose PET-CT for the Diagnosis and Staging of Cholangiocarcinoma

Increased FDG uptake is often present in cholangiocarcinomas, providing a potential means for their identification with PET-CT (**Fig. 10**). FDG

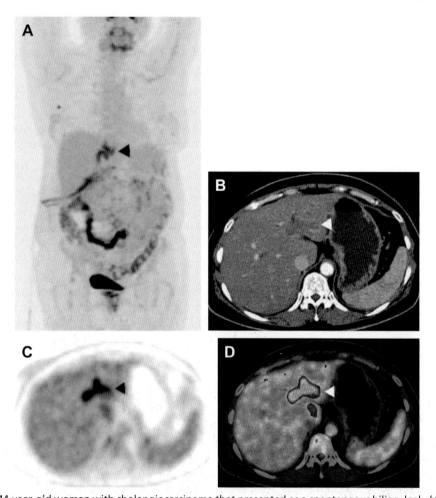

Fig. 10. A 44-year-old woman with cholangiocarcinoma that presented as a spontaneous biliary leak. (*A*) Anterior view of an MIP from FDG PET-CT shows an area of abnormal FDG avidity projecting with a branching configuration (*arrowhead*) in region of the hilum and left hepatic lobe. FDG activity can also be seen draining into the patient's percutaneous subhepatic biliary drain. An incidental reactive lymph node is present in the right axilla. (*B–D*) CECT, PET, and fused PET-CT show the dilated central left hepatic ducts with corresponding intense FDG avidity (*arrowheads*), representing a portion of the cholangiocarcinoma. Lesion was perihilar in location (Klatskin tumor) with intrahepatic extension into the left biliary tree. Morphology was the papillary/intraductal type, which some researchers have found often not to be FDG avid, in contrast to this lesion.

avidity may possibly vary with morphologic sub-type. Anderson and colleagues[113] examined 36 cases of cholangiocarcinoma and found that FDG PET was able to detect 85% of cases involving the mass-forming (exophytic) subtype, but only 18% of cases of the periductal (infiltrating) subtype. A subsequent study of 94 patients showed no such difference in FDG uptake between the differing morphologies.[114] Similarly, some studies have suggested that the sensitivity of FDG PET varies depending on the location of the cholangiocarcinoma, with PET best at detecting intrahepatic lesions (>90%), with a lower sensitivity in perihilar or extrahepatic tumors (<60%).[115,116] Kim and colleagues[114] looked at 123 patients with suspected cholangiocarcinoma with PET-CT and multiple conventional modalities to determine whether the metabolic information gleaned from FDG PET provided any diagnostic advantage. Despite accuracy of 83%, PET-CT did not significantly improve the diagnosis over CT, MR imaging, or MRCP. One exception may exist in the differentiation of benign and malignant strictures. Reinhard and colleagues[117] prospectively evaluated 22 patients and found that there was a significant difference in measured SUV between malignant and benign hilar strictures (6.8 vs 3.3, respectively).

Although PET-CT does not have a significant role in the T-staging of cholangiocarcinoma, it appears to improve the evaluation of N-staging (**Box 9**). In the same study already noted, Kim and colleagues[114] found PET-CT to have a better sensitivity and accuracy in assessing lymph node status in comparison with standard diagnostic CT. PET-CT demonstrated improvement in accuracy of 76% for regional nodal spread of disease compared with that of CT, which was only 61%. Other researchers have affirmed the superiority of PET-CT in this role. Seo and colleagues[118] examined patients with intrahepatic cholangiocarcinoma, and found FDG PET to have an accuracy of 86% for detecting lymph node metastases versus 68% for CT and 58% for MR imaging. Near identical results were obtained by Kato and colleagues[119] when looking at the ability of FDG PET to detect lymph node involvement in patients with extrahepatic cholangiocarcinoma.

Similar to the other GI tumors discussed in this article, M-staging of cholangiocarcinoma benefits greatly from PET-CT. In the 123 cases of cholangiocarcinoma in the study by Kim and colleagues,[114] an accuracy of 88% was demonstrated for PET-CT versus 79% for CT. Jadvar and colleagues[120] retrospectively evaluated 24 patients with suspected recurrent disease, and showed the sensitivity and specificity of PET-CT

Box 9
AJCC TNM staging for intrahepatic cholangiocarcinoma

T1: solitary tumor without vascular invasion

T2a: solitary tumor with vascular invasion

T2b: multiple tumors with or without vascular invasion

T3: tumor perforating the visceral peritoneum or directly invading local extrahepatic structures

T4: tumor with periductal invasion

N0: no regional lymph node metastases

N1: metastases to regional lymph nodes

M0: no distant metastases

M1: distant metastases

Stage I: T1 N0 M0

Stage II: T2 N0 M0

Stage III: T3 N0 M0

Stage IVA: T4 N0 M0 or Any T N1 M0

Stage IVB: Any T, Any N, M1

Both perihilar and extrahepatic cholangiocarcinoma have a separate staging system.

Used with the permission of the American Joint Committee on Cancer (AJCC), Chicago, Illinois. The original source for this material is the AJCC Cancer Staging Manual, Seventh Edition (2010) published by Springer-Verlag, New York, www.springer.com.

---

to be 94% and 100%, respectively, in comparison with 82% and 43% for CT. It is this increased detection of distant disease spread and resultant upstaging that results in a change in management of 17% to 30% in patients who have PET as part of their staging evaluation.[115]

[¹⁸F]Fluorodeoxyglucose PET-CT for the Diagnosis of Recurrent Cholangiocarcinoma

Only 10% of patients with biliary tract tumors are eligible for curative surgery, owing to late presentations of disease. Despite surgery, most patients experience recurrence. As with initial staging, PET-CT appears to have a valuable role in the assessment of patients who present with clinical signs and symptoms concerning for recurrent cholangiocarcinoma. In a prospective study of 50 patients, Lee and colleagues[121] found PET-CT (using low-dose, noncontrast CT) to have a higher, but not statistically significant, sensitivity compared with standard CECT (88% vs 76%). However, the combination of the two modalities significantly improved the sensitivity to 94%

without affecting specificity, supporting the ongoing movement to routinely perform PET-CT using diagnostic-quality CT.

Summary

The accuracy of PET-CT in diagnosing cholangio-carcinoma seems to be reliant on the location of lesions and, possibly, the morphology. Intrahepatic lesions are best detected, in contrast to perihilar or extrahepatic lesions. Some, but not all, investigators have found PET to be most effective for the detection of the mass-forming (exophytic) type of cholangiocarcinoma and less helpful in identifying extrahepatic tumors (**Box 10**). PET-CT appears to outperform CT and MR imaging for the detection of regional lymph node involvement, and clearly improves M-staging. The addition of PET-CT to the staging of cholangiocarcinoma has had a major impact on patient management, altering the treatment plan in up to 30% of patients.

COLORECTAL CANCER

Colorectal cancer is a major health care concern, comprising up to 5% of all cancers in Western countries and accounting for approximately 10% of cancer-related deaths.[3] Its prevalence in developed countries is due to most cases being associated with lifestyle habits (obesity, sedentary lifestyle, smoking, diet rich in fatty foods), whereas very few cases are due to genetic factors such as inflammatory bowel disease (<2% of cases), hereditary nonpolyposis colorectal cancer (approximately 3% of cases), and Gardner syndrome and familial adenomatous polyposis (1% of patients).[122–125]

Because most colorectal cancers arise from adenomatous polyps, the disease is amenable to screening with techniques such as fecal occult blood testing and sigmoidoscopy/colonoscopy. In the United States it is recommended that colorectal cancer screening start at age 50 years, or age 40 years in patients considered at high risk. As a result of these screening techniques the majority of patients (80%) will be diagnosed with locoregional disease, allowing for potential curative resection.[126] Although around half of patients treated with surgery will relapse within 5 years, some are potential candidates for curative second surgeries.[127] Given the success of screening and treatment options, 5-year survival approaches 60%.[128]

[¹⁸F]Fluorodeoxyglucose PET-CT for the Diagnosis and Staging of Colorectal Carcinoma

PET-CT is not routinely recommended for screening or initial diagnosis of colorectal cancer. Even though a malignant or premalignant colonic lesion will occasionally be incidentally first detected by PET-CT during imaging for other indications, this is a relatively rare occurrence, and the vast majority of colorectal malignancies are diagnosed by tissue sampling obtained during sigmoidoscopy or colonoscopy. T-staging, comprising lesion size, mural invasion, and infiltration of adjacent structures, is typically assessed by CT and/or MR imaging with the addition of endorectal ultrasonography for rectal cancers (**Box 11**). PET is unsuitable for this role, mainly because of its limited spatial resolution that precludes differentiation of bowel wall layers.

As seen with esophageal cancer, the ability of PET in accurately assessing regional lymph node involvement can be limited. In the instance of colorectal cancer, this is likely due to obscuration of FDG-avid pericolic lymph nodes by the intense metabolic activity of the adjacent primary tumor. In addition, many involved nodes contain only microscopic disease on histologic assessment; a volume of disease that is usually below detection by PET. In 2 early studies, sensitivity of PET for regional lymph node metastases was only 22% to 29%; however, specificity was 85% to 96%.[129,130] More recent studies have focused specifically on PET-CT and have shown better results. Kwak and colleagues[131] retrospectively

---

Box 10
FDG PET-CT pitfalls in evaluation of primary or recurrent cholangiocarcinoma

False Negatives

Infiltrating morphology (some researchers have found PET sensitivity to be as low as 18% for this subtype, although other studies dispute this finding)

Perihilar/extrahepatic location (sensitivity of FDG PET is less than 60% for tumors arising in these locations)

Mucinous tumors

False Positives

Cholangitis

Hepatic abscess

Granulomatous disease

Biliary stent: approximately 50% of patients will demonstrate FDG avidity along stent tract, likely due to combination of procedural inflammation and attenuation artifact

---

Box 11
AJCC TNM staging for colorectal carcinoma

T1: tumor invades submucosa

T2: tumor invades muscularis propria

T3: tumor invades through muscularis propria and into pericolorectal tissues

T4a: tumor penetrates surface of visceral peritoneum

T4b: tumor directly invades or is adherent to other organs/structures

N0: no regional lymph node metastases

N1: metastases to 1 to 3 regional lymph nodes

    N1a: metastases to 1 locoregional lymph node

    N1b: metastases to 2 to 3 locoregional lymph nodes

    N1c: deposits in subserosa, mesentery, non-peritonized perirectal/pericolic tissues

N2: metastases to 4 or more regional lymph nodes

    N2a: metastases to 4 to 6 locoregional lymph nodes

    N2b: metastases to 7 or more locoregional lymph nodes

M0: no distant metastases

M1: distant metastases

    M1a: metastases confined to 1 organ/site (liver, lung, nonregional node)

    M1b: metastases to more than 1 organ/site or peritoneum

Stage I: T1 N0 M0

Stage II: T2 N0 M0

Stage III: T3 N0 M0

Stage IVA: T4 N0 M0 or any T N1 M0

Stage IVB: Any T, Any N, M1

Used with the permission of the American Joint Committee on Cancer (AJCC), Chicago, Illinois. The original source for this material is the AJCC Cancer Staging Manual, Seventh Edition (2010) published by Springer-Verlag, New York, www.springer.com.

---

reviewed 473 patients with colorectal cancer who underwent preoperative FDG PET-CT followed by curative surgery. PET-CT was found to have sensitivity of 66% and accuracy of 63% for the detection of local lymph node spread of disease, although diagnostic CT still proved superior, with sensitivity of 87% accuracy of 59%. Tsunoda and colleagues[132] reported somewhat similar findings in a prospective study of 88 patients. When using a maximum SUV of greater than 1.5 as criterion for malignant local lymph node spread of disease, they reported sensitivity, specificity, and accuracy of 53%, 91%, and 80%, respectively. Of interest, in their study the visual analysis of FDG uptake for malignant lymph nodes provided a significantly worse sensitivity of 28%.

Of note is the specific value PET-CT brings to the N-staging of low rectal cancers. Gearhart and colleagues[133] showed that, in comparison with traditional CT, PET upstaged nodal disease frequently in these patients (50% of cases) primarily because of the detection of positive inguinal lymph nodes that are characteristic sites of metastatic disease for these lesions.[134]

Spread of colorectal cancer outside the pericolic and mesenteric lymph nodes is considered metastatic. A frequent site of metastases is the liver, with hepatic spread of disease found in 10% to 25% of patients at presentation.[3] Detection of such is critical, because a significant percentage of these patients remain candidates for curative surgery. A recent meta-analysis comparing CT, MR imaging, PET, and PET-CT showed that PET-CT had the highest accuracy for the detection of liver metastases. Niekel and colleagues[135] reported that PET-CT had both sensitivity and specificity of 97%, versus 88% and 93%, respectively, for MR imaging and 84% and 95%, respectively, for CT. Though not shown in this meta-analysis, some believe that subcentimeter liver lesions may be better depicted using MR imaging with liver-specific contrast.[136]

In a broader assessment of PET-CT for staging colorectal cancer, Dirisamer and colleagues[137] looked at 73 patients undergoing either initial staging or restaging. Metastatic sites included distal lymph nodes, liver, lung, peritoneal carcinomatosis, and osseous structures. Using histologic verification or patient follow-up as the reference standard, they identified 232 metastases and found contrast-enhanced PET-CT to have sensitivity, specificity, and accuracy of 100%, 81%, and 99%, respectively. When looking specifically at the added benefit of PET-CT versus PET for the staging of colorectal cancer, Cohade and colleagues[138] evaluated 45 patients retrospectively and found that the overall correct staging increased from 78% with PET to 89% with PET-CT.

[18F]Fluorodeoxyglucose PET-CT for Evaluating the Response of Colorectal Carcinoma to Therapy

Similar to other GI malignancies, studies have shown the ability of PET to predict response to therapy in patients with colorectal cancer. One area of particular utility is monitoring the response of colorectal liver metastases after ablative therapy. Complete surgical resection offers the best chance for cure in patients with liver metastases, although this cannot be achieved in all patients. In these individuals, intrahepatic tumor destruction by means of radiofrequency ablation and other techniques provides alternative treatment options. Evaluation with CT and MR imaging is hampered by the typical posttreatment enhancement pattern that mimics residual/recurrent disease.[139] FDG PET appears to have great usefulness in this scenario. In a study of 56 lesions treated with local tumor ablation, Langenhoff and colleagues[140] found PET-CT performed within 3 weeks of therapy to be 100% accurate for confirming treatment success (51 cases). In the 5 patients with FDG avidity concerning for residual disease, PET-CT was 100% sensitive and 80% specific, with 1 false-positive case from a liver abscess. Donkier and colleagues[141] showed similar success when using PET following radiofrequency ablation. In their study, peripheral uptake of FDG uptake on PET correctly identified 4 patients, with recurrence that was later confirmed by biopsy or CT follow-up. The other 24 patients showed no hypermetabolic activity associated with the ablation site, and remained negative for recurrence over a mean follow-up of 11 months. Two other studies, looking at patients who had undergone cryosurgical ablation and laser-induced thermotherapy, confirmed the accuracy of PET in these scenarios, with a negative predictive value of 96% to 97% and positive predictive value of 88% to 97%.[142,143]

[18F]Fluorodeoxyglucose PET-CT for the Diagnosis of Recurrent Colorectal Carcinoma

Measurement of carcinoembryonic antigen (CEA) concentration is widely used in the surveillance of patients following resection of colorectal cancer, and has sensitivity of approximately 76% and accuracy of approximately 82%.[144] Although an elevated CEA level may indicate recurrence it is not helpful in identifying the site of recurrence, therefore imaging is necessary for localization.

Local recurrence of rectal cancer develops in up to one-third of patients following curative surgery.[145] It is less commonly seen in colon cancer, affecting up to one-fifth of patients after resection.[146] Differentiating recurrence from postsurgical scarring and radiation fibrosis is challenging, particularly in the presacral region. Conventional imaging relies on serial examinations to assess for interval anatomic changes, a technique that has poor accuracy and often results in

a delayed diagnosis. PET with FDG has been shown to be superior to either CT or MR imaging in this regard. In a study of 30 patients with indeterminate presacral lesions following surgical resection of colorectal carcinoma, Evan-Sapir and colleagues[147] found PET-CT to accurately identify all 7 cases of recurrence and 22 of 23 cases of benign postoperative changes (1 false positive) for a sensitivity 100% and specificity of 96% (**Fig. 11**). The excellent utility of PET-CT for detecting local recurrence has been repeated in other studies.[144,148,149]

As with initial staging, identification of metastatic disease is critical in correctly determining therapeutic options, as several studies have shown that surgery with curative intention may be possible even in patients with distant colorectal metastases.[150,151] As mentioned earlier, PET-CT has significant utility in this capacity. Selzner and colleagues[149] looked at 76 patients using CECT and PET-CT. Although they found the 2 modalities to be comparable in the detection of liver metastases (both >90% sensitivity), CECT missed one-third of surgically proven extrahepatic metastases (sensitivity 64%), whereas PET-CT failed to detect these metastatic lesions in only 11% of cases (sensitivity 89%). The additional findings by PET-CT resulted in a change in therapy in 21% of the study patients. In a study of 54 patients referred for restaging of colorectal carcinoma, Soyka and colleagues[152] looked at the value of PET-CT versus CECT, using PET-CT acquired with a standard-dose CECT (cePET-CT) versus PET-CT acquired with a traditional low-dose noncontrast CT (ncPET-CT). The investigators found that, compared with CECT, ncPET-CT provided further relevant information in 50% of patients, because of either inconclusive findings on CECT or identification of additional lesions. Likewise, compared with ncPET-CT, cePET-CT revealed additional information in 72% of cases, primarily because of the correct segmental localization of liver metastases needed for surgical planning. The investigators suggested that cePET-CT be considered the first-line diagnostic tool for restaging patients with recurrent colorectal cancer.

Incidental Colonic Abnormalities

Although considered the hallmark of malignancy, increased FDG uptake can be benign or be due to nonmalignant abnormality such as inflammation and granulomatous diseases (**Box 12**). This situation is particularly common in the GI tract where physiologic uptake is frequently identified, particularly in the proximal stomach, colon, gastroesophageal junction, and anal sphincter. Diffuse or

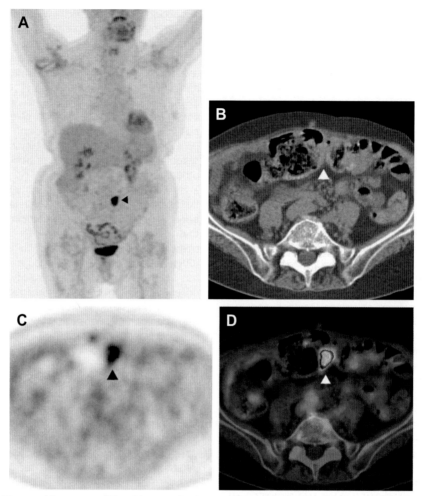

Fig. 11. An 85-year-old woman with a history of colon cancer treated with resection and chemotherapy presented with abdominal pain and diarrhea. Diagnostic CT of abdomen/pelvis was significant solely for diverticulosis. (*A*) Anterior view of an MIP from FDG PET-CT shows an intense abnormal focus of FDG accumulation in the mid abdomen (*arrowhead*). (*B–D*) Noncontrast CT, PET, and fused PET-CT show subtle mural thickening at the suture line, which is markedly hypermetabolic (*arrowheads*). Surgery confirmed local recurrence.

segmental uptake without any anatomic correlate can be deemed benign with a high degree of certainty.[153] By contrast, several large studies have shown that focal areas of increased FDG avidity, with or without an anatomic correlate, raise significant concern for malignancy. Agress and Cooper[154] retrospectively reviewed 1750 PET scans obtained for a variety of known or suspected malignancies, and found 58 abnormal foci of increased FDG uptake throughout the body that did not appear to be related to the primary tumor of concern. Forty-two of the lesions went to biopsy and were found to be malignant or premalignant in 71% of patients, including 3 colonic adenocarcinomas and 18 colonic adenomas. There were 7 false-positive findings in the GI tract in their study: 1 case of focal gastritis,

2 cases of rectal inflammation and/or hemorrhoids, 1 hyperplastic colonic polyp, and 3 cases whereby no lesion was found. In a separate study of 4390 PET-CT examinations, looking specifically at abnormal FDG foci in the GI tract, Israel and colleagues[153] found incidental note of concerning foci of GI uptake in 1.3% of cases. Using long-term follow-up or histology to confirm the benign versus malignant nature of these lesions, they found that 59% of these foci corresponded to malignant or premalignant lesions, which included 4 colon cancers, 1 metastasis to the large bowel, and 9 adenomatous polyps. These studies and others indicate that incidental focal FDG uptake in the GI tract is frequently clinically significant, and such findings should be followed up with appropriate procedures for further assessment.

Box 12
FDG PET-CT pitfalls in evaluation of primary or recurrent colorectal cancer

False Negatives

Mucinous tumors

Locoregional lymph nodes

False Positives

Physiologic

Colitis: typically segmental or diffuse in distribution

Diverticulitis: associated diverticular disease with pericolonic fat stranding

Radiation therapy: most intense during first 4 to 6 weeks following treatment

Anal sphincter uptake (should be circumferential, uniform, and without mass/soft-tissue irregularity)

Summary

PET-CT plays an important role in the assessment of colorectal cancer. It can accurately stage and restage patients with limited disease diagnosed by other imaging modalities. Its value is most notable in the M-staging of both intrahepatic and extrahepatic metastatic disease, which ensures that patients are appropriately treated with surgery for curative intent, or with chemotherapy and/or radiation therapy in those individuals that resection is contraindicated. Its ability to assess response to chemotherapy and/or radiation therapy is well documented, but it also shows excellent usefulness in the assessment of liver metastases treated with local ablative techniques. In comparison with CT and MR imaging, which are both hindered by morphologic changes related to ablation, PET and PET-CT have been extremely accurate in identifying residual/recurrent disease, with the added benefit of much earlier detection compared with anatomic imaging. For assessment of any and all recurrent disease, either suspected by increasing CEA and/or symptoms, PET-CT with diagnostic CECT is emerging as the first-line tool for evaluation, providing the most sensitive means for identifying metastatic lesions for potential liver metastectomies.

SUMMARY

PET-CT has become the standard of care for staging and/or monitoring of many GI malignancies. The physiologic information of PET provides a functional map of abnormal versus normal tissue metabolism while CT provides complementary anatomic data to include accurate localization of PET findings. Together, these two modalities are synergistic and provide valuable information not available from other imaging tests. PET-CT can serve as a means for de novo diagnosis of GI tumors, although this most typically occurs only when PET-CT identifies an incidental focal site of FDG uptake on an examination performed for other reasons. In such a setting, further evaluation is an absolute requirement because the majority of these lesions will be malignant or premalignant. For T-staging, ultrasonography, CT, or postoperative tissue assessment is generally best for GI tumors. The same is true for N-staging, based on the current literature; however, PET-CT is likely to be more useful in this role as more examinations are performed with standard-dose CECT. As for M-staging, PET-CT is clearly the best modality for identifying distant metastases, which is critical in determining the use of appropriate surgical and nonsurgical treatment options. When neoadjuvant therapy is used, the metabolic information derived from FDG PET has been shown by many researchers to serve as an early and accurate noninvasive means of predicting response and potentially directing changes in therapy, helping to avoid the morbidity and expense of chemotherapy and radiation therapy that would be ineffective. In cases of GIST, PET-CT has become the standard for monitoring the response of recurrent/metastatic lesions to treatment with tyrosine kinase inhibitors, revealing a metabolic response as early as 24 hours after start of treatment, whereas anatomic changes may lag weeks to months behind. Although not yet universally accepted, PET-CT is becoming the first-line imaging tool at many institutions for assessing patients with suspected recurrent GI malignancies, as it is able to detect recurrent lesions earlier and with greater accuracy, which, in turn, improves management decisions. Its value when added to conventional imaging evaluations is clear, with the metabolic information obtained from PET-CT resulting in a change in the treatment of a large percentage of patients with GI cancers. Finally, the addition of a dedicated CECT to the PET-CT protocol has been demonstrated to further improve its accuracy, and will likely become the standard of care for most PET-CT examinations in the near future.

REFERENCES

1. Hustinx R. PET-CT in gastrointestinal tumors: fast technologic changes lead to improved patient management. PET Clin 2008;3:xi–xiii.

2. Kamangar F, Dores GM, Anderson WF. Patterns of cancer incidence, mortality and prevalence across five continents: defining priorities to reduce cancer disparities in different geographic regions of the world. J Clin Oncol 2006;24:2137–50.

3. Blodgett TM, Meltzer CC, Townsend DW. PET-CT: form and function. Radiology 2007;242:360–85.

4. Hillner BE, Siegel BA, Shields AF, et al. Relationship between cancer type and impact of PET and PET-CT on intended management: findings of the National Oncologic PET Registry. J Nucl Med 2008;49:1928–35.

5. Czernin J, Allen-Auerbach M, Schelbert HR. Improvements in cancer staging with PET-CT: literature-based evidence as of September 2006. J Nucl Med 2007;48:78S–88S.

6. Townsend DW. Physics and instrumentation for PET in Clinical PET and PET-CT imaging. In: Wahl RL, editor. Categorical Course in Diagnostic Radiology: Clinical PET and PET/CT Imaging. Oak Brook (IL): Radiologic Society of North America, Inc; 2007. p. 9–22.

7. Pfannenberg AC, Aschoff P, Brechtel K. Value of contrast-enhanced multiphase CT in combined PET-CT protocols for oncological imaging. Br J Radiol 2007;80:437–55.

8. Yau YY, Chan WS, Tam YM, et al. Application of intravenous contrast in PET-CT: does it really introduce significant attenuation correction error? J Nucl Med 2005;46:283–91.

9. Cronin CG, Prakash P, Blake MA. Oral and IV contrast agents for the CT portion of PET-CT. AJR Am J Roentgenol 2010;195:W5–13.

10. Groves AM, Kayani I, Dickson JC, et al. Oral contrast medium in PET-CT: should you or shouldn't you? Eur J Nucl Med Mol Imaging 2005;32:1160–6.

11. Hany TF. PET-CT in gastrointestinal cancer: methodological aspects. PET Clin 2008;3:115–22.

12. Pfannenberg AC, Aschoff P, Brechtel K, et al. Low dose non-enhanced CT versus standard dose contrast-enhanced CT in combined PET-CT protocols for staging and therapy planning in non-small cell lung cancer. Eur J Nucl Med Mol Imaging 2007;34:36–44.

13. Bombardieri E. The added value of metabolic imaging with FDG-PET in oesophageal cancer: prognostic role and prediction of response to treatment. Eur J Nucl Med Mol Imaging 2006;33: 753–8.

14. Krause BJ, Herrmann K, Wieder H, et al. ^{18}F-FDG PET and ^{18}F-FDG PET-CT for assessing response to therapy in esophageal cancer. J Nucl Med 2009;50:89S–96S.

15. American Cancer Society. (updated December 26, 2012). Survival rates for esophagus cancer. Retrieved from: http://www.cancer.org/Cancer/EsophagusCancer/OverviewGuide/esophagus-cancer-overview-survival-rates. Accessed June 21, 2013.

16. Flanagan FL, Dehdashti F, Siegal BA, et al. Staging of esophageal cancer with ^{18}F-fluorodeoxyglucose positron emission tomography. AJR Am J Roentgenol 1997;168:417–24.

17. Erasmus JJ, Rohren EM, Hustinx R. PET and PET-CT in the diagnosis and staging of esophageal and gastric cancers. PET Clin 2008;3:135–45.

18. Kato H, Miyazaki T, Nakajima M, et al. The incremental effect of positron emission tomography on diagnostic accuracy in the initial staging of esophageal carcinoma. Cancer 2005;103(1):148–56.

19. Miyata H, Doki Y, Yasuda T, et al. Evaluation of clinical significance of ^{18}F-fluorodeoxyglucose positron emission tomography in superficial squamous cell carcinomas of the thoracic esophagus. Dis Esophagus 2008;21(2):144–50.

20. Little SG, Rice TW, Bybel B, et al. Is FDG-PET indicated for superficial esophageal cancer? Eur J Cardiothorac Surg 2007;31(5):791–6.

21. Walker AJ, Spier BJ, Perlman SB, et al. Integrated PET-CT fusion imaging and endoscopic ultrasound in the pre-operative staging and evaluation of esophageal cancer. Mol Imaging Biol 2011;13: 166–71.

22. Roedl JB, Colen RR, King K, et al. Visual PET-CT scoring for nonspecific ^{18}F-FDG uptake in the differentiation of early malignant and benign esophageal lesions. AJR Am J Roentgenol 2008;191(2):515–21.

23. Bruzzi JF, Munden RF, Truong MT, et al. PET-CT of esophageal cancer: its role in clinical management. Radiographics 2007;27:1635–52.

24. Lowe VJ, Booya F, Fletcher JG, et al. Comparison of positron emission tomography, computed tomography, and endoscopic ultrasound in the initial staging of patients with esophageal cancer. Mol Imaging Biol 2005;7(6):422–30.

25. Bar-Shalom R, Guralnik L, Tsalic M, et al. The additional value of PET-CT over PET in FDG imaging of oesophageal cancer. Eur J Nucl Med Mol Imaging 2005;32(8):918–24.

26. van Westreenen HL, Heeren PA, van Dullemen HM, et al. Systematic review of the staging performance of ^{18}F-fluorodeoxyglucose positron emission tomography in esophageal cancer. J Clin Oncol 2004;18:3805–12.

27. Choi JY, Lee KH, Shim YM, et al. Improved detection of individual nodal involvement in squamous cell carcinoma of the esophagus by FDG PET. J Nucl Med 2000;41:808–15.

28. Yuan S, Yu Y, Chao KS, et al. Additional value of PET-CT over PET in assessment of locoregional lymph nodes in thoracic esophageal squamous cell cancer. J Nucl Med 2006;47:1255–9.

29. Shimizu S, Hosokawa M, Itoh K, et al. Can hybrid FDG-PET-CT detect subclinical lymph node

metastasis of esophageal cancer approximately and contribute to radiation treatment planning? A comparison of image-based and pathological findings. Int J Clin Oncol 2009;14:421–5.

30. Liberale G, Van Laethem JL, Gay F, et al. The role of PET scan in the preoperative management of oesophageal cancer. Eur J Surg Oncol 2004;9:942–7.

31. Flamen P, Lerut A, Van Cutsem E, et al. Utility of positron emission tomography for the staging of patients with potentially operable esophageal carcinoma. J Clin Oncol 2000;18:3202–10.

32. Luketich JD, Friedman DM, Weigel TL, et al. Evaluation of distant metastases in esophageal cancer: 100 consecutive positron emission tomography scans. Ann Thorac Surg 1999;4:1133–6.

33. Quint LE, Hepburn LM, Francis IR, et al. Incidence and distribution of distant metastases from newly diagnosed esophageal carcinoma. Cancer 1995; 76:1120–5.

34. Gananadha S, Haxebroek EJ, Leibman S, et al. The utility of FDG-PET in the preoperative staging of esophageal cancer. Dis Esophagus 2008;21: 389–94.

35. Urschel JD, Vasan H. A meta-analysis of randomized controlled trials that compared neoadjuvant chemoradiation and surgery to surgery alone for resectable esophageal cancer. Am J Surg 2003; 185:538–43.

36. Fiorica F, Di Bona D, Schepis F, et al. Preoperative chemoradiotherapy for oesophageal cancer: a systematic review and meta-analysis. Gut 2004;53: 925–30.

37. Ancona E, Ruol A, Santi S, et al. Only pathologic complete response to neoadjuvant chemotherapy improves significantly the long term survival of patients with resectable esophageal squamous cell carcinoma: final report of a randomized, controlled trial of preoperative chemotherapy versus surgery alone. Cancer 2001;91:2165–74.

38. Law S, Fok M, Chow S, et al. Preoperative chemotherapy versus surgical therapy alone for squamous cell carcinoma of the esophagus: a prospective randomized trial. J Thorac Cardiovasc Surg 1997;114:210–7.

39. Westerterp M, Van Westreenen JL, Hoekstra OS, et al. Esophageal cancer: CT, endoscopic US, and ^{18}F-FDG PET for assessment of response to neoadjuvant therapy—systematic review. Radiology 2005;236:841–51.

40. Wieder HA, Brucher BL, Zimmermann F, et al. Time course of tumor metabolic activity during chemoradiotherapy of esophageal squamous cell carcinoma and response to therapy. J Clin Oncol 2004;22:900–8.

41. Wieder HA, Ott K, Lordick F, et al. Prediction of tumor response by ^{18}F-FDG-PET: comparison of the accuracy of single and sequential studies in patients with adenocarcinomas of the esophagogastric junction. Eur J Nucl Med Mol Imaging 2007;34:1925–32.

42. Lordick F, Ott K, Krause B-J, et al. PET to assess early metabolic response and to guide treatment of adenocarcinoma of the oesophagogastric junction: the MUNICOM phase II trial. Lancet Oncol 2007;8(9):797–805.

43. Law SY, Fok M, Wong J. Pattern of recurrence after oesophageal resection for cancer: clinical implications. Br J Surg 1996;83:107–11.

44. Raoul JL, Le Prise E, Meunier B, et al. Combined radiochemotherapy for postoperative recurrence of oesophageal cancer. Gut 1995;37(2):174–6.

45. Guo H, Zhu H, Xi Y, et al. Diagnostic and prognostic value of ^{18}F-FDG PET-CT for patients with suspected recurrence from squamous cell carcinoma of the esophagus. J Nucl Med 2007;48: 1251–8.

46. Flamen P, Lerut A, Van Cutsem E, et al. The utility of positron emission tomography for the diagnosis and staging of recurrent esophageal cancer. J Thorac Cardiovasc Surg 2000;120(6):1085–92.

47. Parkin DM, Bay F, Ferlay J, et al. Global cancer statistics, 2002. CA Cancer J Clin 2005;55(2):74–108.

48. "Proceedings of the fourth Global Vaccine Research Forum" produced by the Initiative for Vaccine Research team of the Department of Immunization, Vaccines and Biologicals. Seoul, Korea: WHO; 2003.

49. Crane SJ, Locke GR, Harmsen WS, et al. Survival trends in patients with gastric and esophageal adenocarcinomas: a population-based study. Mayo Clin Proc 2008;83(10):1087–94.

50. Paterson HM, McCole D, Auld CD. Impact of open-access endoscopy on detection of early oesophageal and gastric cancer 1994-2003: population-based study. Endoscopy 2006;38(5):503–7.

51. Heise K, Bertran E, Andia ME, et al. Incidence and survival of stomach cancer in a high-risk population of Chile. World J Gastroenterol 2009;15(15):1854–62.

52. Schwarz RE, Zagala-Nevarez PA. Recurrence patterns after radical gastrectomy for gastric cancer: prognostic factors and implications for postoperative adjuvant therapy. Ann Surg Oncol 2002;9(4): 394–400.

53. Stahl A, Ott K, Weber WA, et al. FDG PET imaging of locally advanced gastric carcinomas: correlation with endoscopic and histopathological findings. Eur J Nucl Med 2003;30(2):288–95.

54. Mochiki E, Kuwano H, Katoh H, et al. Evaluation of ^{18}F-2-deoxy-2-fluoro-D-glucose positron emission tomography for gastric cancer. World J Surg 2004;28:247–53.

55. Kim EY, Lee WJ, Choi D, et al. The value of PET-CT for preoperative staging of advanced gastric cancer: comparison with contrast-enhanced CT. Eur J Radiol 2011;79:183–8.

56. Kelly S, Harris KM, Berry E, et al. A systematic review of the staging performance of endoscopic ultrasound in gastro-oesophageal carcinoma. Gut 2001;49:534–9.

57. Willis S, Truong S, Gribnitz S, et al. Endoscopic ultrasonography in the pre-operative staging of gastric cancer: accuracy and impact on surgical therapy. Surg Endosc 2000;14:951–4.

58. Yang QM, Kawamura T, Itoh H, et al. Is PET-CT suitable for predicting lymph node status for gastric cancer? Hepatogastroenterology 2008;55:782–5.

59. Atay-Rosenthal S, Fishman EK, Wahl RL. PET-CT findings in gastric cancer: potential advantages and current limitations. Imag Med 2012;4(2):241–50 Expanded Academic ASAP. Web. 22 May 2012.

60. Oskan E, Araz M, Soydal C, et al. The role of ^{18}F-FDG-PET-CT in the preoperative staging and post-therapy followup of gastric cancer: comparison with spiral CT. World J Surg Oncol 2011;9(75):1–5.

61. Turlakow A, Yeung HW, Salmon AS. Peritoneal carcinomatosis: role of ^{18}F-FDG PET. J Nucl Med 2003;44:1407–12.

62. Hur H, Kim SH, Kim W, et al. The efficacy of preoperative PET/CT for prediction of curability in surgery for locally advanced gastric carcinoma. World J Surg Oncol 2010;8(86):1–7.

63. Krause BJ, Ott K, Herrmann K, et al. Metabolic imaging predicts response and prognosis in neoadjuvant treated, locally advanced gastric cancer: final results of a prospective study. J Nucl Med 2007; 48(Suppl 2):27P.

64. Shah MA, Yeung H, Coit D, et al. A phase II study of preoperative chemotherapy with irinotecan (CPT) and cisplatin (CIS) for gastric cancer (NCI 5917): FDG-PET-CT predicts patient outcome. J Clin Oncol 2007;25(Suppl 18):4502 (meeting abstracts).

65. Park MJ, Lee WJ, Lim HK, et al. Detecting recurrence of gastric cancer: the value of FDG PET-CT. Abdom Imaging 2009;43:441–7.

66. Sim SH, Kim YJ, Oh DY, et al. The role of PET-CT in detection of gastric cancer recurrence. BMC Cancer 2009;9(73):1–7.

67. Miettinen M, Lasota J. Gastrointestinal stromal tumors: definition, clinical, histological, immunohistochemical, and molecular genetic features and differential diagnosis. Virchows Ach 2001;438(1):1–12.

68. Burkill GJ, Badran M, Al-Muderis O, et al. Malignant gastrointestinal stromal tumor: distribution, imaging features, and pattern of metastatic spread. Radiology 2003;226:527–32.

69. Fletcher CD, Berman JJ, Corless C, et al. Diagnosis of gastrointestinal stromal tumors: a consensus approach. Hum Pathol 2002;33(5):459–65.

70. Nishida T, Kumano S, Sugiura T, et al. Multidetector CT of high-risk patients with occult gastrointestinal stromal tumors. AJR Am J Roentgenol 2003;180:185–9.

71. Lau S, Tam KF, Kam CK, et al. Imaging of gastrointestinal stromal tumour (GIST). Clin Radiol 2004; 59(6):487–98.

72. DeMatteo RP, Lewis JJ, Leung D, et al. Two hundred gastrointestinal stromal tumors: recurrence patterns and prognostic factors for survival. Ann Surg 2000;231:51.

73. Ertuk M, Van den Abbeele AD. Infrequent tumors of the gastrointestinal tract including gastrointestinal stromal tumor (GIST). PET Clin 2008;3:207–15.

74. DeMatteo RP. The GIST of targeted cancer therapy: a tumor (gastrointestinal stromal tumor), a mutated gene (c-kit), and a molecular inhibitor (STI571). Ann Surg Oncol 2002;9(9):831–9.

75. Plaat BE, Hollema H, Molenaar WM, et al. Soft tissue leiomyosarcomas and malignant gastrointestinal stromal tumors: differences in clinical outcome and expression of multidrug resistance proteins. J Clin Oncol 2000;18:3211–20.

76. Joensuu H, Robert PJ, Sarlomo-Rikala M, et al. Brief report: effect of the tyrosine kinase inhibitor STI 571 in a patient with a metastatic gastrointestinal stromal tumor. N Engl J Med 2001;344: 1052–6.

77. van den Abbeele AD, Badawi RD. Use of positron emission tomography in oncology and its potential role to assess response to imatinib mesylate therapy in gastrointestinal stromal tumors (GISTs). Eur J Cancer 2002;38:560–5.

78. van Oosterom AT, Judson I, Verweij J, et al, European Organization for Research and Treatment of Cancer Soft Tissue and Bone Sarcoma Group. Safety and efficacy of imatinib (STI571) in metastatic gastrointestinal stromal tumours: a phase I study. Lancet 2001;358(9291):1421–3.

79. Antoch G, Kanja J, Bauer S, et al. Comparison of PET, CT and dual-modality PET-CT imaging for monitoring of imatinib (STI571) therapy in patients with gastrointestinal stromal tumors. J Nucl Med 2004;45:357–65.

80. Hahn S, Bauer S, Heusner TA, et al. Postoperative FDG-PET/CT staging in GIST: is there a benefit following R0 resection? Eur J Radiol 2011;80:670–4.

81. Basu S, Mohandas KM, Peshwe H, et al. FDG-PET and PET-CT in the clinical management of gastrointestinal stromal tumor. Nucl Med Commun 2008;29: 1026–39.

82. Van den Abbeele AD. The lessons of GIST—PET and PET-CT: a new paradigm for imaging. Oncologist 2008;13(Suppl 2):8–13.

83. Chen MY, Bechtold RE, Savage PD. Cystic changes in hepatic metastases from gastrointestinal stromal tumors (GISTs) treated with Gleevac (imatinib mesylate). Am J Roentgenol 2002;179: 1059–62.

84. Goerres GW, Stupp R, Barghouth G, et al. The value of PET, CT and in-line PET/CT in patients

with gastrointestinal stromal tumours: long-term outcome of treatment with imatinib mesylate. Eur J Nucl Med Mol Imaging 2005;32(2):153–62.

85. van den Abbeele AD, Badawi RD, Cliche JP, et al. Response to imatinib mesylate (Gleevac) therapy in patients with advanced gastrointestinal stromal tumors (GIST) is demonstrated by F-18-FDG-PET prior to anatomic imaging with CT. Radiology 2002;225(Suppl):424.

86. Demetri GD, von Mehren M, Blanke CD, et al. Efficacy and safety of imatinib mesylate in advanced gastrointestinal stromal tumors. N Engl J Med 2002;347(7):472–80.

87. Stroobants S, Seegers M, Goeminne J, et al. ¹⁸FDG-positron emission tomography for the early prediction of response in advanced soft tissue sarcoma treated with imatinib mesylate (Glivec). Eur J Cancer 2003;39:2012–20.

88. Jager PL, Gietema JA, van der Graaf WT. Imatinib mesylate for the treatment of gastrointestinal stromal tumours: best monitored with FDG PET. Nucl Med Commun 2004;25(5):433–8.

89. Gayed I, Vu T, Iyer R, et al. The role of ¹⁸F-FDG PET in staging and early prediction of response to therapy of recurrent gastrointestinal stromal tumors. J Nucl Med 2004;45(1):17–21.

90. Delbeke D, Martin WH. PET and PET/CT for pancreatic malignancies. PET Clin 2008;3:155–67.

91. Tempero MA, Arnoletti P, Behrman S, et al. Pancreatic adenocarcinoma. J Natl Compr Canc Netw 2010;8:972–1017.

92. Faria SC, Tamm EP, Loyer EM, et al. Diagnosis and staging of pancreatic tumors. Semin Roentgenol 2004;39(3):397–411.

93. Kitajima K, Murakami K, Yamasaki E, et al. Performance of integrated FDG-PET/contrast-enhanced CT in the diagnosis of recurrent pancreatic cancer: comparison with integrated FDG-PET/non-contrast-enhanced CT and enhanced CT. Mol Imaging Biol 2010;12:452–9.

94. Czernin J. PET-CT: imaging structure and function. J Nucl Med 2004;45(Suppl 1):1S–103S.

95. Kauhanen SP, Komar G, Seppanen MP, et al. A prospective diagnostic accuracy study of ¹⁸F-fluorodeoxyglucose positron emission tomography/computed tomography, multidetector row computed tomography, and magnetic resonance imaging in primary diagnosis and staging of pancreatic cancer. Ann Surg 2009;250(6): 957–63.

96. Farma JM, Santillan AA, Melis M, et al. PET/CT fusion scan enhances CT staging in patients with pancreatic neoplasms. Ann Surg Oncol 2008; 15(9):2465–71.

97. Maldonado A, Gonzalez F, Tamames S, et al. The role of ¹⁸F-FDG PET/CT in the evaluation of pancreatic lesions. J Nucl Med 2007;48(Suppl 2):26P.

98. DeWitt J, Devereaux B, Chriswell M, et al. Comparison of endoscopic ultrasonography and multidetector computed tomography for detecting and staging pancreatic cancer. Ann Intern Med 2004; 141(10):753–63.

99. Kalady MF, Clary BM, Clark LA, et al. Clinical utility of positron emission tomography in the diagnosis and management of periampullary neoplasms. Ann Surg Oncol 2002;9(8):799–806.

100. Strobel K, Heinrich S, Bhure U, et al. Contrast-enhanced ¹⁸F-FDG PET/CT: 1-stop-shop imaging for assessing the respectability of pancreatic cancer. J Nucl Med 2008;49(9):1408–13.

101. Rose DM, Delbeke D, Beauchamp RD, et al. ¹⁸F-Fluorodeoxyglucose-positron emission tomography (¹⁸FDG-PET) in the management of patients with suspected pancreatic cancer. Ann Surg 1998;229:729–38.

102. Heinrich S, Schafer M, Weber A, et al. Neoadjuvant chemotherapy generates a significant tumor response in resectable pancreatic cancer without increasing morbidity: results of a prospective phase II trial. Ann Surg 2008;248(6):1014–22.

103. Chuong MD, Hoffe SE, Shridhar R, et al. PET/CT response predicts histopathologic response after neoadjuvant therapy for borderline resectable pancreatic cancer [abstract]. The ASTRO's Annual Meeting. Miami Beach, Florida. October 2, 2011.

104. Sperti C, Pasquali C, Bissoli S, et al. Tumor relapse after pancreatic cancer resection is detected earlier by 18-FDG PET than by CT. J Gastrointest Surg 2010;14(1):131–40.

105. Sperti C, Bissoli S, Pasquali C, et al. 18-fluorodeoxyglucose positron emission tomography enhances computed tomography diagnosis of malignant intraductal papillary mucinous neoplasms of the pancreas. Ann Surg 2007;246(6):932–7.

106. Baiocchi GL, Portolani N, Bertagna F, et al. Possible additional value of ¹⁸FDG-PET in managing pancreas intraductal papillary mucinous neoplasms: preliminary results. J Exp Clin Cancer Res 2008;27:10.

107. Sainani NI, Catalano OA, Holalkere N-S, et al. Cholangiocarcinoma: current and novel imaging techniques. Radiographics 2008;28:123–8.

108. Singh P, Patel T. Advances in the diagnosis, evaluation and management of cholangiocarcinoma. Curr Opin Gastroenterol 2006;22:294–9.

109. Bloom CM, Langer B, Wilson SR. Role of US in the detection, characterization, and staging of cholangiocarcinoma. Radiographics 1999;19: 1199–218.

110. Lee JD, Kang WJ, Yun M. Primary cancer of the liver and biliary duct. PET Clin 2008;3:169–86.

111. Slattery JM, Sahani DV. What is the current state-of-the-art for detection and staging of cholangiocarcinoma? Oncologist 2006;11:913–22.

112. Oh SW, Yoon YS, Shin SA. Effects of excess weight on cancer incidences depending on cancer sites and histologic findings among men: Korea National Health Insurance Corporation Study. J Clin Oncol 2005;23:4742–54.

113. Anderson CA, Rice MH, Pinson CW, et al. FDG PET imaging in the evaluation of gallbladder carcinoma and cholangiocarcinoma. J Gastrointest Surg 2004;8(1):90–7.

114. Kim JY, Kim MH, Lee TY, et al. Clinical role of ^{18}F-FDG PET-CT in suspected and potentially operable cholangiocarcinoma: a prospective study compared with conventional imaging. Am J Gastroenterol 2008;103:1145–51.

115. Sacks A, Peller PJ, Surasi DS, et al. Value of PET/CT in the management of primary hepatobiliary tumors, part 2. AJR Am J Roentgenol 2011;197:W260–5.

116. Petrowsky H, Wildbrett P, Husarik DB, et al. Impact of integrated positron emission tomography and computed tomography on staging and management of gallbladder cancer and cholangiocarcinoma. J Hepatol 2006;45:43–50.

117. Reinhard MJ, Strunk H, Gerhardt T, et al. Detection of Klatskin's tumour in extrahepatic bile duct strictures using delayed 18-F-FDG PET-CT: preliminary results for 22 patient studies. J Nucl Med 2005;46:1158–63.

118. Seo S, Hatano E, Higashi T, et al. Fluorine-18-fluorodeoxyglucose positron emission tomography predicts lymph node metastasis, P-glycoprotein expression, and recurrence after resection in mass-forming intrahepatic cholangiocarcinoma. Surgery 2008;143:769–77.

119. Kato T, Tsukamoto E, Kuge Y, et al. Clinical role of (18)F-FDG PET for initial staging of patients with extrahepatic bile duct cancer. Eur J Nucl Med Mol Imaging 2002;29:1047–54.

120. Jadvar H, Henderson RW, Conti PS. [F-18]fluorodeoxyglucose positron emission tomography and positron emission tomography in recurrent and metastatic cholangiocarcinoma. J Comput Assist Tomogr 2007;31:223–8.

121. Lee YG, Han SW, Oh DY, et al. Diagnostic performance of contrast enhanced CT and ^{18}F-FDG PET-CT in suspicious recurrence of biliary tract cancer after curative resection. BMC Cancer 2011;11(188):1–7.

122. Watson AJ, Collins PD. Colon cancer: a civilization disorder. Dig Dis 2011;29(2):222–8.

123. Triantafillidis JK, Nasioulas G, Kosmidis PA. Colorectal cancer and inflammatory bowel disease: epidemiology, risk factors, mechanisms of carcinogenesis and prevention strategies. Anticancer Res 2009;29(7):2727–37.

124. Cunningham D, Atkin W, Lenz HJ, et al. Colorectal cancer. Lancet 2010;375:1030–47.

125. Half E, Bercovich D, Rozen P. Familial adenomatous polyposis. Orphanet J Rare Dis 2009;4:22.

126. Siegel R, Naishadham D, Jemal A. Cancer statistics 2012. CA Cancer J Clin 2012;62(1):10–29.

127. Ben-Haim S, Ell P. ^{18}F-FDG PET and PET/CT in the evaluation of cancer treatment response. J Nucl Med 2009;50(1):88–99.

128. Delbeke D. Integrated PET-CT imaging: implications for evaluation of patients with colorectal carcinoma. Semin Colon Rectal Surg 2005;16:69–81.

129. Mukai M, Sadahiro S, Yasuda S, et al. Preoperative evaluation by whole-body ^{18}F-fluorodeoxyglucose positron emission tomography in patients with primary colorectal cancer. Oncol Rep 2000;7(1):85–7.

130. Abdel-Nabi H, Doerr RJ, Lamonica DM, et al. Staging of primary colorectal carcinomas with fluorine-18 fluorodeoxyglucose whole-body PET: correlation with histopathologic and CT findings. Radiology 1998;206(3):755–60.

131. Kwak JY, Kim JS, Kim HJ, et al. Diagnostic value of FDG-PET/CT for lymph node metastasis of colorectal cancer. World J Surg 2012;36(8):1898–905.

132. Tsunoda Y, Ito M, Fujii H, et al. Preoperative diagnosis of lymph node metastases of colorectal cancer by FDG-PET/CT. Jpn J Clin Oncol 2008;38(5):347–53.

133. Gearhart SL, Frassica D, Rosen R, et al. Improved staging with pretreatment positron emission tomography/computed tomography in low rectal cancer. Ann Surg Oncol 2006;13:397–404.

134. Lonneux M. FDG-PET and PET/CT in colorectal cancer. PET Clin 2008;3:147–53.

135. Niekel MC, Bipat S, Stoker J. Diagnostic imaging of colorectal liver metastases with CT, MR imaging, FDG PET, and/or FDG PET/CT: a meta-analysis of prospective studies including patients who have not previously undergone treatment. Radiology 2010;257(3):674–84.

136. Kong G, Jackson C, Koh DM, et al. The use of ^{18}F-FDG PET-CT in colorectal liver metastases-Comparison with CT and liver MRI. Eur J Nucl Med Mol Imaging 2008;35(7):1323–9.

137. Dirisamer A, Halpern BS, Flory D, et al. Performance of integrated FDG-PET/contrast-enhanced CT in the staging and restaging of colorectal cancer: comparison with PET and enhanced CT. Eur J Radiol 2010;73:324–8.

138. Cohade C, Osman M, Leal J, et al. Direct comparison of (18)F-FDG PET and PET/CT in patients with colorectal carcinoma. J Nucl Med 2003;44:1797–803.

139. de Geus-Oei LF, Vriens D, van Laarhoven HW, et al. Monitoring and predicting response to therapy with ^{18}F-FDG PET in colorectal cancer: a systematic review. J Nucl Med 2009;50:43S–54S.

140. Langenhoff BS, Oyen WJ, Jager GJ, et al. Efficacy of fluorine-18-desyglucose positron emission tomography in detecting tumor recurrence after local ablative therapy for liver metastases: a prospective study. J Clin Oncol 2002;20:4453–8.

141. Donkier V, Van Laethem JL, Goldman S, et al. [F-18] fluorodeoxyglucose positron emission tomography as a tool for early recognition of incomplete tumor destruction after radiofrequency ablation for liver metastases. J Surg Oncol 2003;84:215–23.

142. Denecke T, Steffen I, Hildebrandt B, et al. Assessment of local control after laser-induced thermotherapy of liver metastases from colorectal cancer: contribution of FDG-PET in patients with clinical suspicion of progressive disease. Acta Radiol 2007;48:821–30.

143. Joosten J, Jager G, Oyen W, et al. Cryosurgery and radiofrequency ablation for unresectable colorectal liver metastases. Eur J Surg Oncol 2005;31:1152–9.

144. Staib L, Schirrmeister H, Reske SN, et al. Is ^{18}F-fluorodeoxyglucose positron emission tomography in recurrent colorectal cancer a contribution to surgical decision making? Am J Surg 2000;180(1):1–5.

145. Israel O, Kuten A. Early detection of cancer recurrence: ^{18}F-FDG PET/CT can make a difference in diagnosis and patient care. J Nucl Med 2007;48:28S–35S.

146. Turk PS, Wanebo HJ. Results of surgical treatment of nonhepatic recurrence of colorectal carcinoma. Cancer 1993;71(12):4267–77.

147. Evan-Sapir E, Parag Y, Lerman H, et al. Detection of recurrence in patients with rectal cancer: PET/CT after abdominoperineal or anterior resection. Radiology 2004;232:815–22.

148. Chen LB, Tong JL, Song HZ, et al. ^{18}F-DG PET/CT in detection of recurrence and metastasis of colorectal cancer. World J Gastroenterol 2007;13(37):5025–9.

149. Selzner M, Hany TF, Wildbrett P, et al. Does the novel PET/CT imaging modality impact on the treatment of patients with metastatic colorectal cancer of the liver? Ann Surg 2004;240(6):1027–34.

150. Khatri VP, Chee KG, Petrelli NJ. Modern multimodality approach to hepatic colorectal metastases: solutions and controversies. Surg Oncol 2007;16:71–83.

151. Inoue M, Ohta M, Iuchi K, et al. Benefits of surgery for patients with pulmonary metastases from colorectal carcinoma. Ann Thorac Surg 2004;78:238–44.

152. Soyka JD, Veit-Haibach P, Strobel K, et al. Staging pathways in recurrent colorectal carcinoma: is contrast-enhanced ^{18}F-FDG PET/CT the diagnostic tool of choice? J Nucl Med 2008;49:354–61.

153. Israel O, Yefremov N, Bar-Shalom R, et al. PET/CT detection of unexpected gastrointestinal foci of ^{18}F-FDG uptake: incidence, localization patterns, and clinical significance. J Nucl Med 2005;46:758–62.

154. Agress H, Cooper BZ. Detection of clinically unexpected malignant and premalignant tumors with whole-body FDG PET: histopathologic comparison. Radiology 2004;230:417–22.

PET/Computed Tomography and Lymphoma

Martin Allen-Auerbach, MD[a,*], Sven de Vos, MD, PhD[b],
Johannes Czernin, MD[a]

KEYWORDS

- Lymphoma • FDG • PET • PET/CT

KEY POINTS

- Most lymphomas, including low-grade lymphomas, show sufficient fluorodeoxyglucose (FDG) uptake to be reliably staged with FDG-PET/computed tomography (CT).
- PET/CT is the modality of choice for staging and assessment of therapeutic response in patients with lymphoma.
- Physicians interpreting PET/CT scans should make every effort to include the available interpretation guidelines.

INTRODUCTION

This article focuses on the practical applications of PET/computed tomography (CT) in lymphoma.[1–3] In particular, the glucose metabolic phenotype (and by inference fluorodeoxyglucose [FDG] avidity) of the most important lymphoma subtypes, the role of PET/CT for initial and subsequent management decisions, appropriate image acquisition protocols and image interpretation, as well as pitfalls in interpreting studies, are discussed.

FDG UPTAKE AMONG DIFFERENT TYPES OF LYMPHOMA

The increase of glycolytic activity, even under normoxic conditions, as a hallmark of malignant degeneration was initially described by Otto Warburg in 1924.[4] This switch to glycolysis forms the basis of imaging malignant disease with PET and the glucose analogue FDG.[5,6]

FDG is transported into cells by membrane-bound glucose transporters (Glut-1 and Glut-3), where FDG is phosphorylated by hexokinases (HK-1 and HK-2) into FDG-6-phosphate. Glucose transporters[7] and hexokinases are overexpressed in many cancers.[8] Contrary to glucose-6-phosphate, FDG-6-phosphate is no longer a substrate for the glycolytic pathway. Furthermore, glucose-6-phosphatase, which could dephosphorylate FDG-6-phosphate, is present in only limited amounts in most cancers (the most important exceptions being renal cell and hepatocellular cancer).[9] Thus, FDG-6-phosphate is essentially trapped in tumor cells in proportion to the glycolytic activity of the tumor cell (**Fig. 1**). For the clinical interpretation of staging PET/CT scans in patients with lymphoma, a visual assessment is considered sufficient. However, different rules apply to scans performed as part of early treatment response assessment, for which interpretation criteria have been proposed and implemented.[10,11]

For the purpose of quantification, semiquantitative assessment by means of standardized uptake values (SUV) is possible[12] SUV is defined as:

Decay-corrected activity [kBq]/tissue volume [mL]

Injected-FDG activity [kBq]/body weight [g]

[a] Ahmanson Translational Imaging Division/Nuclear Medicine, Department of Molecular and Medical Pharmacology, David Geffen School of Medicine at UCLA, 10833 Le Conte Avenue, Los Angeles, CA 90095-6948, USA;
[b] Division of Hematology/Oncology, Department of Medicine, David Geffen School of Medicine at UCLA, 10833 Le Conte Avenue, Los Angeles, CA 90095-6948, USA
* Corresponding author.
E-mail address: mauerbach@mednet.ucla.edu

Radiol Clin N Am 51 (2013) 833–844
http://dx.doi.org/10.1016/j.rcl.2013.05.004
0033-8389/13/$ – see front matter

Plasma   Lymphoma Cell

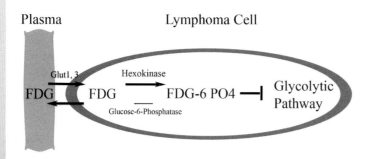

Fig. 1. FDG uptake via glucose transporters Glut-1 and Glut-3, with subsequent phosphorylation and trapping of the phosphorylated FDG (FDG-PO4) in a malignant cell.

Various SUV parameters can be used but SUV_{max} or SUV_{peak} seem to provide the most robust response assessments.[13]

The degree of FDG uptake varies among different lymphoproliferative diseases (Table 1). It is important to recognize the glycolytic phenotypes of various subtypes, because those with a low glycolytic phenotype require a baseline scan for subsequent treatment response assessments. In general, more aggressive lymphomas show higher FDG uptake than indolent lymphomas.[14,15] FDG uptake in diffuse large B-cell lymphoma (DLBCL) and high-grade follicular lymphoma has been reported to be on average 3-fold higher than in indolent lymphomas such as low-grade follicular, lymphocytic, plasmacytic, mantle cell, marginal zone, or small cell lymphoma.[16] Nevertheless, not only high-grade but also most low-grade lymphomas can be staged accurately with FDG-PET.

T-cell lymphomas are frequently primarily extranodal or involve extranodal sites. FDG-PET may be useful in primary extranodal T-cell lymphomas, particularly for the evaluation of systemic involvement.[17] Equivalent to aggressive B-cell

lymphomas, angioimmunoblastic T-cell, natural killer/T-cell, and anaplastic large cell lymphomas usually show high FDG avidity.

Extranodal mucosa-associated lymphoid tissue (MALT) lymphomas consistently show low FDG uptake, resulting in low overall disease detection with PET. Detectability is to some extent site dependent. Gastric MALT is rarely detected, whereas lung involvement is almost always correctly identified.[18,19]

The source of FDG uptake in Hodgkin lymphoma (HL) seems to be different from non-Hodgkin lymphoma (NHL). The atypical cells (Reed-Sternberg cells and variants) represent only 1% to 3% of the tumor bulk in HL. In contrast to NHLs, in which most of the tumor bulk consists of neoplastic cells, the FDG uptake in classic HL mainly reflects glucose metabolic activity in the reactive microenvironment (lymphoid hyperplasia) in which the malignant cells are found.[20] Although FDG uptake has been reported to vary between subtypes, all HLs show significant FDG uptake.[21,22]

The differences in glucose metabolic activity of various lymphomas likely account for their variable detection rates as reported in the literature[16,17,23] and probably result from differing proliferative activity, different activation of oncogenic signaling pathways, and different gene expression profiles. Yet given the large overlap in the degree of FDG uptake between indolent and aggressive lymphomas, it is unlikely that FDG-PET can replace biopsy for proper histologic characterization.[14,15]

The variability in FDG uptake affects staging of disease as well as treatment monitoring. A low baseline FDG uptake renders treatment assessments difficult. However, the role of FDG-PET for the few low-grade lymphomas with very low FDG uptake (mainly marginal cell lymphoma including MALT, as well as small lymphocytic lymphoma) might lie in the detection of transformation to more aggressive lymphomas, because this transformation is associated with a marked increase in glucose metabolic activity (Fig. 2).[24]

Table 1	
FDG uptake in selected lymphomas	
Diffuse large B-cell lymphoma	Moderate to high
Follicular lymphoma	Low to moderate
Small lymphocytic lymphoma	None to low
Mantle cell lymphoma	Low to high
Marginal zone lymphoma (including MALT lymphoma)	None[a] to high
T-cell lymphoma	Low to high
HL	Moderate to high
Burkitt lymphoma	High

[a] Approximately 35% of marginal zone lymphomas have no FDG uptake.

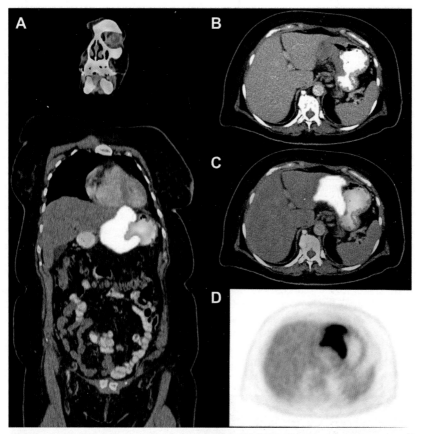

Fig. 2. (A) fused coronal PET/CT, (B) axial CT, (C) fused axial, (D) PET axial. 65-year-old woman diagnosed with MALT transformed to DLBCL. Intense FDG uptake is seen throughout thickened wall of the gastric antrum.

INDICATIONS FOR PET/CT IMAGING IN LYMPHOMA

The important role of FDG-PET imaging in lymphoma is emphasized by the recent report of the International Harmonization Project.[10,11] Their recommendations are among the first to formally acknowledge the importance of FDG-PET for managing patients who have cancer. Taking into account variability among readers and equipment the working group arrived at the following recommendations: (1) FDG-PET is strongly recommended before treatment in patients with routinely FDG avid lymphoma such as DLBCL or HL; (2) treatment effects should be assessed 6 to 8 weeks after completion of chemotherapy; (3) quantification of FDG uptake with SUVs and measurement of SUV changes are not necessary, because visual assessments of treatment effects after completion of therapy are sufficient.[11]

Medicare covers PET/CT imaging for lymphoma in 2 settings defined as initial treatment strategy (formerly known as diagnosis and initial staging) and subsequent treatment strategy (which includes treatment monitoring, restaging, and the detection of suspected recurrence).

Staging usually follows the Ann Arbor classification,[25] which accounts for the number of tumor sites (nodal and extranodal), location, and the presence or absence of systemic (B) symptoms. The disease stage has considerable impact on treatment.[2,26] Therefore, accurate staging is the next important step after tissue diagnosis. Several studies have reported a superior staging accuracy of PET when compared with CT,[27–33] usually resulting in an upward stage migration of patients with HL and NHL.[34] Furthermore, because most patients with lymphoma with potentially curable disease undergo treatment, a baseline PET/CT scan represents a more rational initial staging approach, because it allows not only for staging but also for subsequent treatment monitoring.

One important aspect of staging is the evaluation of bone marrow involvement. Although the specificity of PET for the detection of marrow involvement is high, the sensitivity of PET is not sufficient to replace biopsy for bone marrow staging. However, FDG-PET can provide valuable information in patients with heterogeneous bone marrow involvement in whom biopsy sampling errors can occur. For instance, FDG-PET identified bone marrow involvement in 6 patients with negative bone marrow biopsies (**Fig. 3**).[35–37]

Restaging of patients with PET after completion of therapy has proved to be a valuable tool, especially for DLBCL and HL. Because PET can differentiate active lymphoproliferative disease from necrotic or fibrotic residual tissue, it is more accurate than CT in the evaluation of residual masses.[38–40] The prognosis of patients with a negative PET scan at the end of treatment is excellent.[39,41] The recently established Harmonization criteria provide an easy reference for assessing scans as positive or negative (**Table 2**).[11]

Interval treatment response assessment with PET/CT will likely become the standard of care for response assessments in lymphoma. FDG-PET performed after 1 to 4 cycles of chemotherapy accurately predicted the patient outcome, especially in HL.[42–47] Given the high negative predictive value of interim PET for identifying treatment failure,[48] an additional clinical question being addressed in several clinical trials is whether an interim PET/CT scan can provide the basis for adjusted treatment protocols. Such risk-adapted therapies could help avoid unnecessary toxicities of ineffective therapies, possibly leading to early initiation of more effective treatments. Conversely, in patients showing a good interval response, treatment would be continued as scheduled[49,50] However, recent studies give reason for caution, because in a significant subset of patients, interim positive PET scans did convert to PET negative with ongoing therapy, especially in DLBCL.[51–53] This finding suggests that more sensitive response criteria (such as proposed in PERCIST (Positron Emission tomography Response Criteria In Solid Tumors) or EORTC (European Organization for Research and Treatment of Cancer)[54,55] should be tested for early response assessments.

Surveillance with PET for early detection of recurrence, although widely practiced, is not useful. Given the high false-positive rate, PET/CT scans in the surveillance setting should be reserved for high-risk patients and patients with clinical signs of relapse.[56,57]

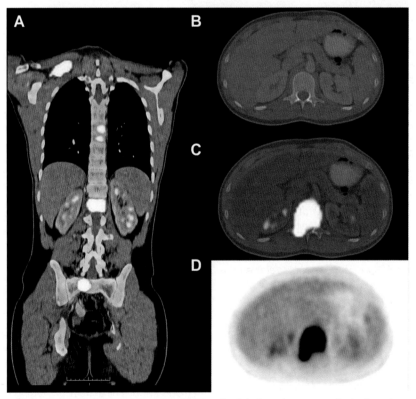

Fig. 3. 27-year-old man with HL. Selected fused and PET and axial slices show supraclavicular adenopathy (*A*) and bone involvement of the spine (*B–D*). Bone involvement would not have been identified on CT alone. Routine bone marrow biopsy of the iliac crest was negative. However, based on the PET/CT findings, the patient was treated for stage IV disease.

Table 2
Harmonization criteria

Criterion	Interpretation
Residual mass ≥2 cm	FDG uptake > mediastinal blood pool is abnormal
Residual mass <2 cm	Any FDG uptake > surrounding background is abnormal
New lung lesions (with or without FDG uptake) and complete response elsewhere	Should be considered negative for lymphoma because these typically represent infectious or inflammatory lesions
Residual hepatic or splenic lesions	>1.5 cm: positive for lymphoma if FDG uptake ≥ liver or spleen FDG uptake <1.5 cm: positive if FDG uptake > liver or spleen FDG uptake
Diffusely increased splenic FDG uptake > liver	Compatible with lymphoma unless the patient has a history of recent cytokine administration
Bone marrow	Focal bone marrow FDG uptake should be interpreted as positive for lymphoma Diffusely increased bone marrow FDG uptake is usually caused by posttherapy marrow hyperplasia

PET/CT PROTOCOLS

Because PET/CT provides comprehensive anatomic and functional information in a single examination of less than 30 minutes, PET/CT has largely replaced stand-alone PET systems.[58] Patient comfort is increased by reducing the need for multiple visits for additional imaging. Diagnostic information is improved by combining the anatomic information from CT with the functional, molecular information of PET. This strategy results in fewer equivocal findings, increased reader confidence,[59] and more accurate assessments of the extent of disease.[60,61] PET/CT interpretations also yield a higher diagnostic accuracy than side-by-side PET and CT interpretations.[59,62] This diagnostic advantage was achieved by using low-dose non–contrast-enhanced CT rather than fully diagnostic contrast CT studies acquired during intravenous (IV) contrast application. However, no consensus exists regarding the best CT protocol for PET/CT studies.

Imaging guidelines have been established by various professional organizations, including the European Association of Nuclear Medicine, the Society of Nuclear Medicine, and the American College of Radiology. None of these guidelines specifically addresses the issue of IV or oral contrast for PET/CT studies.[63–65] Preliminary data suggest that fully diagnostic CT scans result in a more accurate assessment of oncologic diseases than low-dose CT scans.[66–69]

The current University of California at Los Angeles (UCLA) protocol includes diagnostic CT for several reasons: (1) contrast enhancement is the current standard of care in CT imaging; (2) quantification of FDG uptake is generally not significantly affected by the presence of IV or oral contrast[70,71]; (3) most patients with lymphoma who receive a non–contrast-enhanced PET/CT scan would be referred for separate additional contrast CT examinations. This situation adds to the radiation burden and the time spent in imaging clinics, as well as the complexity of image interpretation and comprehension of imaging reports by the referring physician. For these reasons, we suggest a PET/CT protocol that includes oral and IV contrast enhancement (**Fig. 4**).

IMAGE INTERPRETATION
Initial Staging and Restaging After Completion of Therapy

Given the availability of specific criteria (see **Table 2**) for interpreting a PET/CT scan performed for patients with lymphoma in these specific settings, the reporting radiologist should make every effort to include references to mediastinal blood pool activity, as detailed in the Harmonization criteria (**Fig. 5**). A visual comparison is sufficient, although a clear definition of how and where mediastinal blood pool activity should be assessed is not part of the Harmonization criteria. We recommend visual assessment of blood pool FDG activity in the descending aorta. Placing a region of interest (ROI) on axial images in the descending aorta at the approximate level of the carina and recording the SUV_{mean} and SUV_{max} can sometimes aid in assessing the degree of FDG uptake in residual masses relative to mediastinal blood pool FDG activity. For low-grade lymphomas, the report should clearly identify nodes that are disproportionately PET avid, because these might

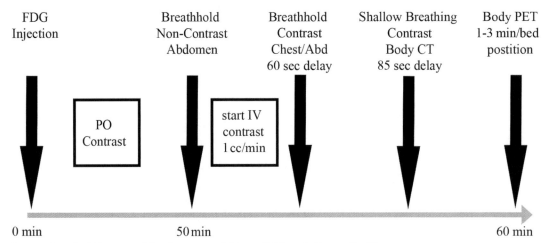

Fig. 4. UCLA PET/CT protocol for 1-stop acquisition of PET and diagnostic CT.

reflect areas of transformed disease that would warrant further evaluations.

For the referring hematologist, the PET scan performed after completion of treatment is the most important. Caution is necessary because not every mildly PET-positive residual finding is caused by persistent disease. It is particularly important to avoid overinterpretation of the images depending on the underlying disease. A complete remission by FDG-PET is more reliable in HLs or DLBCLs, than in follicular lymphomas, small cell lymphomas, or other low-grade NHLs. If a clear response assignment is not possible, then that should be stated and the patient may require a biopsy or close follow-up.

Interval treatment response assessment: although guidelines of how to interpret these interval scans visually are available (Deauville criteria, **Table 3**), the guidelines do state that they should be used only in the setting of clinical trials.

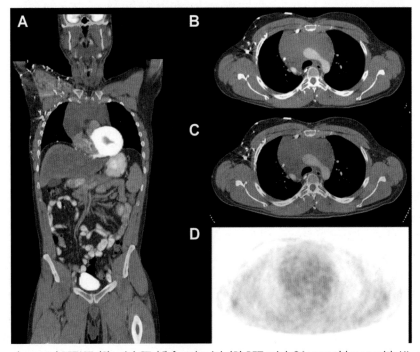

Fig. 5. (A) fused coronal PET/CT, (B) axial CT, (C) fused axial, (D) PET axial. 34-year-old man with HL, status after 6 cycles of chemotherapy. FDG uptake in the residual anterior mediastinal mass is lower than mediastinal blood pool activity, consistent with no residual active lymphoproliferative disease.

Table 3
Deauville criteria

Score	Definition	Interpretation
1	No FDG uptake	Negative
2	FDG uptake ≤ mediastinal blood pool	
3	FDG uptake > mediastinum ≤ liver	
4	FDG uptake moderately > liver	Positive
5	FDG uptake markedly > liver or new sites of disease	

Ongoing trials such as the PETAL and IVS trial in DLBCL are investigating the use of SUV changes for interim PET scans. Data suggest a Δ SUV$_{max}$ with a cutoff at 66% for optimal identification of good versus poor responders after 2 cycles of chemotherapy. To this end, the recent Third International Workshop on Interim Positron Emission Tomography in Lymphoma also discussed guidelines for ROI drawing. The experts agreed that to measure Δ SUV with the highest reproducibility, the hottest lesion should be identified on baseline PET and on interim PET. In residual active lesions, the tumor with the highest uptake FDG should be considered the target, even although its location might differ from the hottest lesion on baseline PET. The SUV$_{max}$ should be identified by making use of 3 to 5 contiguous slices and choosing the slice with the maximal FDG uptake.[72,73]

ARTIFACTS, PITFALLS AND POTENTIALLY FALSE-POSITIVE STUDIES

Dense materials including IV and oral contrast and metallic implants result in potential overcorrection of photon attenuation, which can result in artificially increased FDG uptake on attenuation-corrected images.[74,75] Clinically, this situation does not represent a significant problem because these artifacts are readily identified on the CT images. In cases of persistent ambiguity, non–attenuation-corrected images, which do not show artifact-induced increased FDG uptake, are always available for inspection (**Fig. 6**).

Nonmalignant conditions such as inflammation, infection, granulomatous disease, and sarcoid-like reaction after chemotherapy[76,77] (**Fig. 7**) and

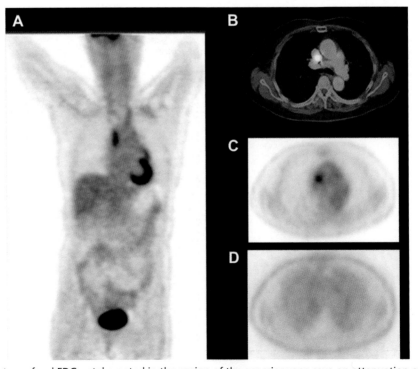

Fig. 6. The intense focal FDG uptake noted in the region of the superior vena cava on attenuation-corrected coronal (A) and axial (B, C) images is not seen on non–attenuation-corrected images (D). The apparent FDG uptake seen on the corrected images constitutes an attenuation-correction artifact caused by high-density material (IV contrast bolus).

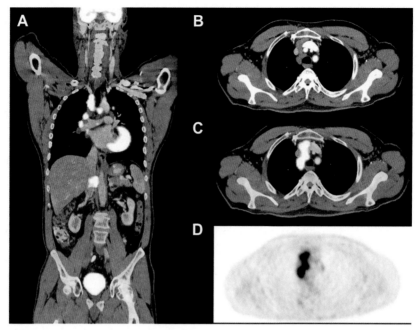

Fig. 7. 50-year-old man with generalized adenopathy. Intense FDG uptake is noted in multiple lymph node stations seen on coronal fused (*A*) and selected axial fused, (*B*) axial CT, (*C*) PET/CT and PET (*D*) images. Subsequent biopsy results were consistent with sarcoidosis.

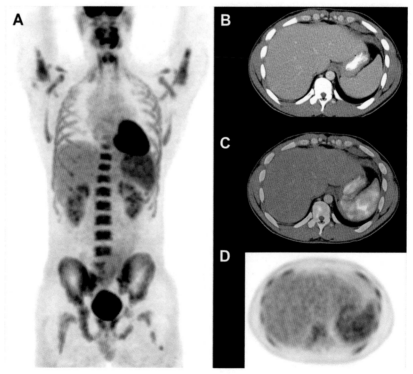

Fig. 8. (*A*) PET MIP, (*B*) axial CT, (*C*) fused axial, (*D*) PET axial. 31-year-old man with DLBCL undergoing chemotherapy with granulocyte colony-stimulating factor support. Diffuse FDG uptake above liver FDG uptake can be seen in the spleen as well as the bone marrow.

physiologic variants of FDG uptake such as in brown adipose tissue,[78] activated muscle, or hyperplasia of the thymus[79] can cause focal FDG uptake and can result in a false-positive reading of a study by less experienced radiologists. Diffusely increased FDG uptake has been associated with reactive changes in the bone marrow and spleen after chemotherapy, especially in patients receiving colony-stimulating factors (granulocyte colony-stimulating factor, erythropoietin) as supportive measures after chemotherapy (**Fig. 8**).[80,81] The most common causes of false-negative PET findings are lesions that fall below the resolution of the scanner because of their small size. Conservatively, FDG-negative lesions less than 10 mm in size should be regarded as too small to be reliably evaluated by PET.[82]

SUMMARY

Most lymphomas, including low-grade lymphomas, show sufficient FDG uptake to be reliably staged with FDG-PET/CT.

PET/CT is the modality of choice for staging and assessment of therapeutic response in patients with lymphoma. Physicians interpreting PET/CT scans should make every effort to include the available interpretation guidelines.

REFERENCES

1. Seam P, Juweid ME, Cheson BD. The role of FDG-PET scans in patients with lymphoma. Blood 2007; 110(10):3507–16.
2. Jerusalem G, Hustinx R, Beguin Y, et al. Evaluation of therapy for lymphoma. Semin Nucl Med 2005; 35(3):186–96.
3. Kasamon YL, Jones RJ, Wahl RL. Integrating PET and PET/CT into the risk-adapted therapy of lymphoma. J Nucl Med 2007;48(Suppl 1):19S–27S.
4. Warburg O, Posener K, Negelein E VIII. The metabolism of cancer cells. Biochem Z 1924;152: 129–69.
5. Phelps M. Positron emission tomography provides molecular imaging of biological processes. Proc Natl Acad Sci U S A 2000;97(16):9226–33.
6. Czernin J, Phelps ME. Positron emission tomography scanning: current and future applications. Annu Rev Med 2002;53:89–112.
7. Calvo MB, Figueroa A, Pulido EG, et al. Potential role of sugar transporters in cancer and their relationship with anticancer therapy. Int J Endocrinol 2010;2010. pii:205357.
8. Flier J, Mueckler M, Usher P, et al. Elevated levels of glucose transport and transporter messenger RNA are induced by ras and sarc oncogenes. Science 1987;235:1492–5.
9. Pauwels EK, Ribeiro MJ, Stoot JH, et al. FDG accumulation and tumor biology. Nucl Med Biol 1998; 25(4):317–22.
10. Cheson BD, Pfistner B, Juweid ME, et al. Revised response criteria for malignant lymphoma. J Clin Oncol 2007;25(5):579–86.
11. Juweid ME, Stroobants S, Hoekstra OS, et al. Use of positron emission tomography for response assessment of lymphoma: consensus of the Imaging Subcommittee of International Harmonization Project in Lymphoma. J Clin Oncol 2007;25(5):571–8.
12. Huang SC. Anatomy of SUV. Standardized uptake value. Nucl Med Biol 2000;27(7):643–6.
13. Vanderhoek M, Perlman SB, Jeraj R. Impact of the definition of peak standardized uptake value on quantification of treatment response. J Nucl Med 2012;53(1):4–11.
14. Schoder H, Noy A, Gonen M, et al. Intensity of 18fluorodeoxyglucose uptake in positron emission tomography distinguishes between indolent and aggressive non-Hodgkin's lymphoma. J Clin Oncol 2005;23(21):4643–51.
15. Papajik T, Myslivecek M, Sedova Z, et al. Standardised uptake value of 18F-FDG on staging PET/CT in newly diagnosed patients with different subtypes of non-Hodgkin's lymphoma. Eur J Haematol 2011; 86(1):32–7.
16. Elstrom R, Guan L, Baker G, et al. Utility of FDG-PET scanning in lymphoma by WHO classification. Blood 2003;101(10):3875–6.
17. Bishu S, Quigley JM, Schmitz J, et al. F-18-fluoro-deoxy-glucose positron emission tomography in the assessment of peripheral T-cell lymphomas. Leuk Lymphoma 2007;48(8):1531–8.
18. Perry C, Herishanu Y, Metzer U, et al. Diagnostic accuracy of PET/CT in patients with extranodal marginal zone MALT lymphoma. Eur J Haematol 2007;79(3):205–9.
19. Beal KP, Yeung HW, Yahalom J. FDG-PET scanning for detection and staging of extranodal marginal zone lymphomas of the MALT type: a report of 42 cases. Ann Oncol 2005;16(3):473–80.
20. Allen-Auerbach M, de Vos S, Czernin J. The impact of fluorodeoxyglucose-positron emission tomography in primary staging and patient management in lymphoma patients. Radiol Clin North Am 2008; 46(2):199–211, vii.
21. Dobert N, Menzel C, Berner U, et al. Positron emission tomography in patients with Hodgkin's disease: correlation to histopathologic subtypes. Cancer Biother Radiopharm 2003;18(4):565–71.
22. Hutchings M, Loft A, Hansen M, et al. Position emission tomography with or without computed tomography in the primary staging of Hodgkin's lymphoma. Haematologica 2006;91(4):482–9.
23. Jerusalem G, Beguin Y, Najjar F, et al. Positron emission tomography (PET) with

18F-fluorodeoxyglucose (18F-FDG) for the staging of low-grade non-Hodgkin's lymphoma (NHL). Ann Oncol 2001;12(6):825–30.

24. Rodriguez M, Rehn S, Ahlstrom H, et al. Predicting malignancy grade with PET in non-Hodgkin's lymphoma. J Nucl Med 1995;36:1790–6.

25. Carbone P, Kaplan H, Musshoff K, et al. Report of the committee on Hodgkin's disease staging classification. Cancer Res 1971;31:1860–1.

26. Ansell SM, Armitage JM. Non-Hodgkin lymphoma: diagnosis and treatment. Mayo Clin Proc 2005; 80(8):1087–97.

27. Hernandez-Maraver D, Hernandez-Navarro F, Gomez-Leon N, et al. Positron emission tomography/computed tomography: diagnostic accuracy in lymphoma. Br J Haematol 2006;135(3): 293–302.

28. Kostakoglu L, Leonard JP, Kuji I, et al. Comparison of fluorine-18 fluorodeoxyglucose positron emission tomography and Ga-67 scintigraphy in evaluation of lymphoma. Cancer 2002;94(4):879–88.

29. la Fougere C, Hundt W, Brockel N, et al. Value of PET/CT versus PET and CT performed as separate investigations in patients with Hodgkin's disease and non-Hodgkin's lymphoma. Eur J Nucl Med Mol Imaging 2006;33(12):1417–25.

30. Wirth A, Seymour JF, Hicks RJ, et al. Fluorine-18 fluorodeoxyglucose positron emission tomography, gallium-67 scintigraphy, and conventional staging for Hodgkin's disease and non-Hodgkin's lymphoma. Am J Med 2002;112(4):262–8.

31. Freudenberg LS, Antoch G, Schutt P, et al. FDG-PET/CT in re-staging of patients with lymphoma. Eur J Nucl Med Mol Imaging 2004;31(3):325–9.

32. Tsukamoto N, Kojima M, Hasegawa M, et al. The usefulness of (18)F-fluorodeoxyglucose positron emission tomography ((18)F-FDG-PET) and a comparison of (18)F-FDG-pet with (67)gallium scintigraphy in the evaluation of lymphoma: relation to histologic subtypes based on the World Health Organization classification. Cancer 2007;110(3): 652–9.

33. Nogami M, Nakamoto Y, Sakamoto S, et al. Diagnostic performance of CT, PET, side-by-side, and fused image interpretations for restaging of non-Hodgkin lymphoma. Ann Nucl Med 2007;21(4): 189–96.

34. Hutchings M, Specht L. PET/CT in the management of haematological malignancies. Eur J Haematol 2008;80(5):369–80.

35. Pakos EE, Fotopoulos AD, Ioannidis JP. 18F-FDG PET for evaluation of bone marrow infiltration in staging of lymphoma: a meta-analysis. J Nucl Med 2005;46(6):958–63.

36. Kabickova E, Sumerauer D, Cumlivska E, et al. Comparison of 18F-FDG-PET and standard procedures for the pretreatment staging of children and adolescents with Hodgkin's disease. Eur J Nucl Med Mol Imaging 2006;33(9):1025–31.

37. Ribrag V, Vanel D, Leboulleux S, et al. Prospective study of bone marrow infiltration in aggressive lymphoma by three independent methods: whole-body MRI, PET/CT and bone marrow biopsy. Eur J Radiol 2008;66(2):325–31.

38. Jerusalem G, Beguin Y, Fasotte M, et al. Whole body positron emission tomography using 18 F-fluorodeoxyglucose for posttreatment evaluation in Hodgkin's disease and non-Hodgkin's lymphoma has higher diagnostic and prognostic value than classical computed tomography scan imaging. Blood 1999;94:429–33.

39. Spaepen K, Stoobants S, Dupont P, et al. Prognostic value of positron emission tomography with fluorine-18 fluorodeoxyglucose ([18F]FDG) after first line chemotherapy in non-Hodgkin's lymphoma: is [18F]FDG-PET a valid alternative to conventional diagnostic methods? J Clin Oncol 2001;19:414–9.

40. Zinzani P, Magagnoli M, Chierichetti F, et al. The role of positron emission tomography (PET) in the management of lymphoma patients. Ann Oncol 1999;10:1181–4.

41. Spaepen K, Stroobants S, Dupont P, et al. Can positron emission tomography with [(18)F]-fluorodeoxyglucose after first-line treatment distinguish Hodgkin's disease patients who need additional therapy from others in whom additional therapy would mean avoidable toxicity? Br J Haematol 2001;115(2):272–8.

42. Jerusalem G, Beguin Y, Fassotte MF, et al. Persistent tumor 18F-FDG uptake after a few cycles of polychemotherapy is predictive of treatment failure in non-Hodgkin's lymphoma. Haematologica 2000; 85(6):613–8.

43. Zinzani PL, Gandolfi L, Broccoli A, et al. Midtreatment 18F-fluorodeoxyglucose positron-emission tomography in aggressive non-Hodgkin lymphoma. Cancer 2011;117(5):1010–8.

44. Gallamini A, Rigacci L, Merli F, et al. The predictive value of positron emission tomography scanning performed after two courses of standard therapy on treatment outcome in advanced stage Hodgkin's disease. Haematologica 2006;91(4):475–81.

45. Hutchings M, Loft A, Hansen M, et al. FDG-PET after two cycles of chemotherapy predicts treatment failure and progression-free survival in Hodgkin lymphoma. Blood 2006;107(1):52–9.

46. Safar V, Dupuis J, Itti E, et al. Interim [18F]fluorodeoxyglucose positron emission tomography scan in diffuse large B-cell lymphoma treated with anthracycline-based chemotherapy plus rituximab. J Clin Oncol 2012;30(2):184–90.

47. Zinzani PL, Rigacci L, Stefoni V, et al. Early interim 18F-FDG PET in Hodgkin's lymphoma: evaluation

on 304 patients. Eur J Nucl Med Mol Imaging 2012; 39(1):4–12.

48. Ziakas PD, Poulou LS, Voulgarelis M, et al. The Gordian knot of interim 18-fluorodeoxyglucose positron emission tomography for Hodgkin lymphoma: a meta-analysis and commentary on published studies. Leuk Lymphoma 2012;53(11):2166–74.

49. Engert A, Haverkamp H, Kobe C, et al. Reduced-intensity chemotherapy and PET-guided radiotherapy in patients with advanced stage Hodgkin's lymphoma (HD15 trial): a randomised, open-label, phase 3 non-inferiority trial. Lancet 2012; 379(9828):1791–9.

50. Kasamon YL, Wahl RL, Ziessman HA, et al. Phase II study of risk-adapted therapy of newly diagnosed, aggressive non-Hodgkin lymphoma based on midtreatment FDG-PET scanning. Biol Blood Marrow Transplant 2009;15(2):242–8.

51. Cox MC, Ambrogi V, Lanni V, et al. Use of interim [18F]fluorodeoxyglucose-positron emission tomography is not justified in diffuse large B-cell lymphoma during first-line immunochemotherapy. Leuk Lymphoma 2012;53(2):263–9.

52. Pregno P, Chiappella A, Bello M, et al. Interim 18-FDG-PET/CT failed to predict the outcome in diffuse large B-cell lymphoma patients treated at the diagnosis with rituximab-CHOP. Blood 2012; 119(9):2066–73.

53. Barnes JA, LaCasce AS, Zukotynski K, et al. End-of-treatment but not interim PET scan predicts outcome in nonbulky limited-stage Hodgkin's lymphoma. Ann Oncol 2011;22(4):910–5.

54. Wahl RL, Jacene H, Kasamon Y, et al. From RECIST to PERCIST: evolving considerations for PET response criteria in solid tumors. J Nucl Med 2009;50(Suppl 1):122S–50S.

55. Young H, Baum R, Cremerius U, et al. Measurement of clinical and subclinical tumour response using [18F]-fluorodeoxyglucose and positron emission tomography: review and 1999 EORTC recommendations. European Organization for Research and Treatment of Cancer (EORTC) PET Study Group. Eur J Cancer 1999;35(13):1773–82.

56. El-Galaly TC, Mylam KJ, Brown P, et al. Positron emission tomography/computed tomography surveillance in patients with Hodgkin lymphoma in first remission has a low positive predictive value and high costs. Haematologica 2012;97(6):931–6.

57. Petrausch U, Samaras P, Haile SR, et al. Risk-adapted FDG-PET/CT-based follow-up in patients with diffuse large B-cell lymphoma after first-line therapy. Ann Oncol 2010;21(8):1694–8.

58. Lonsdale MN, Beyer T. Dual-modality PET/CT instrumentation–today and tomorrow. Eur J Radiol 2010;73(3):452–60.

59. Lardinois D, Weder W, Hany T, et al. Staging of non–small-cell lung cancer with integrated

positron-emission tomography and computed tomography. G Batteriol Virol Immunol 2003;348: 2500–7.

60. Antoch G, Freudenberg L, Nemat A, et al. Preoperative staging of non-small cell lung cancer with dual modality PET/CT imaging: a comparison with PET and CT. J Nucl Med 2003;44(Suppl 5):172P.

61. Allen-Auerbach M, Quon A, Weber WA, et al. Comparison between 2-deoxy-2-[18F]fluoro-D-glucose positron emission tomography and positron emission tomography/computed tomography hardware fusion for staging of patients with lymphoma. Mol Imaging Biol 2004;6(6):411–6.

62. Veit-Haibach P, Luczak C, Wanke I, et al. TNM staging with FDG-PET/CT in patients with primary head and neck cancer. Eur J Nucl Med Mol Imaging 2007;34(12):1953–62.

63. Boellaard R, O'Doherty MJ, Weber WA, et al. FDG PET and PET/CT: EANM procedure guidelines for tumour PET imaging: version 1.0. Eur J Nucl Med Mol Imaging 2010;37(1):181–200.

64. Delbeke D, Coleman RE, Guiberteau MJ, et al. Procedure guideline for tumor imaging with 18F-FDG PET/CT 1.0. J Nucl Med 2006;47(5):885–95.

65. American College of Radiology. ACR practice guideline for performing FDG-PET/CT in oncology 2007.

66. Pfannenberg AC, Aschoff P, Brechtel K, et al. Value of contrast-enhanced multiphase CT in combined PET/CT protocols for oncological imaging. Br J Radiol 2007;80(954):437–45.

67. Morimoto T, Tateishi U, Maeda T, et al. Nodal status of malignant lymphoma in pelvic and retroperitoneal lymphatic pathways: comparison of integrated PET/CT with or without contrast enhancement. Eur J Radiol 2008;67(3):508–13.

68. Kitajima K, Murakami K, Yamasaki E, et al. Performance of integrated FDG PET/contrast-enhanced CT in the diagnosis of recurrent colorectal cancer: comparison with integrated FDG PET/non-contrast-enhanced CT and enhanced CT. Eur J Nucl Med Mol Imaging 2009;36(9):1388–96.

69. Rodriguez-Vigil B, Gomez-Leon N, Pinilla I, et al. PET/CT in lymphoma: prospective study of enhanced full-dose PET/CT versus unenhanced low-dose PET/CT. J Nucl Med 2006;47(10):1643–8.

70. Yau YY, Chan WS, Tam YM, et al. Application of intravenous contrast in PET/CT: does it really introduce significant attenuation correction error? J Nucl Med 2005;46(2):283–91.

71. Dizendorf E, Hany TF, Buck A, et al. Cause and magnitude of the error induced by oral CT contrast agent in CT-based attenuation correction of PET emission studies. J Nucl Med 2003;44(5):732–8.

72. Meignan M, Gallamini A, Haioun C, et al. Report on the Second International Workshop on interim positron emission tomography in lymphoma held in

Menton, France, 8-9 April 2010. Leuk Lymphoma 2010;51(12):2171–80.

73. Meignan M, Gallamini A, Itti E, et al. Report on the Third International Workshop on Interim Positron Emission Tomography in Lymphoma held in Menton, France, 26–27 September 2011 and Menton 2011 consensus. Leuk Lymphoma 2012;53(10):1876–81.

74. Kinahan PE, Townsend DW, Beyer T, et al. Attenuation correction for a combined 3D PET/CT scanner. Med Phys 1998;25(10):2046–53.

75. Halpern BS, Dahlbom M, Waldherr C, et al. Cardiac pacemakers and central venous lines can induce focal artifacts on CT-corrected PET images. J Nucl Med 2004;45(2):290–3.

76. Teirstein AS, Machac J, Almeida O, et al. Results of 188 whole-body fluorodeoxyglucose positron emission tomography scans in 137 patients with sarcoidosis. Chest 2007;132(6):1949–53.

77. de Hemricourt E, De Boeck K, Hilte F, et al. Sarcoidosis and sarcoid-like reaction following Hodgkin's disease. Report of two cases. Mol Imaging Biol 2003;5(1):15–9.

78. Yeung HW, Grewal RK, Gonen M, et al. Patterns of (18)F-FDG uptake in adipose tissue and muscle: a potential source of false-positives for PET. J Nucl Med 2003;44(11):1789–96.

79. Jerushalmi J, Frenkel A, Bar-Shalom R, et al. Physiologic thymic uptake of 18F-FDG in children and young adults: a PET/CT evaluation of incidence, patterns, and relationship to treatment. J Nucl Med 2009;50(6):849–53.

80. Sugawara Y, Fisher SJ, Zasadny KR, et al. Preclinical and clinical studies of bone marrow uptake of fluorine-1-fluorodeoxyglucose with or without granulocyte colony-stimulating factor during chemotherapy. J Clin Oncol 1998;16(1):173–80.

81. Sugawara Y, Zasadny KR, Kison PV, et al. Splenic fluorodeoxyglucose uptake increased by granulocyte colony-stimulating factor therapy: PET imaging results. J Nucl Med 1999;40(9):1456–62.

82. Reinhardt MJ, Wiethoelter N, Matthies A, et al. PET recognition of pulmonary metastases on PET/CT imaging: impact of attenuation-corrected and non-attenuation-corrected PET images. Eur J Nucl Med Mol Imaging 2006;33(2):134–9.

Role of Positron Emission Tomography/Computed Tomography in Bone Malignancies

Patrick J. Peller, MD[a,b,*]

KEYWORDS

- Fluorodeoxyglucose • Positron emission tomography • PET/CT • Osteosarcoma • Bony metastasis
- Multiple myeloma

KEY POINTS

- Positron emission tomography combined with computed tomography (PET/CT) is useful in characterizing bone lesions that require biopsy.
- PET/CT is and important adjunct in the staging of primary bone tumors, identifying favorable response to therapy and detecting recurrence.
- In the evaluation of patients with common carcinomas, especially those arising from the lung, breast, and prostate, PET/CT is highly sensitive and specific for the detection of osseous metastases.
- Multiple myeloma is a heterogeneous disease process exhibiting a wide range of biological behavior, which is reflected by the uptake of ^{18}F-labeled fluorodeoxyglucose (FDG) in skeletal and extraosseous lesions.
- Some benign bone tumors are very metabolically active, and low-grade primary bone tumors demonstrate low FDG accumulation on PET/CT scans.

INTRODUCTION

Malignancies in the bone can arise from skeletal tissue itself (primary bone tumors), from a distant site (secondary or metastatic tumors), or from within the marrow space impinging primarily on the bone (multiple myeloma [MM]). Primary bone tumors are a heterogeneous group of sarcomas: osteosarcoma, Ewing sarcoma, chondrosarcoma, fibrosarcoma, and malignant fibrous histiocytoma. Their mesenchymal tissue of origin defines them. Bony metastases are the most common malignant bone tumor, and lung, breast, and prostate are the major primary cancer sites.[1] MM arises from a single clone of differentiated plasma cells, usually producing high levels of a monoclonal immunoglobulin. These malignant plasma cells proliferate within the marrow space and commonly produce osseous lesions.[2]

Diagnostic imaging plays a critical role in the evaluation of patients with known or possible bone malignancies. Conventional anatomic imaging with plain film radiographs, ultrasonography, computed tomography (CT), and magnetic resonance (MR) imaging, and functional ^{99m}Tc–methyl diphosphonate bone scintigraphy are established

Disclosures: Dr Peller is a consultant for Eli Lilly and Company.
[a] Nuclear Radiology, Mayo Clinic, 200 1st Street Southwest, Rochester, MN 55905, USA; [b] Department of Radiology, College of Medicine, Mayo Clinic, 200 1st Street Southwest, Rochester, MN 55905, USA
* Department of Radiology, College of Medicine, Mayo Clinic, 200 1st Street Southwest, Rochester, MN 55905.
E-mail address: peller.patrick@mayo.edu

Radiol Clin N Am 51 (2013) 845–864
http://dx.doi.org/10.1016/j.rcl.2013.05.005

components in the multidisciplinary management of bone tumors.[3–5] ^{18}F-fluorodeoxyglucose (FDG) positron emission tomography (PET) has developed an increasing presence in the evaluation of patients with malignancies, including primary and secondary bone tumors.[6] The integration of PET and CT into a single scanner has yielded a diagnostic modality that identifies metabolically active lesions and accurate localization.[7–9] The current generation of PET/CT scanners can detect primary and metastatic disease, guide biopsies, evaluate response to therapy, and assess for recurrence.[10–13]

This article reviews the use of FDG PET/CT in the evaluation of primary bone tumors and detection of osseous metastases. The growing clinical role of FDG PET/CT in patients with MM is examined.

PRIMARY BONE TUMORS

Primary bone tumors are uncommon malignancies that account for less than 1% of all cancers in adults and nearly 5% of childhood malignancies. In the United States, it is estimated that 2890 primary bone tumors are diagnosed annually, resulting in 1410 deaths.[14] Primary bone tumors have a bimodal distribution, the first peak occurring during the second decade of life and the second peak in patients older than 60 years. Primary bone tumors represent the third most common neoplasm in adolescents and young adults.[15] Although a second peak of primary tumors is seen late in life, it is much more common beyond the age of 40 years for a bone lesion to be secondary to metastases or MM (Table 1). Patient age is one of the most the most important factors in the initial differential diagnosis of a primary bone tumor.[16] Multimodality therapy, including a combination of chemotherapy, radiation, and surgery, has become the norm.

Specific Primary Bone Tumors

Osteosarcoma

The most common primary bone tumor of bone is osteosarcoma, which characteristically produces osteoid tissue or immature bone.[17,18] Approximately 900 patients develop an osteosarcoma each year in the United States. The majority arise in children, adolescents, and young adults in their 20s.[19] Osteosarcomas typically exhibit aggressive biological behavior, and on histology most are high-grade tumors. Osteosarcomas begin in or adjacent to regions of high bone growth.[17–19] The survival has improved markedly over the past 20 years, with improved chemotherapeutic agents. Neoadjuvant chemotherapy attacks

Table 1
Malignant bone tumors: age at presentation

Age (y)	Diagnosis
<20	Ewing sarcoma Osteosarcoma
20–40	Osteosarcoma Fibrosarcoma Chordoma Angiosarcoma
>40	Metastases Multiple myeloma Chondrosarcoma Malignant fibrous histiocytoma Secondary osteosarcoma (Paget disease, radiation) Fibrosarcoma Lymphoma

Data from Roodman GD. Skeletal imaging and management of bone disease. Hematology Am Soc Hematol Educ Program 2008;313–9; and Miller TT. Bone tumors and tumorlike conditions: analysis with conventional radiography. Radiology 2008;246(3):662–74.

presumed micrometastases while shrinking the primary tumor. Presurgical chemotherapy has led to a growth of surgical and reconstruction options, including limb-sparing procedures.[20,21]

Ewing sarcoma

In children and teenagers, Ewing sarcoma is the second most common primary bone tumor. The Ewing sarcoma family of tumors (ESFT) is histologically similar, consisting of primitive, small, round blue cells, and demonstrate translocations involving the same gene on chromosome 22.[19,22,23] Virtually all ESFTs are detected in patients 5 to 25 years old. ESFT most often arises in the long bones of the extremities and the bones of the pelvis.[22,23] Similar to osteosarcomas, ESFTs exhibit aggressive biological behavior. Chemotherapy is the initial treatment, with surgery and radiotherapy focused on the primary tumor depending on its size and location. Ewing tumors were uniformly fatal 30 years ago, but nowadays patients with localized disease have a 5-year survival from 25% to 86% depending on the primary site.[19,22–26]

Chondrosarcoma

This heterogeneous group of malignant bone tumors characteristically produces a chondroid (cartilaginous) matrix.[27] Chondrosarcoma is the third most common primary malignancy of bone, accounting for more than 20% of the total.[28] Only osteosarcoma and MM are more frequent.[16]

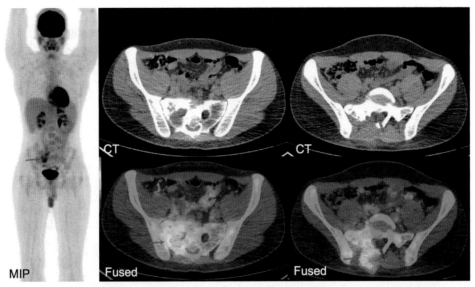

Fig. 1. A 21-year-old man who presented for back pain and initial imaging demonstrated a destructive right sacral abnormality. Staging PET/CT scan demonstrates an intensely FDG-avid (maximum standardized uptake value [SUV_{max}] = 8.3) destructive lesion in the right sacrum (*arrow*). There is extension into the adjacent soft tissues with heterogeneous FDG uptake. No metastases were identified. Biopsy yielded Ewing sarcoma, and the patient underwent chemotherapy. MIP, maximum-intensity projection.

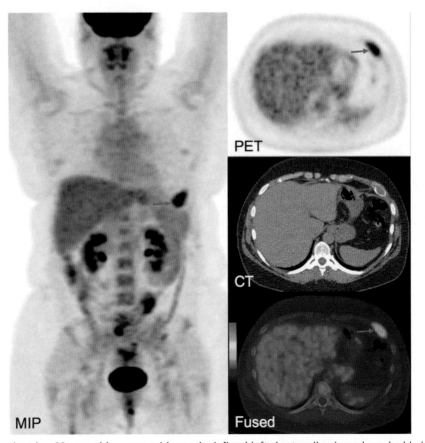

Fig. 2. This patient is a 23-year-old woman with poorly defined left chest wall pain and a palpable left sixth rib abnormality. Staging PET/CT scan demonstrated an expansile, peripherally calcifying lesion with intense FDG uptake (SUV_{max} = 7.4) (*arrow*). No metastatic disease was identified. Needle biopsy demonstrated chondroblastic osteosarcoma. The patient received 4 cycles of chemotherapy and underwent successful chest-wall resection.

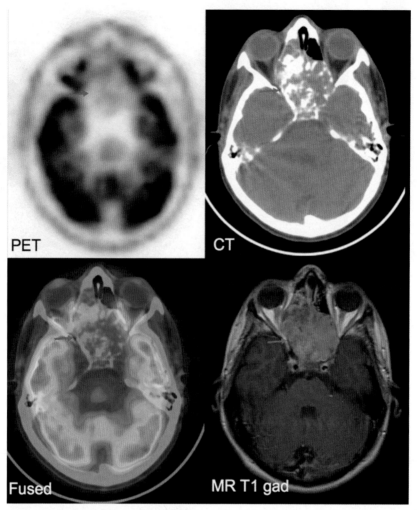

Fig. 3. This patient is a 21-year-old man presenting for persistent headaches. Staging PET/CT scan demonstrated minor FDG uptake (SUV$_{max}$ = 2.0) within a 6.5-cm mass arising from the paranasal sinuses and demonstrating typical chondroid calcification on corresponding CT images (*arrow*). MR imaging shows significant gadolinium (gad) enhancement of the mass. Surgical resection showed chondrosarcoma at pathologic examination.

Chondrosarcomas exhibit variable biological behavior. Most are low-grade to intermediate-grade tumors and are initially slow growing with a low metastatic potential.[29,30] The biology of chondrosarcoma makes it relatively refractory to chemotherapy and radiation therapy. Surgery is the primary therapy for chondrosarcomas.[30,31] The 5-year relative survival has remained stable for the past 30 years, ranging from 52% to 87% depending on histologic subtype.[31–33]

In primary bone tumors the presenting symptoms are nonspecific. Patients relate pain and/or swelling for a duration of weeks or months. Diagnosis is frequently delayed for several weeks to months, and often presentation is associated with minor or possible trauma.[19] The rarity of primary bone tumors, especially in an otherwise healthy child or adolescent, leads to locally advanced disease. On physical examination a palpable soft-tissue mass is often identified. After detection of a potential primary bone malignancy,

---

Box 1
Clinical roles of PET/CT: primary bone tumors

Clinically suspected malignant bone tumor–guided biopsy

Staging/assess biological aggressiveness

Surgical and radiation planning

Response assessment after chemotherapy

Detect/stage recurrence

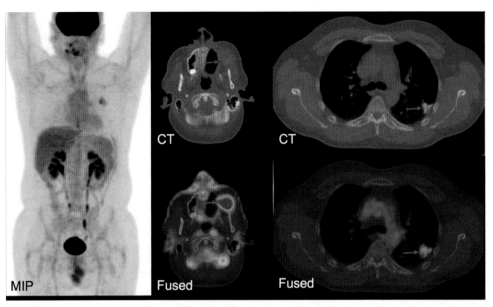

Fig. 4. This 67-year-old man had a history of head and neck cancer treated with radiation therapy 17 years prior. He sought medical attention for left facial pain. Staging PET/CT scan demonstrated a destructive lesion at the junction of the left zygomatic arch and orbital rim (*arrow*). This poorly defined mass has intense FDG accumulation (SUV$_{max}$ = 11.0). There are multiple calcified nodules scattered throughout both lungs. The largest nodule is located within the posterior left lung measuring 1.9 cm in greatest dimension with moderate activity (SUV$_{max}$ = 4.0) (*arrow*). Histology of the primary lesion returned as osteosarcoma, possibly resulting from the patient's prior radiation therapy.

imaging plays a crucial role in assessing malignant potential and staging.[19,21,33]

Staging is important in selection and, often, sequencing of proper therapy. The American Joint Commission on Cancer (AJCC) system for staging primary bone tumors focuses on the tumor size, nodal involvement, and metastatic disease, but also the tumor grade.[34] The surgical staging system developed by Enneking uses the grade of the tumor to separate nonmetastatic malignant bone tumors into stage I (low grade) and stage II (high grade).[35] In both systems, patients with distant metastases are stage III.[34,35] Both systems are incomplete because tumor location, tumor biology, patient age, and genetic abnormalities often are used to select the intensity of therapy and to define prognosis.[19,21,23,31]

PET/CT Imaging

A growing body of published literature supports FDG PET/CT imaging of primary bone tumors.[11,13,36–42] The imaging technique is similar to that used for other oncologic indications, except that PET/CT scanning for sarcomas requires axial coverage from vertex to toes. The FDG avidity of primary bone tumors and sarcoma metastases is commonly high, which significantly aids detection (**Figs. 1** and **2**).[11,13,37,39,41,42] Chondrosarcomas

are the exception, with mild to moderate FDG uptake mirroring histologic grade (**Fig. 3**).[36,40] PET/CT has multiple clinical roles in primary bone tumors (**Box 1**).

Initial Imaging

Initial imaging of primary bone tumors is ideally performed before biopsy. PET/CT is used as an

---

Box 2
Key report features: primary bone tumors

Primary lesion:

   Size

   Intensity of FDG uptake (SUV$_{max}$)

   FDG heterogeneity

   Presence of necrosis

   Location within the bone

   Local extent

   Soft-tissue extension

   Involvement of adjacent of vessel or nerve

Presence of skip lesions

Distant metastases

adjunct to MR imaging in evaluating the primary tumor site. PET/CT imaging of the primary lesion is focused on identifying the biological aggressiveness, and the locoregional extent and involvement of adjacent tissues. The magnitude of FDG uptake within a region of tumor corresponds to the histologic grade.[10–13,39,42–44] Many primary sarcomas exhibit significant heterogeneity in FDG accumulation (see **Figs. 1–3**). Tumor heterogeneity may be a negative prognostic factor.[45] Biopsy directed at the area of maximum activity improves biopsy sampling. Primary bone tumors often are locally advanced, exceeding 10 cm in size at the time of presentation. Large tumors frequently outgrow their blood supply and areas of necrosis centrally. FDG uptake is absent necrotic areas, and PET/CT may be helpful in directing biopsy toward viable tumor regions.[10,46,47]

The major role of PET/CT in initial imaging is to identify distant metastatic disease, commonly in the skeleton and lungs (**Fig. 4**). In patients with Ewing sarcoma, FDG PET/CT has been shown to be significantly more sensitive for the detection of osseous metastasis compared with conventional imaging, whereas the results in patients with osteosarcoma are similar to those for conventional imaging.[10–13,40,42] Performing a high-quality, breath-hold CT evaluation of the lungs in conjunction with the PET/CT scan permits identification of subcentimeter nodular pulmonary metastases (**Box 2**).[41,48]

Therapy Assessment

FDG PET/CT is frequently used to assess the response to initial chemotherapy (**Fig. 5**). Because the response to initial chemotherapy is so tightly associated with progression-free survival, much of the PET/CT literature is focused on this aspect. The measured change in FDG uptake has been used in correlation with histologic response. Most commonly the maximum standardized uptake value (SUV_{max}) is utilized. Different primary bone tumor histologies respond to different rates and magnitudes of chemotherapy Ewing sarcoma usually develops a more profound reduction in size and activity with chemotherapy than does osteosarcoma. Researchers have combined size and activity to create measurements of metabolic tumor volume, which may improve correlation with histologic response in comparison with SUV_{max}. In general, a greater than 50% reduction is associated with a favorable response in osteosarcoma, whereas an 80% to 90% reduction in metabolism is sought in Ewing sarcoma.[12,13,49–57]

Detecting and Staging Recurrence

Advances in the treatment of primary bone tumors have significantly improved survival in patients with primary bone tumors; nonetheless, up to 40% of patients will develop local and/or distant recurrent disease within the first 3 years after diagnosis.[22,24–26] PET/CT plays an important role in the

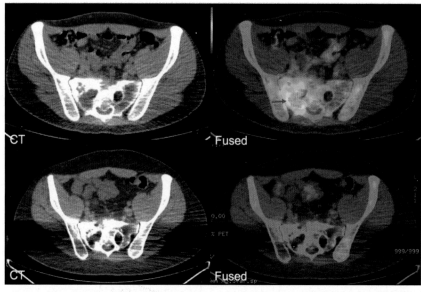

Fig. 5. The patient in **Fig. 1** underwent 6 cycles of systemic chemotherapy. As part of the reevaluation, a PET/CT scan was performed to assess the metabolic response of the right sacral sarcoma (*arrow*). The activity within the tumor mass has decreased, with an SUV_{max} of 1.9 compared with 8.3 initially. No new lesions were identified.

restaging of high-risk patients. FDG PET/CT can provide an assessment of local disease despite structural changes induced by treatment and the presence of a metallic prosthesis. PET/CT from vertex to toes locates distant metastases, characterizes the abnormalities and likelihood of malignancy, and can direct biopsy. Initial studies suggest that the sensitivity and specificity of FDG PET/CT for the detection of a recurrence exceeds those of conventional imaging.[10–13,42]

Pitfalls

- The degree of FDG uptake can be helpful in distinguishing benign from malignant lesions.
- Osseous lesions with high FDG uptake are far more likely to be neoplastic; however, increased FDG uptake in the skeletal lesion is not pathognomonic for a malignancy (Table 2).
- Increased tracer accumulation has been described in several benign bone lesions, including giant cell tumors, fibrous dysplasia, fracture, or infection (Fig. 6).[58,59]
- In the evaluation bony lesions care must be taken to integrate both PET and CT data with clinical information and prior imaging tests.

SECONDARY BONE TUMORS

Malignancies in the bone most commonly arise from an extraskeletal site.[60–62] Bone metastases are common in patients with cancer, and more than 50% of people who die of cancer have osseous involvement.[63–65] Most bone metastases have been present for a considerable length of time before symptoms develop. Pain is the most frequent presenting manifestation of a bone metastasis.[63,66,67] Breast, lung, prostate, renal cell, and colorectal cancers are the most common cause of bony metastases. In adults, more than 90% of all osseous metastases are found in the axial and proximal appendicular skeleton where there is residual red marrow. Bone metastases are typically multiple at the time of diagnosis.[66,68]

PET/CT Imaging

FDG PET/CT has been found to be more sensitive than bone scintigraphy and diagnostic CT in detecting osseous metastases.[63,69–72] Typically osteolytic metastatic disease is intensely FDG avid (Fig. 7). The reason that PET/CT is more sensitive

Table 2
Bone tumors: relative FDG uptake

Bone Tumors	FDG Uptake
Malignant	
Osteosarcoma	High
Ewing sarcoma	High
Metastasis	Moderate to high
Chondrosarcoma	Low to moderate
Multiple myeloma	Variable/heterogeneous
Benign	
Giant cell tumor	High
Fibrous dysplasia	Moderate
Chondromyxoid fibroma	Moderate
Fracture	Low to moderate
Osteochondroma	Low
Enchondroma	Low
Osteoid osteoma	Low

Data from Hamada K, Tomita Y, Konishi E, et al. FDG-PET evaluation of chondromyxoid fibroma of left ilium. Clin Nucl Med 2009;34(1):15–7; and Dimitrakopoulou-Strauss A. Dynamic PET ^{18}F-FDG studies in patients with primary and recurrent soft-tissue sarcomas: impact on diagnosis and correlation with grading. J Nucl Med 2002;178:510–8.

than conventional bone scintigraphy and diagnostic CT imaging is that many early tumor deposits fail to trigger either an osteolytic or osteoblastic response (Fig. 8).[63,70,73] Many metastatic lesions have mixed lytic and blastic properties, which are uniformly FDG avid if patients are untreated. In patients with lung cancer, the overall sensitivity and specificity FDG PET/CT for the detection of bone metastasis was reported as 93% and 95%, respectively, in a recent meta-analysis.[74]

Pitfalls

- In most cancer, FDG accumulates within the tumor and can help in identifying bone metastases at an early stage before host osteoblasts begin the bony reparative response.
- Sclerotic metastatic disease, especially if caused by prostate cancer, often exhibits limited FDG uptake (Fig. 9).
- Osteoblastic metastases are often only visible on the CT component of the PET/CT scan, and can be better visualized on a bone scan.[70,73]
- Bone lesions that measure less than 3 mm have limited detectability on PET.[63,73]

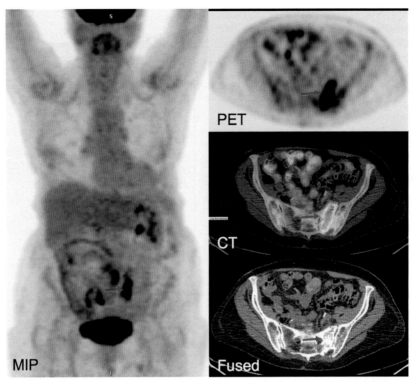

Fig. 6. This patient is a 92-year-old woman who presented for evaluation of a left lower lobe lung nodule. The left lung nodule exhibited negligible FDG uptake. In the left sacrum there was linear intense FDG uptake (SUV$_{max}$ = 8.9), which corresponds to an area of sclerosis (*arrow*). A thin-cut CT supported the diagnosis of a healing insufficiency fracture. The follow-up imaging at 9 months showed continued healing.

Therapy Assessment

Imaging techniques used to visualize skeletal metastases often have limitations when assessing response to therapy.[75,76] Theoretically, integration of PET and CT should lead to the synergy of CT (measuring changes in lesion size and morphology) and FDG PET (assessing tumor glycolysis).[75] Most of the studies have been performed in patients with breast cancer with osseous metastases. Most patients received combinations of hormonal therapy, chemotherapy, and radiotherapy, in different amounts, sequences, and timing. The baseline PET/CT has to be performed before or quite distant, likely 4 to 6 months, for valid results. The majority of lesions become FDG negative, with the best response in lytic metastases. Despite resolution of FDG uptake, the CT scan commonly remains abnormal. The osteoblastic CT appearance corresponds with persistently positive bone scans. The FDG accumulation correlates with the biological behavior of the tumor cells in the bony metastases.[77–79] Additional research is needed in this area.

MULTIPLE MYELOMA

MM is the most common malignant bone neoplasm in adults, the incidence of which increases with age. A monoclonal proliferation of terminally differentiated plasma cells excessively produces immunoglobulins from the marrow space. The great majority of myeloma patients are diagnosed initially when 50 to 70 years old.[14,80] Patients with MM present with a variety of symptoms: bone pain, fatigue and lethargy from anemia, renal failure, and hypercalcemia.[81,82] Many patients are detected incidentally, with laboratory tests showing a monoclonal gammopathy or Bence-Jones proteins in urine. The treatment of myeloma consists of thalidomide and bortezomib (a protease inhibitor) combined with chemotherapy and prednisolone. Stem cell transplantation plays an important role in patients with aggressive and/or advanced disease.[83,84]

Classically MM results from a proliferating, malignant clone of plasma cells secreting a paraprotein. The diagnosis requires specific evidence of end-organ damage caused by the plasma cells (**Box 3**). Multiple myeloma typically is preceded

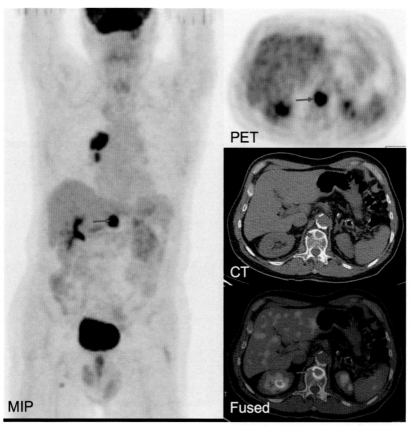

Fig. 7. This 74-year-old man (a smoker) presented for evaluation of a cough, and his chest radiograph suggested a right hilar mass. A staging PET/CT scan demonstrated a 3.2 cm right parahilar mass and hilar lymph nodes with intense FDG uptake (SUV$_{max}$ = 10.2). There was a 1.8-cm lytic metastasis in the L1 vertebral body also with intense FDG uptake (*arrow*). A biopsy of the right hilar mass demonstrated non–small cell lung cancer. The patient was treated with chemotherapy with radiation therapy to the lumbar spine.

by a solitary plasmacytoma of bone (SPB), monoclonal gammopathy of undetermined significance (MGUS), or smoldering (asymptomatic) multiple myeloma (SMM) (**Table 3**). SPB is a lytic bone lesion composed of malignant plasma cells, most commonly located in a vertebral body or the pelvis, and when truly solitary is treated with radiation therapy. About 80% of SPB patients subsequently develop MM within 5 years of treatment.[85] SMM is very similar to MM, but evidence of end-organ damage is not present. Patients with SMM convert to MM at a rate of approximately 10% per year for the first 5 years.[86,87] Patients with MGUS are detected incidentally on routine laboratory tests. The progression from MGUS to MM is slow but long term, approximately 1% per year for the next 15 years.[88,89]

There are 3 staging systems for myeloma: the International Staging System (ISS), the Durie-Salmon staging system, and the Mayo Stratification of Myeloma and Risk-Adapted Therapy (mSMART). The ISS is simple, easy to use, and requires serum levels of β2-microglobulin and albumin. The ISS is better at predicting group than individual patient outcomes.[90] The Durie-Salmon system uses laboratory and imaging data (**Box 4**). It is predictive of patient outcome with standard chemotherapy, but may be less predictive with newer treatment schemes.[91] The mSMART measures individual genetic risk profiles, and its role in managing myeloma patients is still evolving.[92] Recently, Durie added advanced imaging with MR or PET/CT to the staging schema (**Table 4**).[93]

PET/CT Imaging

PET/CT has a growing role to play in the management of MM and in the evaluation of precursor states (**Box 5**). The axial coverage in patients

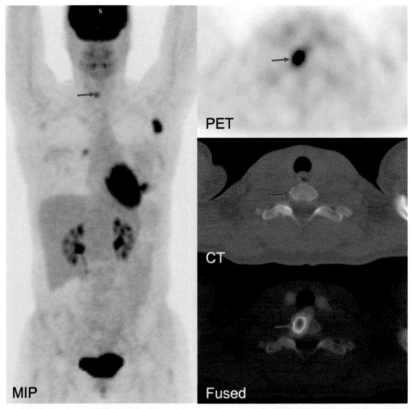

Fig. 8. This 37-year-old woman presented with palpable left axillary adenopathy. Initial imaging demonstrated bilateral breast implants and a left subareolar breast mass. The staging PET/CT scan showed hypermetabolic left axillary lymph and right hilar nodal metastases. The 1.1-cm focus of intense activity in the right aspect of the C7 vertebral body has no corresponding lesion on CT (*arrow*). Needle biopsy of the left axillary lymph nodes showed infiltrating ductal carcinoma. MR imaging of the cervical spine confirmed the C7 metastasis. The patient underwent neoadjuvant chemotherapy before surgical resection.

with MM should be vertex to at least the knees. The integrated PET/CT scanners leverage the high spatial resolution of CT for small lytic bone lesions and high sensitivity of FDG for malignant cells in a focal, multifocal, or diffuse infiltrative pattern.[94–96] Durie[93] specifically added FDG PET/CT to the staging system because he thought that PET/CT would provide an imaging test of the metabolism and bony destruction.

For almost all patients with MGUS and most with SMM, PET/CT has no role until there is clinical evidence of progression. The PET/CT scan of patients with stable MGUS and SMM will typically be normal or show nonspecific low-grade, diffuse marrow uptake (**Fig. 10**). The major dividing line between MGUS and SMM is the presence of end-organ damage. Some MGUS and SMM patients have anemia, hypercalcemia, lytic bone, or renal failure, and the clinical concern is whether the plasma cells are the cause. PET/CT is used

to identify FDG-avid or lytic bone lesions to establish the diagnosis of MM (**Box 6**).[97–100]

The single bone lesion in an SPB is composed of malignant plasma cells whose histology is virtually identical to that of MM. Unfortunately, most patients with an SPB will go on to have MM with the next 5 to 10 years. PET/CT is used as initial imaging to identify the presence of additional, often smaller, FDG-avid lytic lesions in patients with an SPB (**Fig. 11**). When additional myeloma lesions are established, systemic MM therapy is used instead of local radiation therapy. Published studies show that 33% to 47% of patients with an SPB have multiple bony abnormalities that indicate MM.[101,102]

FDG PET/CT is used as a single procedure to drive clinical decision making. Low-dose CT can replace traditional bone surveys in MM patients. MM is a very heterogeneous disease on PET/CT, varying greatly from one patient to the next

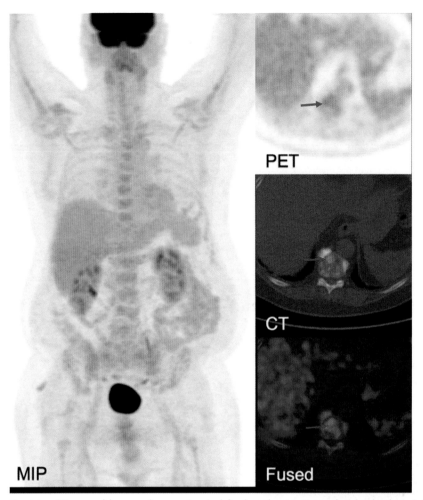

Fig. 9. This patient is a 74-year-old man who was treated for lymphoma at another institution. A PET/CT scan, obtained to evaluate treatment efficacy, demonstrated numerous blastic lesions throughout the axial skeleton. There was very mild FDG uptake within the spine (SUV_{max} = 2.3) corresponding to the blastic lesion on CT (*arrow*). The patient's prostate-specific antigen level was found to be 49.2 ng/dL, and subsequent workup confirmed metastatic prostate cancer.

Box 3
End-organ damage: CRAB

C = elevated calcium level (Ca >11.5 mg/dL)

R = renal insufficiency (Cr >2.0 mg/dL)

A = anemia (hemoglobin <10 g/dL)

B = lytic bony lesions

Adapted from Kyle RA, Rajkumar SV. Criteria for diagnosis, staging, risk stratification and response assessment of multiple myeloma. Leukemia 2009;23(1):3–9.

(**Fig. 12**). Many patients demonstrate significant heterogeneity in their own MM lytic lesions (**Fig. 13**). PET/CT is very sensitive in detecting the hypermetabolism commonly produced by multifocal bone marrow involvement. Studies suggest that MR imaging is more sensitive than FDG PET/CT in detecting infiltrative patterns of MM in the spine. The higher sensitivity of PET/CT likely results in upstaging and earlier treatment in some patients, but more individualized data are now available for all patients.[95–97,103]

Extramedullary deposits of plasma cells are not uncommon in myeloma patients (**Fig. 14**). The frequency of extraosseous disease in MM is not well documented. Initial reports suggest that

Table 3
Diagnostic criteria for multiple myeloma and precedent disorders

	SPB	MGUS	SMM	MM
Monoclonal protein	<3 g/dL	<3 g/dL	≥3 g/dL	Present
Marrow plasma cells	<10%	<10%	≥10% to <60% clonal	Present
End-organ damage	None	None	None	Present from MM cells
Annual MM progression	15%–20%	1%–2%	10%	

Abbreviations: MGUS, monoclonal gammopathy of undetermined significance; MM, multiple myeloma; SMM, smoldering (asymptomatic) multiple myeloma; SPB, solitary plasmacytoma of bone.

Data from Rajkumar SV, Dispenzieri A, Fonseca R, et al. Thalidomide for previously untreated indolent or smoldering multiple myeloma. Leukemia 2001;15(8):1274–6; and Rajkumar SV, Larson D, Kyle RA. Diagnosis of smoldering multiple myeloma. N Engl J Med 2011;365(5):474–5.

Box 4
Durie-Salmon staging system

Stage 1 (all criteria need to be met)

- Hemoglobin >100 g/L
- Normal serum calcium
- Normal bone radiograph or single bone plasmacytoma
- Low M protein levels: immunoglobulin (Ig)G <50 g/L, IgA <30 g/L, urine light chain <4 g/24 h

Stage 2: Neither Stage 1 nor Stage 3

Stage 3 (1 or more criteria need to be met)

- Hemoglobin <85 g/L
- Serum calcium >12 mg/dL
- Multiple lytic bone lesions
- High M protein levels: IgG >70 g/L, IgA >50 g/L, urine light chain >12 g/24 h

Adapted from Durie BG, Salmon SE. A clinical staging system for multiple myeloma. Correlation of measured myeloma cell mass with presenting clinical features, response to treatment, and survival. Cancer 1975;36(3):842–54.

Table 4
Durie-Salmon plus staging

Classification	MR or PET/CT
MGUS	All negative
Stage 1A (smoldering MM)	Negative or single plasmacytoma
Stage 1B (MM)	<5 focal lesions/mildly diffuse
Stage 2A/B (MM)	5–20 focal lesions/moderately diffuse
Stage 3A/B (MM)	>20 focal lesions/severely diffuse

A = serum creatinine <2 mg/dL + no extramedullary disease.
B = serum creatinine >2 mg/dL or extramedullary disease.

Adapted from Durie BG. The role of anatomic and functional staging in myeloma: description of Durie/Salmon plus staging system. Eur J Cancer 2006;42(11):1539–43.

Box 5
Clinical roles of PET/CT: multiple myeloma
Clinically suspected MM in MGUS or SMM patient
Evaluate for additional lesions in SPB patient
Staging/assess for aggressive features
Assessment of therapy response
Detect/stage recurrence

Box 6
Key report features: multiple myeloma
Number and intensity (SUV_{max}) of FDG avid foci
Presence of diffuse increased marrow activity
Number and extent of lytic lesions
Presence of significant osteopenia
Overall assessment of marrow replacement by MM
Areas concerning for pathologic fracture
Spine abnormalities: collapse, epidural extension, cord compromise

extramedullary disease is a marker for more aggressive MM. Extramedullary disease with bony disease is most common in the lymph nodes, spleen, and liver. Almost any organ or tissue can be involved with extraosseous plasmacytomas. Patients with extraosseous disease tend to respond less well to traditional myeloma regimens.[98,104,105]

The treatment selection for newly diagnosed MM depends on the patient's comorbidities, the patient's ability to medically tolerate stem cell transplantation, and the presence of high-risk genetic characteristics.[83,91] Patients for transplantation typically receive 3 to 4 months of combination chemotherapy to markedly decrease the number of plasma cells residing within the bone marrow. At this time point the treatment response is evaluated, with a goal of at least a 50% decrease in clinical, laboratory, and PET/CT measurements (**Fig. 15**). Recent published data suggest that PET/CT-based measurements can have prognostic value.[106–108] Patients with only mildly decreased or increased laboratory or

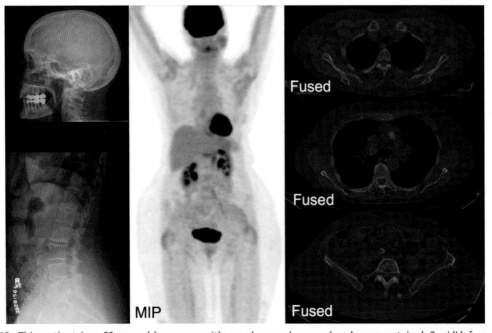

Fig. 10. This patient is a 69-year-old woman with an abnormal monoclonal paraprotein (<3 g/dL) found on routine blood work, which triggered complaints of fatigue. She also had a moderately severe anemia. No lytic lesions were identified on bony survey. A PET/CT scan, ordered to evaluate for possible multiple myeloma (MM), revealed no FDG-avid abnormalities and no lytic lesions within the skeleton. The patient had a monoclonal gammopathy of undetermined significance.

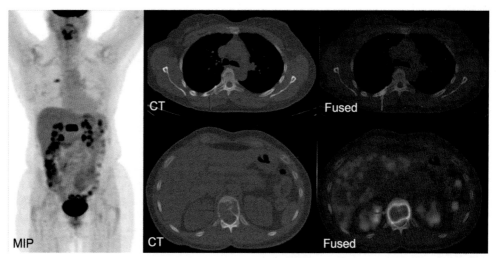

Fig. 11. This patient was a 55-year-old man who presented for back pain. A spine radiograph demonstrated a destructive lesion at T12, and a biopsy obtained clonal plasma cells. A PET/CT scan showed intense FDG uptake in the lytic lesion filling the T12 vertebral body (*arrows*-bottom images). In addition, an FDG-avid lytic abnormality was noted on the right, posterior third rib (*arrows*-top images). Bone marrow biopsy of the posterior iliac crest showed more than 30% plasma cells. The patient was treated with systemic chemotherapy for MM in preparation for a stem cell transplant.

PET/CT data will require additional or alternative chemotherapy in preparation for transplantation. Nontransplant patients typically receive 6 cycles of chemotherapy and then undergo therapy evaluation. The goal in these myeloma patients is for all clinical and imaging evidence to show that the MM has become quiescent. This plateau or quiescent phase occurs in approximately half of the patients and typically lasts 6 or more months.[109,110]

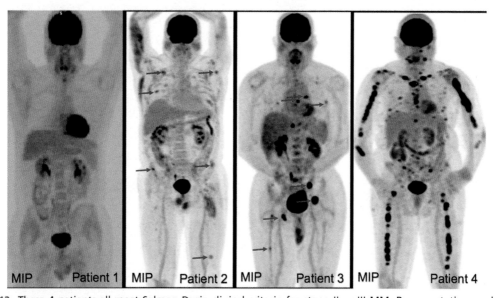

Fig. 12. These 4 patients all meet Salmon-Durie clinical criteria for stage II or III MM. Representative myeloma lesions are marked on each PET MIP image (*arrows*). Patient 1 had no significant PET or CT bone abnormalities. Patient 2 had numerous small, mildly FDG-avid lytic lesions scattered throughout the axial and appendicular skeleton, an SUV_{max} of 3.8. Patient 4 had innumerable large, very FDG-avid lesions with an SUV_{max} of 8.9. The PET/CT of patient 4 shows marked filling of the bone marrow spaces, especially in the appendicular skeleton. There is a wide spectrum of disease identified on PET/CT in MM patients.

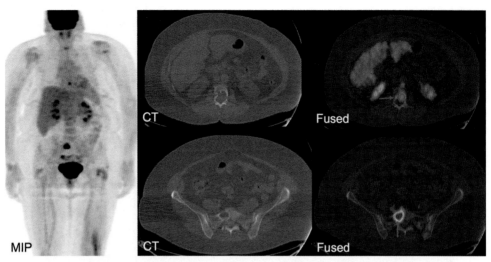

Fig. 13. This patient is a 69-year-old woman presenting for staging of MM. The PET/CT scan demonstrated numerous lytic lesions scattered throughout the axial and appendicular skeleton (*arrow*). The FDG uptake in the osseous lesions ranged from minimal to intense (SUV_{max} = 1.3–9.1). The patient underwent chemotherapy and transplantation.

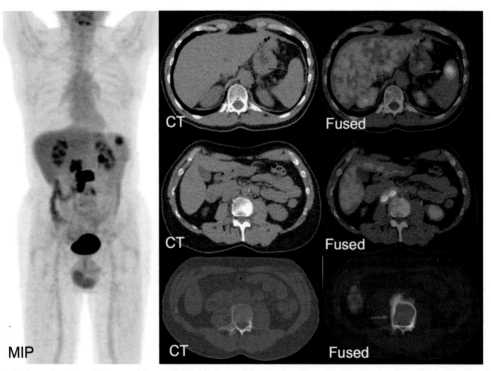

Fig. 14. This patient is a 51-year-old man who presented for evaluation of a biopsy-proven plasmacytoma in the vertebral body of L1. The PET/CT scan demonstrates intense FDG uptake (SUV_{max} = 13.3) in the L1 vertebrae (*arrow*-bottom images). There are mildly enlarged left retroperitoneal lymph nodes with moderate activity (*arrow*-middle images). There is also a single 2.4-cm FDG-avid focus in the spleen (*arrow*-top images). A CT-guided needle biopsy of the retroperitoneal nodes confirmed extramedullary MM. The patient was treated with chemotherapy and bone marrow transplantation.

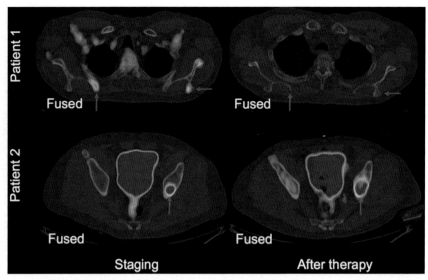

Fig. 15. These patients both had aggressive MM with cytogenic abnormalities, and received aggressive treatment in preparation for bone marrow transplantation. Each patient underwent a staging and then a follow-up PET/CT for the purpose of therapy assessment. The PET/CT scans for patient 1 showed a substantial decrease in FDG uptake within known lytic bone lesions (*arrows*). He was referred for bone marrow transplantation. PET/CT for patient 2 demonstrated increased size and activity of the bony lesions despite treatment (*arrow*). Patient 2 was placed on an experimental treatment protocol.

REFERENCES

1. Resnick DL. Skeletal metastases. In: Resnick DL, editor. Diagnosis of bone and joint disorders. 4th edition. Philadelphia: WB Saunders Co; 2002. p. 4274–351.
2. Roodman GD. Skeletal imaging and management of bone disease. Hematology Am Soc Hematol Educ Program 2008;1:313.
3. Miller TT. Bone tumors and tumorlike conditions: analysis with conventional radiography. Radiology 2008;246:662–74.
4. Patel SR, Zagars GK, Pisters PW. The follow-up of adult soft-tissue sarcomas. Semin Oncol 2003; 30(3):413–6.
5. Abdel-Dayem HM. The role of nuclear medicine in primary bone and soft tissue tumors. Semin Nucl Med 1997;27:355.
6. Gambhir SS. Molecular imaging of cancer with positron emission tomography. Nat Rev Cancer 2002;2:683.
7. Beyer T, Townsend DW, Blodgett TM. Dual-modality PET/CT tomography for clinical oncology. Q J Nucl Med 2002;46:24.
8. Bruzzi JF, Munden RF, Truong MT, et al. PET/CT of esophageal cancer: its role in clinical management. Radiographics 2007;27:1635–52.
9. Truong MT, Erasmus JJ, Macapinlac HA, et al. Integrated positron emission tomography/computed tomography in patients with non-small cell lung cancer: normal variants and pitfalls. J Comput Assist Tomogr 2005;29:205–9.
10. Gerth HU, Juergens KU, Dirksen U, et al. Significant benefit of multimodal imaging: PET/CT compared with PET alone in staging and follow-up of patients with Ewing tumors. J Nucl Med 2007;48(12):1932–9.
11. Kumar R, Chauhan A, Vellimana AK, et al. Role of PET/PET-CT in the management of sarcomas. Expert Rev Anticancer Ther 2006;6:1241.
12. Peterson JJ. F-18 FDG-PET for detection of osseous metastatic disease and staging, restaging, and monitoring response to therapy of musculoskeletal tumors. Semin Musculoskelet Radiol 2007;11:246–60.
13. Bastiannnet E, Groen H, Jager PL, et al. The value of FDG-PET in the detection, grading, and response to therapy of soft tissue and bone sarcomas; a systematic review and meta-analysis. Cancer Treat Rev 2004;30:83–101.
14. Siegel R, Naishadham D, Jemal A. Cancer statistics, 2012. CA Cancer J Clin 2012;62:10.
15. Smith MA, Gurney JG, Ries LA. Cancer in adolescents 15 to 19 years old. In: Ries LA, Smith MA, Gurney JG, et al, editors. Cancer incidence and survival among children and adolescents: United States SEER Program 1975-1995. Bethesda (MD): SEER program, National Cancer Institute; 1999 (Pub #99-4649).
16. Dorfman HD, Czerniak B. Bone cancers. Cancer 1995;75(Suppl 1):203–10.

17. Murphey MD, Robbin MR, Mcrae GA, et al. The many faces of osteosarcoma. Radiographics 1997;17(5):1205–31.

18. McKenna R, Schwinn C, Soong K, et al. Sarcomas of the osteogenic series (osteosarcoma, chondrosarcoma, parosteal osteogenic sarcoma, and sarcomata arising in abnormal bone): an analysis of 552 cases. J Bone Joint Surg Am 1966;48:1.

19. Heare T, Hensley MA, Dell'Orfano S. Bone tumors: osteosarcoma and Ewing's sarcoma. Curr Opin Pediatr 2009;21:365.

20. Bruland OS, Høifødt H, Saeter G, et al. Hematogenous micrometastases in osteosarcoma patients. Clin Cancer Res 2005;11:4666.

21. Federman N, Bernthal N, Eilber FC, et al. The multidisciplinary management of osteosarcoma. Curr Treat Options Oncol 2009;10(1–2):82–93.

22. Burchill SA. Ewing's sarcoma: diagnostic, prognostic, and therapeutic implications of molecular abnormalities. J Clin Pathol 2003;56(2):96–102.

23. Ludwig JA. Ewing sarcoma: historical perspectives, current state-of-the-art, and opportunities for targeted therapy in the future. Curr Opin Oncol 2008;20(4):412–8.

24. Granowetter L, Womer R, Devidas M, et al. Dose-intensified compared with standard chemotherapy for nonmetastatic Ewing sarcoma family of tumors: a Children's Oncology Group Study. J Clin Oncol 2009;27:2536.

25. Gatta G, Capocaccia R, Stiller C, et al. Childhood cancer survival trends in Europe: a EUROCARE Working Group study. J Clin Oncol 2005; 23:3742.

26. Cotterill SJ, Ahrens S, Paulussen M, et al. Prognostic factors in Ewing's tumor of bone: analysis of 975 patients from the European Intergroup Cooperative Ewing's Sarcoma Study Group. J Clin Oncol 2000;18:3108.

27. Bertoni F, Bacchini P, Hogendoorn PCW. Chondrosarcoma. In: Fletcher CD, Unni KK, Mertens F, editors. World Health Organization classification of tumours. Pathology and Genetics of Tumours of Soft Tissue and Bone. Lyon: IARC Press; 2002. p. 247–51.

28. Murphey MD, Walker EA, Wilson AJ, et al. From the archives of the AFIP: imaging of primary chondrosarcoma: radiologic-pathologic correlation. Radiographics 2003;23:1245.

29. Evans HL, Ayala AG, Romsdahl MM. Prognostic factors in chondrosarcoma of bone: a clinicopathologic analysis with emphasis on histologic grading. Cancer 1977;40:818.

30. Pring ME, Weber KL, Unni KK, et al. Chondrosarcoma of the pelvis. A review of sixty-four cases. J Bone Joint Surg Am 2001;83-A:1630.

31. Fiorenza F, Abudu A, Grimer RJ, et al. Risk factors for survival and local control in chondrosarcoma of bone. J Bone Joint Surg Br 2002;84:93.

32. Giuffrida AY, Burgueno JE, Koniaris LG, et al. Chondrosarcoma in the United States (1973 to 2003): an analysis of 2890 cases from the SEER database. J Bone Joint Surg Am 2009;91(5):1063–72.

33. Riedel RF, Larrier N, Dodd L, et al. The clinical management of chondrosarcoma. Curr Treat Options Oncol 2009;10(1–2):94–106.

34. Edge SB, Byrd DR, Compton CC, et al, editors. American Joint Committee on Cancer Staging manual. 7th edition. New York: Spring; 2010. p. 281.

35. Wolf RE, Enneking WF. The staging and surgery of musculoskeletal neoplasms. Orthop Clin North Am 1996;27(3):473–81.

36. Feldman F, Van HR, Saxena C, et al. [18]FDG-PET applications for cartilage neoplasms. Skeletal Radiol 2005;34(7):367–74.

37. Franzius C, Bielack S, Flege S, et al. Prognostic significance of (18)F-FDG and (99m)Tc-methylene diphosphonate uptake in primary osteosarcoma. J Nucl Med 2002;43(8):1012–7.

38. Franzius C, Sciuk J, Daldrup-Link HE, et al. FDG PET for detection of osseous metastases from malignant primary bone tumours: comparison with bone scintigraphy. Eur J Nucl Med 2000;27(9): 1305–11.

39. Brenner W, Conrad EU, Eary JF. FDG PET imaging for grading and prediction of outcome in chondrosarcoma patients. Eur J Nucl Med Mol Imaging 2004;31(2):189–95.

40. Lee FY, Yu J, Chang SS, et al. Diagnostic value and limitations of fluorine-18 fluorodeoxyglucose positron emission tomography for cartilaginous tumors of bone. J Bone Joint Surg Am 2004; 86(12):2677–85.

41. Franzius C, Daldrup-Link HE, Sciuk J, et al. FDG PET for detection of pulmonary metastases from malignant primary bone tumors: comparison with spiral CT. Ann Oncol 2001;12(4): 479–86.

42. McCarville MB, Christie R, Daw NC, et al. PET/CT in the evaluation of childhood sarcomas. AJR Am J Roentgenol 2005;184:1293.

43. Ioannidis JP, Lau J. ^{18}F-FDG PET for the diagnosis and grading of soft-tissue sarcoma: a meta-analysis. J Nucl Med 2003;44(5):717–24.

44. Zwaga T, Bovée JV, Kroon HM. Osteosarcoma of the femur with skip, lymph node, and lung metastases. Radiographics 2008;28(1):277–83.

45. Eary JF, O'Sullivan F, O'Sullivan J, et al. Spatial heterogeneity in sarcoma ^{18}F-FDG uptake as a predictor of patient outcome. J Nucl Med 2008;49(12): 1973–9.

46. O'Sullivan PJ, Rohren EM, Madewell JE. Positron emission tomography-CT imaging in guiding musculoskeletal biopsy. Radiol Clin North Am 2008;46(3):475–86.

47. Bestic JM, Peterson JJ, Bancroft LW. Use of FDG PET in staging, restaging, and assessment of therapy response in Ewing sarcoma. Radiographics 2009;29:1487–501.

48. Iagaru A, Chawla S, Menendez L, et al. ^{18}F-FDG PET and PET/CT for detection of pulmonary metastases from musculoskeletal sarcomas. Nucl Med Commun 2006;27(10):795–802.

49. Bredella MA, Caputo GR, Steinbach LS. Value of FDG positron emission tomography in conjunction with MR imaging for evaluating therapy response in patients with musculoskeletal sarcomas. AJR Am J Roentgenol 2002;179(5):1145–50.

50. Costelloe CM, Macapinlac HA, Madewell JE, et al. ^{18}F-FDG PET/CT as an indicator of progression-free and overall survival in osteosarcoma. J Nucl Med 2009;50(3):340–7.

51. Hamada K, Tomita Y, Inoue A, et al. Evaluation of chemotherapy response in osteosarcoma with FDG-PET. Ann Nucl Med 2009;23(1):89–95.

52. Hawkins DS, Rajendran JG, Conrad U, et al. Evaluation of chemotherapy response in pediatric bone sarcomas by [F-18]-fluorodeoxy-D-glucose positron emission tomography. Cancer 2002;94:3277–84.

53. Hawkins DS, Schuetze SM, Butrynski JE, et al. [F-18]-fluorodeoxy-D-glucose positron emission tomography predicts outcome for Ewing sarcoma family of tumors. J Clin Oncol 2005;23:8828–34.

54. Hawkins DS, Conrad EU, Butrynski JE, et al. [F-18]-fluorodeoxy-D-glucose positron emission tomography response is associated with outcome for extremity osteosarcoma in children and young adults. Cancer 2009;115:3519–25.

55. Schulte M, Brecht-Krauss D, Werner M, et al. Evaluation of neoadjuvant therapy response of osteogenic sarcoma using FDG PET. J Nucl Med 1999;40:1637–43.

56. Ye Z, Zhu J, Tian M, et al. Response of osteogenic sarcoma to neoadjuvant therapy: evaluated by ^{18}F-FDG-PET. Ann Nucl Med 2008;22:475–80.

57. Cheon GJ, Kim MS, Lee JA, et al. Prediction model of chemotherapy response in osteosarcoma by ^{18}F-FDG PET and MRI. J Nucl Med 2009;50(9):1435–40.

58. Dimitrakopoulou-Strauss A, Strauss LG, Heichel T, et al. The role of quantitative (18)F-FDG PET studies for the differentiation of malignant and benign bone lesions. J Nucl Med 2002;43(4):510–8.

59. Hamada K, Tomita Y, Konishi E, et al. FDG-PET evaluation of chondromyxoid fibroma of left ilium. Clin Nucl Med 2009;34(1):15–7.

60. Mundy GR. Metastasis to bone: causes, consequences and therapeutic opportunities. Nat Rev Cancer 2002;2:584.

61. Yin JJ, Pollock CB, Kelly K. Mechanisms of cancer metastasis to the bone. Cell Res 2005;15:57.

62. Salmon JM, Kilpatrick SE. Pathology of skeletal metastases. Orthop Clin North Am 2000;31:537–44.

63. Even-Sapir E. Imaging of malignant bone involvement by morphologic, scintigraphic, and hybrid modalities. J Nucl Med 2005;46(8):1356–67.

64. Hamaoka T, Madewell JE, Podoloff DA, et al. Bone imaging in metastatic breast cancer. J Clin Oncol 2004;22(14):2942–53.

65. Rybak LD, Rosenthal DI. Radiological imaging for the diagnosis of bone metastases. Q J Nucl Med 2001;45(1):53–64.

66. Coleman RE. Metastatic bone disease: clinical features, pathophysiology and treatment strategies. Cancer Treat Rev 2001;27:165.

67. Nielsen OS, Munro AJ, Tannock IF. Bone metastases: pathophysiology and management policy. J Clin Oncol 1991;9(3):509–24.

68. Coleman RE, Rubens RD. The clinical course of bone metastases from breast cancer. Br J Cancer 1987;55:61.

69. Uematsu T, Yuen S, Yukisawa S, et al. Comparison of FDG PET and SPECT for detection of bone metastases in breast cancer. AJR Am J Roentgenol 2005;184:1266–73.

70. Even-Sapir E, Metser U, Mishani E, et al. The detection of bone metastases in patients with high-risk prostate cancer: ^{99m}Tc-MDP planar bone scintigraphy, single- and multi-field-of-view SPECT, ^{18}F-fluoride PET, and ^{18}F-fluoride PET/CT. J Nucl Med 2006;47:287–97.

71. Yoon KT, Kim JK, Kim do Y, et al. Role of ^{18}F-fluorodeoxyglucose positron emission tomography in detecting extrahepatic metastasis in pretreatment staging of hepatocellular carcinoma. Oncology 2007;72(Suppl 1):104–10.

72. Ng SH, Chan SC, Yen TC, et al. Staging of untreated nasopharyngeal carcinoma with PET/CT: comparison with conventional imaging work-up. Eur J Nucl Med Mol Imaging 2009;36:12–22.

73. Cook GJ, Houston S, Rubens R, et al. Detection of bone metastases in breast cancer by [18]FDG PET: differing metabolic activity in osteoblastic and osteolytic lesions. J Clin Oncol 1998;16:3375–9.

74. Chang MC, Chen JH, Liang JA, et al. Meta-analysis comparison of F-18 fluorodeoxyglucose-positron emission tomography and bone scintigraphy in the detection of bone metastasis in patients with lung cancer. Acad Radiol 2012;19(3):349–57.

75. Fogelman I, Cook G, Israel O, et al. Positron emission tomography and bone metastases. Semin Nucl Med 2005;35:135–42.

76. Weber WA. Assessing tumor response to therapy. J Nucl Med 2009;50(Suppl 1):1S–10S.

77. Tateishi U, Gamez C, Dawood S, et al. Bone metastases in patients with metastatic breast cancer: morphologic and metabolic monitoring of response

to systemic therapy with integrated PET/CT. Radiology 2008;247:189–96.

78. Specht JM, Tam SL, Kurland BF, et al. Serial 2-[18F] fluoro-2-deoxy-D-glucose positron emission tomography (FDG-PET) to monitor treatment of bone-dominant metastatic breast cancer predicts time to progression (TTP). Breast Cancer Res Treat 2007;105:87–94.

79. Du Y, Cullum I, Illidge TM, et al. Fusion of metabolic function and morphology: sequential [18F]fluorodeoxyglucose positron-emission tomography/computed tomography studies yield new insights into the natural history of bone metastases in breast cancer. J Clin Oncol 2007;25:3440–7.

80. Kyle RA, Therneau TM, Rajkumar SV, et al. Incidence of multiple myeloma in Olmsted County, Minnesota: Trend over 6 decades. Cancer 2004; 101:2667.

81. Kyle RA, Gertz MA, Witzig TE, et al. Review of 1027 patients with newly diagnosed multiple myeloma. Mayo Clin Proc 2003;78:21.

82. Turesson I, Velez R, Kristinsson SY, et al. Patterns of multiple myeloma during the past 5 decades: stable incidence rates for all age groups in the population but rapidly changing age distribution in the clinic. Mayo Clin Proc 2010;85:225.

83. Kumar SK, Dingli D, Lacy MQ, et al. Autologous stem cell transplantation in patients of 70 years and older with multiple myeloma: results from a matched pair analysis. Am J Hematol 2008; 83:614.

84. Barlogie B, Kyle RA, Anderson KC, et al. Standard chemotherapy compared with high-dose chemoradiotherapy for multiple myeloma: final results of phase III US Intergroup Trial S9321. J Clin Oncol 2006;24:929.

85. Warsame R, Gertz MA, Lacy MQ, et al. Trends and outcomes of modern staging of solitary plasmacytoma of bone. Am J Hematol 2012;87(7):647–51.

86. Kyle RA, Greipp PR. Smoldering multiple myeloma. N Engl J Med 1980;302:1347.

87. Kyle RA, Remstein ED, Therneau TM, et al. Clinical course and prognosis of smoldering (asymptomatic) multiple myeloma. N Engl J Med 2007;356: 2582.

88. Kyle RA, Therneau TM, Rajkumar SV, et al. Long-term follow-up of 241 patients with monoclonal gammopathy of undetermined significance: the original Mayo Clinic series 25 years later. Mayo Clin Proc 2004;79:859.

89. Kyle RA, Therneau TM, Rajkumar SV, et al. A long-term study of prognosis in monoclonal gammopathy of undetermined significance. N Engl J Med 2002;346:564.

90. Greipp PR, San Miguel J, Durie BG, et al. International staging system for multiple myeloma. J Clin Oncol 2005;23:3412.

91. Durie BG, Salmon SE. A clinical staging system for multiple myeloma. Correlation of measured myeloma cell mass with presenting clinical features, response to treatment, and survival. Cancer 1975;36:842.

92. Dispenzieri A, Rajkumar SV, Gertz MA, et al. Treatment of newly diagnosed multiple myeloma based on Mayo Stratification of Myeloma and Risk-adapted Therapy (mSMART): consensus statement. Mayo Clin Proc 2007;82:323.

93. Durie BG. The role of anatomic and functional staging in myeloma: description of Durie/Salmon plus staging system. Eur J Cancer 2006;42:1539–43.

94. Nanni C, Zamagni E, Farsad M, et al. Role of 18F-FDG PET/CT in the assessment of bone involvement in newly diagnosed multiple myeloma: preliminary results. Eur J Nucl Med Mol Imaging 2006;33:525–31.

95. Fonti R, Salvatore B, Quarantelli M, et al. 18F-FDG PET/CT, 99mTc-MIBI, and MRI in evaluation of patients with multiple myeloma. J Nucl Med 2008; 49:195–200.

96. Zamagni E, Nanni C, Patriarca F, et al. A prospective comparison of 18F-fluorodeoxyglucose positron emission tomography-computed tomography, magnetic resonance imaging and whole-body planar radiographs in the assessment of bone disease in newly diagnosed multiple myeloma. Haematologica 2007;92:50–5.

97. Tan E, Weiss BM, Mena E, et al. Current and future imaging modalities for multiple myeloma and its precursor states. Leuk Lymphoma 2011;52(9): 1630–40.

98. Mulligan ME, Badros AZ. PET/CT and MR imaging in myeloma. Skeletal Radiol 2007;36(1):5–16.

99. Mulligan ME. Imaging techniques used in the diagnosis, staging, and follow-up of patients with myeloma. Acta Radiol 2005;46(7):716–24.

100. Durie BG, Waxman AD, D'Agnolo A, et al. Whole-body (18)F-FDG PET identifies high-risk myeloma. J Nucl Med 2002;43(11):1457–63.

101. Kim PJ, Hicks RJ, Wirth A, et al. Impact of 18F-fluorodeoxyglucose positron emission tomography before and after definitive radiation therapy in patients with apparently solitary plasmacytoma. Int J Radiat Oncol Biol Phys 2009;74(3): 740–6.

102. Schirrmeister H, Buck AK, Bergmann L, et al. Positron emission tomography (PET) for staging of solitary plasmacytoma. Cancer Biother Radiopharm 2003;18(5):841–5.

103. Hur J, Yoon CS, Ryu YH, et al. Efficacy of multidetector row computed tomography of the spine in patients with multiple myeloma: comparison with magnetic resonance imaging and fluorodeoxyglucose-positron emission tomography. J Comput Assist Tomogr 2007;31:342–7.

104. Hall MN, Jagannathan JP, Ramaiya NH, et al. Imaging of extraosseous myeloma: CT, PET/CT, and MRI features. AJR Am J Roentgenol 2010;195(5):1057–65.

105. Varettoni M, Corso A, Pica G, et al. Incidence, presenting features and outcome of extraosseous disease in multiple myeloma: a longitudinal study on 1003 consecutive patients. Ann Oncol 2010;21: 325–30.

106. Bartel TB, Haessler J, Brown TL, et al. ^{18}F-fluorodeoxyglucose positron emission tomography in the context of other imaging techniques and prognostic factors in multiple myeloma. Blood 2009; 114:2068–76.

107. Dimitrakopoulou-Strauss A, Hoffmann M, Bergner R, et al. Prediction of progression-free survival in patients with multiple myeloma following anthracycline-based chemotherapy based on dynamic FDG-PET. Clin Nucl Med 2009;34:576–84.

108. Zamagni F, Patriarca C, Nanni C, et al. Prognostic relevance of 18-F FDG PET/CT in newly diagnosed multiple myeloma patients treated with upfront autologous transplantation. Blood 2011;118: 5989–95.

109. Zamagni E, Cavo M. The role of imaging techniques in the management of multiple myeloma. Br J Haematol 2012;159(5):499–513. http://dx.doi.org/10.1111/bjh.12007.

110. van Lammeren-Venema D, Regelink JC, Riphagen II, et al. ^{18}F-fluoro-deoxyglucose positron emission tomography in assessment of myeloma-related bone disease: a systematic review. Cancer 2012;118(8):1971–81.

Positron Emission Tomography/ Computed Tomography in Melanoma

Austin C. Bourgeois, MD, Ted T. Chang, MD,
Lindsay M. Fish, MD, Yong C. Bradley, MD*

KEYWORDS

- Melanoma • PET • CT • Cutaneous melanoma

KEY POINTS

- Fludeoxyglucose–positron emission tomography/computed tomography (PET/CT) has poor sensitivity for regional lymph node metastasis and not a suitable alternative to sentinel lymph node biopsy.
- PET/CT is most sensitive in detecting macrometastatic disease or distant metastatic disease and as a surgical planning tool.
- Dedicated interpretation of coregistered CT increases PET/CT sensitivity.

INTRODUCTION

Malignant melanoma is the sixth most common cause of cancer, responsible for 4.5% of malignancies and 1.5% of cancer-related deaths in the United States. It represents the fifth and sixth most common malignancies affecting men and women, respectively.[1] The National Institutes of Health estimates 76,250 new diagnoses of cutaneous melanoma (CM) with 9180 deaths in the United States in 2012. CM accounts for only 5% of skin cancers but represents more than 50% of skin cancer–related deaths.[2] Although its incidence is highest in the elderly population, melanoma causes disproportional mortality in young and middle-aged individuals.[1,3,4]

Alarmingly, the age-adjusted incidence of melanoma has continued to increase since the mid-1960s at a rate of 3% to 8% per year.[1,3,5,6] Melanoma now represents the fastest growing malignancy to affect men and the second fastest growing malignancy to affect women, second only to primary lung neoplasms.[2] The cause of this increased incidence remains incompletely explored, although the trends of increased sunlight exposure and increased screening vigilance have been implicated.[5] Progressive advances in melanoma therapy, clinical screening, and imaging have provided steadily improved 5-year survival, which now tops 75% for all demographics.[7]

Several factors affect the survival of patients with melanoma. Current literature suggests that the most important of these is thorough clinical screening, which allows for the early detection of CM at a stage when surgical cure may be readily achieved.[6] Thorough history and physical examination have proven to play a critical role in follow-up surveillance.[2,8,9]

The use of imaging in appropriate high-risk patients offers an indispensible adjunct to clinical, pathologic, and surgical staging. The current literature examines the role of computed tomography (CT), magnetic resonance (MR) imaging, ultrasound, positron emission tomography (PET), and PET/CT.[10] Although no consensus guidelines have set forth the proper utilization of these various imaging modalities, PET/CT plays a prominent role in melanoma imaging.

This article aims to examine the utilization of PET/CT in the staging, prognostication,

University of Tennessee Medical Center, 1924 Alcoa Highway, Knoxville, TN 37920, USA
* Corresponding author.
E-mail address: YBradley@mc.utmck.edu

Radiol Clin N Am 51 (2013) 865–879
http://dx.doi.org/10.1016/j.rcl.2013.06.004
0033-8389/13/$ – see front matter © 2013 Elsevier Inc. All rights reserved.

and follow-up of melanoma while providing the physicians who order and interpret these studies practical guidelines and interpretive pitfalls.

CM STAGING

The American Joint Committee on Cancer (AJCC) provides a staging system for CM incorporating clinical and pathologic criteria (**Table 1**).[6] By

Table 1
Clinical staging of melanoma

Primary Tumor

TX	Primary tumor cannot be assessed (regression, curettage)	
T0	No evidence of primary tumor	
Tis	Melanoma in situ	
T1	Melanomas ≤1.0 mm in thickness	a. W/o ulceration and mitosis <1/mm^2 b. With ulceration or mitosis ≥1/mm^2
T2	Melanomas 1.01–2.0 mm	a. W/o ulceration b. With ulceration
T3	Melanomas 2.01–4.0 mm	a. W/o ulceration b. With ulceration
T4	Melanomas >4.0 mm	a. W/o ulceration b. With ulceration

Regional Lymph Nodes

NX	Regional nodes cannot be assessed (previously removed for other reason)	
N0	No regional nodes detected	
N1	1 node	a. Micrometastasis b. Macrometastasis
N2	2–3 nodes	a. Micrometastasis b. Macrometastasis c. In transit mets/satellites *without* metastatic nodes
N3	≥4 nodes	Or matted nodes or in transit mets/satellites *with* metastatic nodes

Distant Metastasis

		Serum LDH
M0	No detectable evidence of any distant metastases	Normal
M1a	Metastases to skin, subcutaneous, or distant lymph nodes	Normal
M1b	Metastases to lung	Normal
M1c	Metastases to all other visceral sites	Elevated

Clinical Staging of Melanoma

Stage 0	Tis	N0	M0
Stage IA	T1a	N0	M0
Stage IB	T1b	N0	M0
	T2a	N0	M0
Stage IIA	T2b	N0	M0
	T3a	N0	M0
Stage IIB	T3b	N0	M0
	T4a	N0	M0
Stage IIC	T4b	N0	M0
Stage III	Any T	≥N1	M0
Stage IV	Any T	Any N	M1

Abbreviations: M, distant metastasis; N, regional lymph nodes; T, primary tumor; W/o, without.
   Used with the permission of the American Joint Committee on Cancer (AJCC), Chicago, Illinois. The original source for this material is the AJCC Cancer Staging Manual, Seventh Edition (2010) published by Springer-Verlag New York, www.springer.com.

convention, staging is performed after surgical primary tumor excision and includes clinical, radiological, and pathologic factors.[6] Five factors most significantly impact staging criteria: (1) primary tumor thickness, (2) primary tumor ulceration, (3) presence of regional or satellite metastasis, (4) presence of distant metastasis, and (5) serum lactate dehydrogenase (LDH) levels.[11] Several other factors have shown prognostic significance but are not included in the AJCC's most recent staging criteria: radial and vertical growth phases, regression, angiolymphatic invasion, angiotropism, perineural invasion, and tumor-infiltrating lymphocytes.[12,13]

Stage I disease includes low-risk primaries that are 2 mm or less in thickness that are without ulceration, invasive features, or evidence of metastasis.[11] Primary tumor thickness is of critical importance (regardless of stage) and is the single best predictor of overall survival.

Stage II disease refers to high-risk primary tumors without evidence of regional or distant metastasis. This stage includes ulcerated tumors from 1 to 2 mm in thickness and other primary tumors with and without ulceration that are 2 mm or more in thickness.[11] Overall, localized disease carries a favorable prognosis, with approximately 98% expected 5-year survival.

Stage III disease conventionally refers to histologically confirmed satellite metastasis and/or metastatic involvement of the regional lymph node basin.[11] Patients with clinical evidence of regional lymph node metastasis who have not yet undergone lymph node dissection are referred to as clinical stage III disease and are not assigned a staging subtype. Factors affecting stage III subtype designation include the following: number of affected lymph nodes, presence or absence of primary tumor ulceration, satellite or in-transit metastasis, and macroscopic or microscopic lymph node involvement. Primary tumor ulceration remains an independent negative prognostic factor, even in the presence of regional metastatic disease. The presence of regional metastatic disease denotes a considerable decrease in 5-year survival, which is approximately 62%.[1]

Stage IV disease refers to the presence of distant metastasis and is subcategorized based on the 3 major sites of metastasis: (1) distant skin, lymph nodes, or subcutaneous tissues; (2) lung metastasis; and (3) other visceral metastasis.[11] An elevated serum LDH in the presence of any distant metastatic disease denotes more advanced disease and suggests a less favorable prognosis.[12] Despite the continued evolution in melanoma therapy, the life expectancy for patients with distant melanoma metastasis remains low, with overall 5-year survival of 15%.[1] Of note, the African American population, which demonstrates below-average survival for stage I to III disease, has an estimated 5-year survival that is nearly double (29%) that of the overall population.[1]

TUMOR MARKERS

Although considerable advancements have been made in melanoma detection and imaging, treatment of advanced disease remains limited by a relative lack of effective systemic therapies. Thus, the desire to decrease melanoma mortality and morbidity has emphasized the study of tumor markers, which hope to improve detection, prognostic considerations, and the monitoring of the treatment response. Several serum tumor markers have been studied, including LDH, S-100B; melanoma-inhibiting activity (MIA); vascular endothelial growth factor (VEGF); and various interleukins (IL), including IL-6 and IL-10.[12,14]

LDH is the most widely adopted melanoma tumor marker and serves as an indirect marker of melanoma cellular ischemia from outgrowing its blood supply.[12] It is the only serum marker formally included in the AJCC's staging guidelines. LDH serves as a strong independent prognostic factor and has proven to be effective in monitoring the treatment response to systemic chemotherapy.[12]

S-100B is a widely distributed protein that directly interacts with the p-53 tumor suppressor gene. Numerous investigators have suggested a role for S-100B as an inexpensive, convenient surveillance tool.[10,12] However, several studies have failed to prove the efficacy of S-100B in melanoma screening.[10,12,15–17] A study published by Strobel and colleagues showed that of the 41 patients studied, S-100B was unsuitable in 15 (37%) patients because baseline and posttreatment values remained normal. In comparison, PET/CT was suitable for all 41 studied patients, and prognosis by S-100B values in the remaining 26 patients showed concordance with semiquantitative PET/CT findings. A later study by Strobel and colleagues[18] showed superiority of PET/CT and CT over S-100B values at following stage IV melanoma response (Table 2). Aukema and colleagues[10] only found positive S-100B values to have a 50% positive predictive value in a study following 46 asymptomatic patients with elevated S-100B values.

Additional serum tumor markers, such as IL-6, show preliminary efficacy in predicting survival; but these findings have yet to be corroborated over a larger patient subset.[14] A detailed discussion of additional serum tumor markers and their clinical application is outside of the scope of this article; however, they are likely to play an

Table 2
Circulating serologic and molecular markers in malignant melanoma

Marker	Role	Significance
LDH	Staging, prognosis	Poor prognosis and response to treatment
S-100B proteins	Diagnosis (tissue), prognosis (serum)	Confirmation of diagnosis, nonspecific
MIA	Prognosis	Poor prognosis and response to treatment
VEGF	Prognosis	Equivocal
BRAF V600E gene mutation	Prognosis, treatment	Negative prognostic factor, therapeutic target

increasing role in the ordering and interpretation of imaging studies in the future.

APPROACH TO INITIAL WORK-UP

In December 2011, the National Comprehensive Cancer Network (NCCN) updated guidelines for staging and follow-up of patients with melanoma. Although these current guidelines stop short of asserting stage-specific imaging policies, they are based on the principle that melanoma staging generally influences the utility of imaging studies. Clinical work-up usually begins with the biopsy of a suspicious pigmented cutaneous lesion and a focused history and physical with attention to locoregional areas (NCCN).

The mainstay of melanoma staging is wide surgical excision of the primary lesion for pathologic analysis and sentinel lymph node (SLN) biopsy. SLN biopsy carries a relatively low risk of morbidity and is considered the standard of care under the AJCC's current guidelines. There are no current high-level data showing an overall survival benefit for those undergoing SLN biopsy; however, it remains the most highly sensitive and specific nodal staging test available.[19–21] Multiple studies have verified that SLN node sampling using dye and radiotracer accurately identifies the SLN and that SLNs are the first lymph nodes to contain metastasis.[2] SLN sampling performed in this fashion has a reported false-negative rate of less than 4% and a negative predicted value of 99%.[19,20] Subsequent complete lymph node dissection may be considered depending on the SLN status (NCCN); see **Fig. 1**.

Imaging with PET and PET/CT has been demonstrated to add little clinically relevant information in stage I and II disease and provides a high false-positive rate.[21–24] In a study by Crippa and colleagues,[25] 38 patients with stage III disease had an evaluation of a total of 56 lymph node basins by both lymph node dissection and fludeoxyglucose (FDG)-PET. PET had a sensitivity of 95% and specificity of 84% for detecting nodal

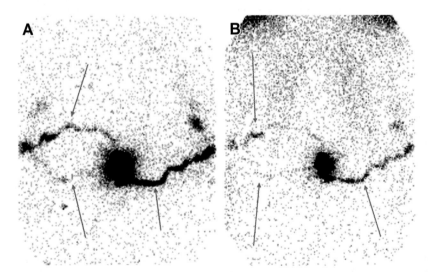

Fig. 1. Melanoma lymphoscintigraphies. (*A*, *B*) Lymphoscintigraphy of the same patient with and without a transmission source. Injection of Tc99m SCOL just left of the midline with 2 different lymphatic drainage pathway. Tc99m SCOL injections centrally with 3 different drainage pathways complicating surgeries. This illustrates the importance of lymphoscintigraphies before surgeries in patients with melanoma.

metastasis. The investigators also compared these PET findings with 114 lymph nodes with histologic evidence of metastasis and found that PET sensitivity is highly correlated with lymph node size. PET detected all metastatic nodes that were greater than 10 mm, 83% of lymph nodes greater than 5 mm, and 23% of nodes less than 5 mm in diameter.[25] Veit-Haibach and colleagues[26] compared PET, CT, and PET/CT findings in 56 patients using histopathology and follow-up as a reference and found that the sensitivity for evaluating lymph node metastasis was less than 50% for each imaging modality. Another study by Singh and colleagues[27] examined 52 patients with stage I or stage II melanoma and concluded that FDG-PET/CT provided a sensitivity for malignant lymph node detection of only 14.3%, far inferior to SLN biopsy (100%). Therefore, PET and PET/CT are of low relative sensitivity in evaluating microscopic regional metastasis, and SLN biopsy may be more appropriate in the evaluation of patients without clinical evidence of nodal metastasis.[21,23,28–31]

FDG-PET/CT offers a range of clinical benefits for patients with palpable regional lymphadenopathy (clinical stage III), macroscopic lymph nodal metastasis (stage IIIB), and those with evident or suspected distant metastasis (stage IV). A retrospective study of 106 patients by Iagaru and colleagues[22] showed sensitivity and specificity of 100% and 83.3%, respectively, in patients with stage IIIC and IV disease, leading to treatment changes in 4 of 30 patients because of unexpected metastatic disease. A study by Aukema and colleagues[32] used PET/CT to examine 70 patients with palpable regional lymphadenopathy and determined 87% sensitivity and 98% specificity for detecting metastasis.

The ability of PET/CT to change the management in patients with stage III disease has been corroborated in several additional studies, with reported rates as high as 49% (Gulec), with averages rates in the 10% to 19% range.[33,34] In addition to preoperative planning for stage III patients, PET/CT also aids prognostic considerations in patients with distant metastasis.[28] Although stage IV melanoma is associated with a dismal prognosis, resection of all radiologically and clinically apparent disease is associated with a survival benefit.[6] Disease localization is also of importance because metastasis to the skin carries a more favorable prognosis to visceral metastasis.[6] For these reasons, PET/CT plays an increasingly prominent role in melanoma work-up and staging.

CT and MR imaging have also proven diagnostic utility in the evaluation of melanoma. MR imaging is often used to address specific clinical questions and helps to delineate the anatomic relationship between the tumor and surrounding tissue. MR imaging is also the modality of choice and has documented superiority to PET/CT in evaluating lesions in the liver and brain, where background metabolic activity is a limiting factor.[2] It should be noted that brain MR imaging has little proven utility in asymptomatic patients and, therefore, is not relied on as a screening tool.[2]

In contrast, CT alone is not as accurate as combined PET/CT and has a very high false-positive rate. One study examining 347 patients with clinical stage III disease showed that CT identified twice as many false-positive findings than metastasis.[35] Relative to CT and PET alone, integrated PET/CT offers a significant benefit in characterizing and localizing lesions.[15] Strobel and colleagues[17] also demonstrated that dedicated imaging review of the coregistered CT images significantly improves the accuracy of PET/CT (instead of using CT for attenuation correction purposes alone) by detecting non–metabolically active metastasis. This finding is of particular importance in the evaluation of pulmonary lesions whereby respiration artifact decreases PET accuracy.

THE ROLE OF PET/CT IN RESTAGING

Once patients have undergone initial clinical and surgical staging, longitudinal follow-up involves a multidisciplinary approach based on clinical and imaging findings. Currently no consensus guidelines exist to dictate routine follow-up with PET/CT, although close clinical observation is recommended (NCCN). A study from the Yale Melanoma Unit of 373 patients showed a survival benefit of patients who were asymptomatic at the time of recurrence, suggesting that disease outcomes can be influenced by early detection.[2] Although utilization of PET/CT as a surveillance tool remains incompletely explored, it may have a role in the follow-up of high-risk patients. In one study, 34 patients with stage III melanoma were followed at least annually with PET/CT, which detected 6 of 7 recurrence and 2 cosynchronous metastasis.[12] The only undetected recurrence in this study was a clinically evident local recurrence, perhaps obscured by regional postsurgical changes.[35] However, the utility of PET/CT as a standard of care requires further confirmation; this application currently remains largely institution specific.

In patients with clinical evidence of recurrence, PET/CT has been shown to influence treatment planning, particularly in those patients with locoregional recurrence or suspected distant metastasis. Camargo and colleagues[35] illustrated this in a review of 78 patients with other evidence of recurrence and concluded that 27% of management plans were changed following PET/CT.[30,36] Upstaging (22%) from stage III to stage IV disease was the most common cause of changes to management, and PET showed a 95% sensitivity for detecting metastatic lesions. Even in patients with distant recurrence, information provided by PET/CT led to a change in the overall management of approximately 30% regarding planned surgical, radiotherapy, or chemotherapy. Restaging based on false-positive findings remains a concern for this application. False positives have proven most prevalent in patients with suspected local recurrence only, which suggests a higher interpretative threshold may be warranted in this subset.[37]

In addition to the initial staging and management of recurrence, the information provided by PET/CT plays an important role in several other aspects of management. It has been reported that PET/CT data lead to alteration of the radiation field for up to 60% of patients undergoing radiation.[37] The metabolic activity information provided by PET also allows for noninvasive treatment response. This information has been used in the process of tailoring treatment strategies and aids the development of potential melanoma therapies.[37] However, the utilization of PET/CT for these applications has not been proven to be cost-effective; whereas is likely cost-effective when used for surgical planning in addition to its documented clinical benefit.[37]

PET/CT TECHNIQUE

Most 18F-FDG–PET/CT oncology protocols image from the skull base to the midfemur. Because melanoma has the potential to metastasize in a relatively unpredictable fashion to virtually anywhere in the body, whole-body PET/CT may be used to characterize the usually excluded lower extremities and skull. Full-body PET/CT extends the scan by 6 to 7 positions, which nearly doubles emission scanning time and limits scanner throughput; although transmission scanning times are negligible with the use of PET/CT, the radiation dose to patients is increased as a result of the increased field of view.[38] Niederkohr and colleagues[39] examined the added benefit of including the skull and extremities in PET/CT for melanoma in 296 patients. In none of these cases were unexpected isolated metastasis detected in the skull or lower extremity. The investigators concluded that imaging the skull and lower extremities provides little clinical benefit but did suggest that PET/CT may be useful in 3 categories of patients: (1) primary melanoma in the head and neck or lower extremities, (2) clinical suspicion of widespread or aggressive disease, and (3) known or suspected head and

neck or lower extremity metastasis. Querellou and colleagues[40] corroborated these findings with a study of 122 patients without known involvement of the lower extremities. In their study, only 28 patients were found to have metastatic foci; of these 28, only 5 had abnormal findings in the lower extremities that were found to be equivocal or suggestive of metastatic involvement. These lower extremity findings were, on further clinical follow-up, found to represent benign processes unrelated to melanoma, thus representing false positives in regard to the lower extremities.

The decision to use intravenous and oral contrast in routine PET/CT protocol for melanoma directly affects the burden of time placed on patients and the safety profile of the study. Although contrast administration aims to increase imaging accuracy, its role in melanoma remains controversial. A study by Pfluger and colleagues[41] examined 50 patients with non–contrast-enhanced CT (NECT) and subsequent intravenous (IV) contrast-enhanced CT (CECT). The investigators concluded that CECT offers greater sensitivity of 97% compared with 90% with NECT. However, in none of these cases did additional sensitivity of CECT change staging or affect clinical management. Oral contrast, on the other hand, is commonly used in PET/CT but is reported to cause standardized uptake value (SUV) overestimation of up to 125%.[41] However, subsequent studies suggest that oral contrast introduces only a small, clinically insignificant effect.[42,43] Interpreting physicians should be aware of these concerns and interpret studies with oral contrast based on CT findings and nonattenuation corrected images when indicated. An alternative is the use of low-density neutral oral contrast agents. A study by Otero and colleagues[44] showed that its use caused no effect on the attenuation correction images and improved visualization of bowel structures.

Elevated serum insulin levels and blood can impair the accuracy of PET/CT. Elevated blood glucose competes with FDG and limits cellular uptake. Insulin, whether administered exogenously or intrinsically produced by patients, promotes preferential FDG deposition in insulin-sensitive tissues. Both of these factors can limit the relative tumor uptake of FDG, impairing PET/CT sensitivity and providing inconsistent comparison examinations.[42]

APPROACH TO PET/CT INTERPRETATION

It is well known that metastatic melanoma generally displays increased glucose metabolism that is readily identified with 18F-FDG–PET/CT, with a reported sensitivity and specificity of 92% and

90%.[45] One potential pitfall to PET/CT interpretation is the lack of standardized interpretation criteria.[39] Most interpreting physicians identify malignant lesions as a focal area with a relative increase in FDG avidity. However, a variety of technique and patient factors affect background metabolic physiology and study interpretation. Therefore, differing standards of interpretation by readers of PET/CT can lead to varying degrees of diagnostic accuracy. For example, a study by Falk and colleagues[36] explored high-threshold versus low-threshold PET/CT interpretations in patients with CM undergoing imaging for surveillance, staging, and restaging. In their retrospective study of 76 patients, they found that the inclusion of equivocal findings on PET/CT did not increase sensitivity for distant metastatic disease and only resulted in decreased diagnostic accuracy.

A focused discussion of factors influencing melanoma PET/CT interpretation is included in this section, using an organ-based approach.

Head and Neck

Brain
Background cerebral metabolic activity limits PET/CT evaluation for brain metastasis. A study by Rohren and colleagues[46] showed only 75% sensitivity and 83% specificity for the detection of cerebral metastases when comparing FDG-PET with MR imaging in a retrospective study of 40 patients. A later study by Kitajima and colleagues[47] compared FDG-PET, CT, and FDG-PET/CT and showed poor sensitivity for cerebral metastases 13%, 20%, and 20%, respectively, when compared with contrast-enhanced MR imaging. Therefore, brain MR imaging has remained the gold standard in evaluating cerebral melanoma metastasis.[2] The rate of cerebral metastases ranks only behind lung and breast cancer, and some studies have shown up to 10% involvement in stage IV patients.[48] The paramagnetic properties of melanin result in a characteristic intermediate or high MR imaging T1 signal. An enhancing cerebral or scalp lesion with these MR imaging features should be considered suspicious for melanoma metastasis. Although routine surveillance with brain MR imaging rarely affects management, the presence of brain metastasis carries a poor prognosis; see **Fig. 2**.

Uvea
Primary uveal melanoma is the most common primary intraocular tumor in adults.[49] Because its location precludes early detection, it has a high rate of stage IV metastatic disease when diagnosed (up to 50%).[50] Treatment options include surgical enucleation, brachytherapy, proton

therapy, and gamma knife; the median survival ranges from 2 to 9 months.[51] Because uveal melanoma has an unusually high incidence of hepatic metastasis at diagnosis, dedicated hepatic imaging may be warranted.[52] PET/CT has been proven to be both highly sensitive and specific in staging patients with uveal metastasis. PET/CT has also shown efficacy in diagnosis evaluating patients with metastasis to the uvea, lessening the need for uveal biopsy.[53]

Cervical lymphatics
Cervical lymphatic draining is notoriously unpredictable, making the identification of the true SLN particularly challenging (**Fig. 3**).[54] Close evaluation of all cervical lymph nodes should be performed in the setting of primary head and neck melanoma, with close attention paid to morphologic and metabolic abnormalities.

Cervical musculature/hybridoma
FDG uptake within skeletal muscle is variable and depends on patient and technique factors. Voluntary and subconscious muscle contractions during the FDG uptake phase may increase the apparent metabolic activity, limiting the study accuracy.[42] Anxiety is a known precipitant of these findings, which generally manifests as a symmetric paravertebral increase in paravertebral muscle activity. Imaging is especially treacherous with diffuse brown fat uptake, which seems to dominate the neck and supraclavicular regions (see **Fig. 3**). Imaging should be used alongside a thorough clinical examination to evaluate this region because metastatic involvement of the cervical musculature may be occult by PET/CT.

Thyroid
Diffuse, moderate to intense FDG uptake may be demonstrated in a normal thyroid gland in approximately 2% of patients.[55] Inflammatory conditions, such as thyroiditis, and benign tumors may mimic malignancy. On rare occasions, melanoma has been known to metastasize to the thyroid, usually deriving from a primary head and neck origin.[56] In the absence of regional primary melanoma or widespread stage IV disease, a focal region of intense FDG thyroid uptake may indicate cosynchronous primary thyroid cancer. A study that reviewed PET/CT findings in 125,754 patients concluded that focal thyroid uptake with intense FDG uptake had a high likelihood of representing thyroid cancer (SUVmax 6.9 vs 4.8 in benign lesions).[55]

Other
Rare incidences of melanoma arising from the iris, choroid, sinonasal mucosa, and esophagus have been reported. The few number of cases limits

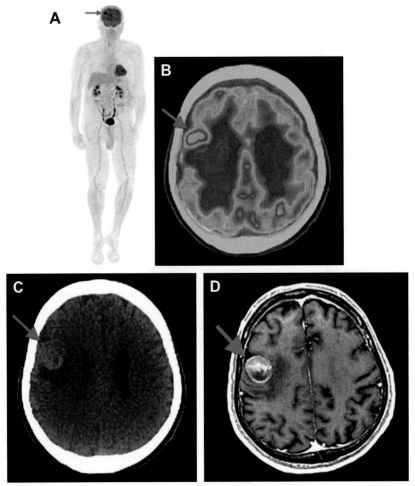

Fig. 2. (*A*) Whole-body MIP reveals a single brain metastasis in the right parietal lobe. (*B*) Fused PET/CT localizes the lesion. (*C*) Hyperdense melanoma metastasis is seen on the attenuation CT. (*D*) Postcontrast MR imaging demonstrates the hypermetabolic component of the metastatic lesion corresponds to the enhancing portion of the study.

the ability to accurately predict the clinical course and choose among treatment strategies. PET/CT is reportedly efficacious for staging patients with choroidal melnoma.[53] Sinonasal primary melanoma accounts for 0.8% to 1.3% of all melanomas and most commonly involves the head and neck. Although a limited number of reports are available, PET/CT has also been proven to be accurate for staging sinonasal melanoma, with superior accuracy to conventional imaging modalities (CT and MR imaging).[57]

Skin

Combining CT with 18F-FDG–PET not only allows improved anatomic characterization but also provides attenuation correction of PET findings. PET imaging requires 2 photons to escape the patients

and be detected simultaneously to register as a true event. Loss of counts caused by attenuation significantly contributes to both image noise and artifacts, limiting quantitative (SUV) and qualitative evaluation. Because relatively little attenuation is present at the patients' surface, attenuation correction *subtracts counts* from these regions to adjust for the relative lack of regional attenuation.

However, in the setting of melanoma, cutaneous evaluation is of relatively high importance. Thus, when evaluating the superficial soft tissues for local recurrence or cutaneous metastasis, the non–attenuation-corrected PET/CT images should be windowed properly and thoroughly examined. This technique may provide more accurate characterization of the superficial soft tissues because lesions closer to the PET crystals are easier to identify without attenuation correction (**Fig. 4**).

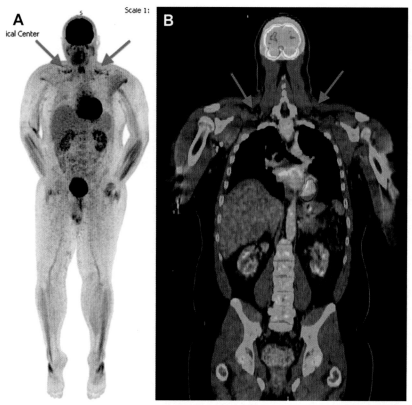

Fig. 3. (*A*) Whole-body MIP demonstrating brown fat in the usual supraclavicular region. (*B*) Coronal fused PET/CT confirms brown fat uptake as the PET is toggled off the CT.

Postoperative Changes

Evaluating postsurgical sites should primarily involve clinical examination because PET/CT findings may be variable and nonspecific. Postsurgical granulation tissue contains an inflammatory reaction with increased cellular activity mediating wound repair. Although the granulation process may present as relatively intense FDG uptake and, thus, easily confused with recurrent neoplasm, typically the uptake is more diffuse involving a larger area with mildly increased uptake.[42] Thus, previous surgical sites of melanoma resection, prior trauma, ostomy sites, or indwelling catheters should be interpreted with caution in the immediate and recent postsurgical periods.

Lymphatics

Conventional imaging is not as sensitive as intraoperative hand gamma probe in the detection of lymphatic locoregional melanoma metastasis, particularly for microscopic nodal disease. Also, FDG uptake in lymph nodes is not specific for malignancy because many non-neoplastic disease processes may result in intense FDG uptake. Granulomatous disease, such as histoplasmosis,

tuberculosis, and sarcoidosis, are widely prevalent and can cause intense FDG uptake. The response of regional lymph nodes to infectious and inflammatory conditions also commonly causes increased nodal FDG activity.[42] In contrast, PET is limited in the evaluation of necrotic lymph nodes and mucinous tumors. In these cases, anatomic characterization with coregistered CT images may provide more diagnostic utility.

Interferon-alfa (IFN-α) is commonly used as a systemic chemotherapy agent for melanoma and may produce findings that mimic metastasis. In 2006, Cone and colleagues[58] reported a case of IFN-α therapy causing hyperstimulation marrow pattern and diffuse hypermetabolic adenopathy (pseudolymphoma) imaged by PET/CT. A thorough examination for non-nodal metastasis may help assess the cause of widespread FDG-avid lymphadenopathy representing metastasis in such cases.

Accidental extravasation of contrast at the IV insertion site may produce increased nodal FDG uptake in the regional soft tissues and lymph nodes. For this reason, IV injection of FDG should be performed in the extremity contralateral that with know melanoma or suspected metastasis.

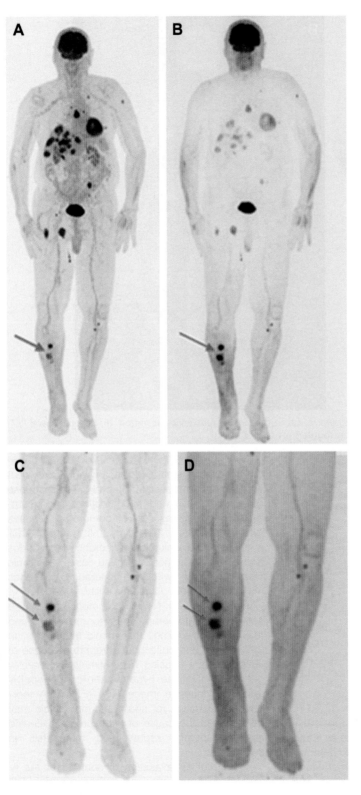

Fig. 4. (*A*) Whole-body MIP attenuation corrected (AC) image reveals extensive metastases. (*B*) Whole-body MIP nonattenuation corrected (NAC) image reveals that the noncutaneous metastases are not as apparent. (*C*) Limited AC MIP of the lower extremity reveals the cutaneous lesions that are not as apparent as the NAC MIP (*D*).

Documentation of the IV insertion site and suspected extravasation may prevent false-positive findings as a result of this phenomenon.

Musculoskeletal

Bone marrow
Under normal conditions, relatively modest FDG uptake is found in the bone marrow. Physiologic states producing an increased rate of myeloproliferative cellular division may result in increased marrow FDG uptake. Patients treated with granulocyte colony-stimulating factor or those who have recently undergone chemotherapy may have globally increased FDG accumulation in the marrow. Cessation of therapy with interferon, a known myelosuppressant, may produce compensatory marrow hyperstimulation (the so-called rebound phenomenon).[58] Evidence of diffusely increased FDG uptake in the bone marrow and spleen in this clinical context should suggest this condition rather than global metastasis.

Detecting osseous metastasis with PET/CT may prevent the need for work-up with other time-consuming, costly imaging modalities, such as MR imaging. One study that compared MR imaging to PET/CT showed no statistically significant difference in sensitivity of detecting metastasis.[59,60] However, sensitivity for detecting metastasis remained relatively low for both modalities, reportedly only 45% and 64% for PET/CT and MR imaging, respectively. This high false-negative rate underscores the need for close follow-up for patients with suspected bone metastasis.

Bone fractures and degenerative and inflammatory joint conditions may also mimic metastatic disease. Healing rib fractures are a well-known cause of increased FDG uptake but, with the addition of the CT and clinical history of trauma, will help differentiate from metastasis in most cases.

Chest

Lungs
The incidence of pulmonary melanoma metastasis to the lung is associated with a bleak prognosis, with only 53% 1-year survival. Early detection is important to both staging and the likelihood of surgical cure. PET imaging is of relatively low sensitivity for characterizing thoracic lesions seen on the coregistered CT, with rates ranging from 57% to 70%.[61] This low sensitivity is accounted for by relatively poor spatial resolution and increased motion artifacts, which are particularly problematic in the lung bases. The pulmonary metastatic size is highly correlated with the sensitivity of detection with PET. In one study of 183 patients, PET sensitivity for 4- to 5-mm nodules was only 7.9% and was 100% for lesions greater than 11 mm. Thus, PET cannot accurately characterize pulmonary nodules less than 12 mm in size.[61]

A variety of infectious and inflammatory conditions may mimic thoracic metastasis. Radiation pneumonitis, pneumonia, and granulomatous disease are common reasons for false-positive PET/CT findings. Metabolic activity of respiratory muscles and the diaphragmatic crura may also be mistaken for pathology and should be examined with caution.

Heart
Cardiac metastases are not uncommon in the setting of widespread melanoma metastasis but are rarely detected antemortem.[62] Background cardiac metabolic activity is a likely explanation for this, which may limit the evaluation of the myocardium. FDG activity in patients who have fasted for 4 to 18 hours is highly variable, ranging from intense to virtually absent. Cheng and colleagues present a case of myocardial metastasis detected by FDG-PET/CT resulting in heart block.[62] Therefore, particularly in symptomatic patients with a high likelihood of melanoma metastasis and abnormal PET findings, cardiac metastasis may be considered (Fig. 5).

Abdomen

Liver and spleen
Metastatic melanoma to the liver occurs significantly less often than to lymph nodes but occurs with relatively high frequency. PET/CT may detect a liver metastasis, but anatomic characterization is usually limited by background hepatic metabolic activity. Because MR imaging has proven superiority in detecting melanoma metastasis, it may a beneficial adjunct to PET/CT in several scenarios. If isolated hepatic metastatic disease is present, which may be the case in up to 50% of ocular melanomas, surgical cure may be achieved. In this setting, the improved spatial resolution of MR imaging may aid presurgical planning.[63] In the setting of clinical symptoms of liver metastasis and a negative PET/CT, the increased sensitivity of MR imaging may assist detection. Because the reduction of tumor burden prolongs life expectance, surgical tumor resection, radiofrequency ablation, or several other management options may be considered.

Spleen
Two known disease entities are of relevance in the setting of splenic evaluation of patients with melanoma with PET/CT: rebound splenic hyperstimulation syndrome and metastasis. Rebound splenic

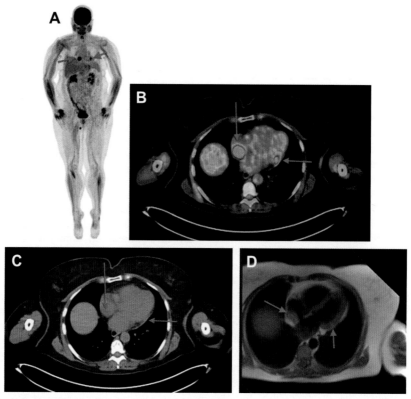

Fig. 5. (*A*) Whole-body MIP reveals 2 cardiac metastases. (*B*) Fused PET/CT confirms location of the lesions in the right atrium (RA) and left ventricle (LV) lateral wall. (*C*) Attenuation correction CT does not clearly demonstrate the lesions. (*D*) MR imaging confirms the lesions in the RA and involvement of the LV wall.

hyperstimulation manifests following chemotherapy as diffusely hypermetabolic bone marrow and splenic parenchyma. Metastasis presents as focal hypermetabolic splenic disease. Quarles and colleagues[64] reported a case of an isolated splenic melanoma metastasis exceeding 10 cm in size.

Adrenals

Both malignant and nonmalignant adrenal processes can produce hypermetabolic adrenal nodules. A study of 689 patients with various primary malignancies showed that minor morphologic abnormalities of the adrenals had little ability in the detection of early metastasis.[65] However, metastasis has well-documented correlation with intense levels of FDG uptake. Benign processes, such as adenomas and adrenal hyperplasia, can increase FDG uptake, although usually to a lesser degree than metastasis. A study by Ozcan and colleagues[66,67] demonstrated that an SUVmax lower limit cutoff of 4.2 has a 88.6% sensitivity and 88.2% specificity for metastasis. It should be noted that the authors of this article advise against using absolute SUV limits because of the high

variability of patient and technical factors that produce SUVmax.

Genitourinary system

PET/CT evaluation of the genitourinary (GU) tract is limited by the excretion of radiotracer into the ureters and bladder. Although excreted contrast permits the identification of pathology under normal conditions, the pooling of excreted tracer in the calices, extrarenal pelvic, or diverticulum of the bladder or calyx can confound the evaluation. Good hydration and furosemide can improve the clearance of the radiopharmaceutical from the renal collecting system. However, in the setting of melanoma, in which isolated GU metastases are exceedingly rare and unlikely to change management, this has little utility.

Bowel

Melanoma is the most common metastatic tumor to the bowel and may present as gastrointestinal bleed, bowel obstruction, or be asymptomatic.[68] Although rare, melanoma may arise from the small bowel.[69] Findings of increased FDG in metastatic melanoma must be differentiated from physiologic bowel activity. Normal bowel uptake is variable and can be patchy or diffuse, with variable causes of bowel activity to include swallowed secretions, smooth muscle metabolic activity, and lymphoid activity.[42]

Pelvis

Gynecologic
The vagina is a known site of primary melanoma formation, usually associated with late detection and poor prognosis. Vaginal melanoma typically occurs in the sixth and seventh decades and presents with symptoms of bleeding, mass, or dyspareunia. FDG-PET is used in the process of staging these patients, and MR imaging is often used as an adjuvant. Stage IV patients typically receive systemic chemotherapy, whereas stage III disease is treated with surgery and high-dose radiation therapy.[70]

Distinguishing metastasis from physiologic pelvic structures is important. Uterine fibroids are a common entity showing variable FDG uptake. In premenopausal women, inflammatory changes in the endometrium associated with menstruation and the ovary associated with ovulation may show increased FDG uptake.

SUMMARY

F18-FDG–PET/CT has been invaluable in the assessment of melanoma throughout the course of the disease. As with any modality, the studies are incomplete and more information will be gleaned as our experience progresses. Additionally, it is hoped that a newer PET agent in the pipeline will give us even greater success in the identification and subsequent treatment of melanoma.

REFERENCES

1. Siegel R, Naishadham D, Jemal A. Cancer statistics, 2012. CA Cancer J Clin 2012;62(1):10–29.
2. Choi EA, Gershenwald JE. Imaging studies in patients with melanoma. Surg Oncol Clin N Am 2007;16(2):403–30.
3. Bevona C, Sober AJ. Melanoma incidence trends. Dermatol Clin 2002;20(4):589–95, vii.
4. Balch CM, Buzaid AC, Soong SJ, et al. Final version of the American Joint Committee on cancer staging system for cutaneous melanoma. J Clin Oncol 2001;19(16):3635–48.
5. Erdmann F, Tieulent JL, Schüz J. International trends in the incidence of malignant melanoma 1953-2008—are recent generations at higher or lower risk? Int J Cancer 2013;132(2):385–400.
6. Ho Shon IA, Chung DK, Saw RP, et al. Imaging in cutaneous melanoma. Nucl Med Commun 2008; 29(10):847–76.
7. Lens MB, Dawes M. Global perspectives of contemporary epidemiological trends of cutaneous malignant melanoma. Br J Dermatol 2004;150(2): 179–85.
8. Weiss M, Loprinzi CL, Creagan ET, et al. Utility of follow-up tests for detecting recurrent disease in patients with malignant melanomas. JAMA 1995; 274(21):1703–5.
9. Hofmann U, Szedlak M, Rittgen W, et al. Primary staging and follow-up in melanoma patients–monocenter evaluation of methods, costs and patient survival. Br J Cancer 2002;87(2):151–7.
10. Aukema TS, Olmos RA, Korse CM, et al. Utility of FDG PET/CT and brain MRI in melanoma patients with increased serum S-100B level during follow-up. Ann Surg Oncol 2010;17(6):1657–61.
11. Mohr P, Eggermont AM, Hauschild A, et al. Staging of cutaneous melanoma. Ann Oncol 2009;20(Suppl 6):vi14–21.
12. Abbott RA, Acland KM, Harries M, et al. The role of positron emission tomography with computed tomography in the follow-up of asymptomatic cutaneous malignant melanoma patients with a high risk of disease recurrence. Melanoma Res 2011;21(5):446–9.
13. Palmer SR, Erickson LA, Ichetovkin I, et al. Circulating serologic and molecular biomarkers in malignant melanoma. Mayo Clin Proc 2011;86(10):981–90.
14. Hoejberg L, Bastholt L, Johansen JS, et al. Serum interleukin-6 as a prognostic biomarker in patients with metastatic melanoma. Melanoma Res 2012; 22(4):287–93.
15. Mottaghy FM, Sunderkötter C, Schubert R, et al. Direct comparison of [18F]FDG PET/CT with PET alone and with side-by-side PET and CT in patients with malignant melanoma. Eur J Nucl Med Mol Imaging 2007;34(9):1355–64. Available at: http://www.springerlink.com.prospero.mc.utmck.edu:2048/content/q61942k722480814/fulltext.pdf.
16. Strobel K, Skalsky J, Steinert HC, et al. S-100B and FDG-PET/CT in therapy response assessment of melanoma patients. Dermatology 2007;215(3): 192–201.
17. Strobel K, Dummer R, Husarik DB, et al. High-risk melanoma: accuracy of FDG PET/CT with added CT morphologic information for detection of metastases. Radiology 2007;244(2):566–74.
18. Strobel K, Dummer R, Steinert HC, et al. Chemotherapy response assessment in stage IV melanoma patients—comparison of 18F-FDG-PET/CT, CT, brain MRI, and tumormarker S-100B. Eur J Nucl Med Mol Imaging 2008;35(10):1786–95. Available at: http://www.springerlink.com.prospero.mc.utmck.edu:2048/content/t04m526851381337/fulltext.pdf.
19. Morton DL, Thompson JF, Cochran AJ, et al. Sentinel-node biopsy or nodal observation in melanoma. N Engl J Med 2006;355(13):1307–17.

20. Baldwin BT, Cherpelis BS, Sondak V, et al. Sentinel lymph node biopsy in melanoma: facts and controversies. Clin Dermatol 2010;28(3):319–23.

21. El-Maraghi RH, Kielar AZ. PET vs sentinel lymph node biopsy for staging melanoma: a patient intervention, comparison, outcome analysis. J Am Coll Radiol 2008;5(8):924–31.

22. Iagaru A, Quon A, Johnson D, et al. 2-Deoxy-2-[F-18] fluoro-D-glucose positron emission tomography/computed tomography in the management of melanoma. Mol Imaging Biol 2007;9(1):50–7.

23. Yancovitz M, Finelt N, Warycha MA, et al. Role of radiologic imaging at the time of initial diagnosis of stage T1b-T3b melanoma. Cancer 2007;110(5):1107–14.

24. Sabel MS, Wong SL. Review of evidence-based support for pretreatment imaging in melanoma. J Natl Compr Canc Netw 2009;7(3):281–9.

25. Crippa F, Leutner M, Belli F, et al. Which kinds of lymph node metastases can FDG PET detect? A clinical study in melanoma. J Nucl Med 2000;41(9):1491–4.

26. Veit-Haibach P, Vogt FM, Jablonka R, et al. Diagnostic accuracy of contrast-enhanced FDG-PET/CT in primary staging of cutaneous malignant melanoma. Eur J Nucl Med Mol Imaging 2009;36(6):910–8.

27. Singh B, Ezziddin S, Palmedo H, et al. Preoperative 18F-FDG-PET/CT imaging and sentinel node biopsy in the detection of regional lymph node metastases in malignant melanoma. Melanoma Res 2008;18(5):346–52.

28. Macapinlac HA. FDG PET and PET/CT imaging in lymphoma and melanoma. Cancer J 2004;10(4):262–70.

29. Dancey AL, Mahon BS, Rayatt SS. A review of diagnostic imaging in melanoma. Br J Plast Surg 2008;61(11):1275–83.

30. Tyler DS, Onaitis M, Kherani A, et al. Positron emission tomography scanning in malignant melanoma. Cancer 2000;89(5):1019–25.

31. Acland KM, Healy C, Calonje E, et al. Comparison of positron emission tomography scanning and sentinel node biopsy in the detection of micrometastases of primary cutaneous malignant melanoma. J Clin Oncol 2001;19(10):2674–8.

32. Aukema TS, Valdés Olmos RA, Wouters WM, et al. Utility of preoperative 18F-FDG PET/CT and brain MRI in melanoma patients with palpable lymph node metastases. Ann Surg Oncol 2010;17(10):2773–8.

33. Bronstein Y, Tummala S, Rohren E. F-18 FDG PET/CT for detection of malignant involvement of peripheral nerves: case series and literature review. Clin Nucl Med 2011;36(2):96.

34. Gulec SA, Faries MB, Lee CC, et al. The role of fluorine-18 deoxyglucose positron emission tomography in the management of patients with metastatic melanoma: impact on surgical decision making. Clin Nucl Med 2003;28(12):961–5.

35. Camargo Etchebehere EC, Romanato JS, Santos AO, et al. Impact of [F-18] FDG-PET/CT in the restaging and management of patients with malignant melanoma. Nucl Med Commun 2010;31(11):925–30. Available at: http://graphics.tx.ovid.com.prospero.mc.utmck.edu:2048/ovftpdfs/FPDDNCFBAALFLG00/fs046/ovft/live/gv023/00006231/00006231-201011000-00001.pdf.

36. Falk MS, Truitt AK, Coakley FV, et al. Interpretation, accuracy and management implications of FDG PET/CT in cutaneous malignant melanoma. Nucl Med Commun 2007;28(4):273–80. Available at: http://graphics.tx.ovid.com.prospero.mc.utmck.edu:2048/ovftpdfs/FPDDNCFBAALFLG00/fs046/ovft/live/gv023/00006231/00006231-200704000-00008.pdf.

37. Buck AK, Herrmann K, Stargardt T, et al. Economic evaluation of PET and PET/CT in oncology: evidence and methodologic approaches. J Nucl Med Technol 2010;38(1):6–17.

38. Niederkohr RD, Rosenberg J, Shabo G, et al. Clinical value of including the head and lower extremities in 18F-FDG PET/CT imaging for patients with malignant melanoma. Nucl Med Commun 2007;28(9):688–95.

39. Bastiaannet E, Hoekstra HJ, Hoekstra OS. Methods in molecular biology. In: Juweid ME, Hoekstra OS, editors. Totowa (NJ): Humana Press; 2011. p. 123–39.

40. Querellou S, Keromnes N, Abgral R, et al. Clinical and therapeutic impact of 18F-FDG PET/CT whole-body acquisition including lower limbs in patients with malignant melanoma. Nucl Med Commun 2010;31(9):766–72.

41. Pfluger T, Melzer HI, Schneider V, et al. PET/CT in malignant melanoma: contrast-enhanced CT versus plain low-dose CT. Eur J Nucl Med Mol Imaging 2011;38(5):822–31.

42. Gorospe L, Raman S, Echeveste J, et al. Whole-body PET/CT: spectrum of physiological variants, artifacts and interpretative pitfalls in cancer patients. Nucl Med Commun 2005;26(8):671–87.

43. Dizendorf EV, Treyer V, Van Schulthess GK, et al. Application of oral contrast media in coregistered positron emission tomography-CT. Am J Roentgenol 2002;179(2):477–81.

44. Otero HJ, Yap JT, Patak MA, et al. Evaluation of low-density neutral oral contrast material in PET/CT for tumor imaging: results of a randomized clinical trial. AJR Am J Roentgenol 2009;193(2):326–32.

45. Prichard RS, Hill AD, Skehan SJ, et al. Positron emission tomography for staging and management of malignant melanoma. Br J Surg 2002;89(4):389–96.

46. Rohren EM, Provenzale JM, Barboriak DP, et al. Screening for cerebral metastases with FDG PET in patients undergoing whole-body staging of non–central nervous system malignancy1. Radiology 2003;226(1):181–7.

47. Kitajima K, Nakamoto Y, Okizuka H, et al. Accuracy of whole-body FDG-PET/CT for detecting brain metastases from non-central nervous system tumors. Ann Nucl Med 2008;22(7):595–602.

48. Barnholtz-Sloan JS, Sloan AE, Davis FG, et al. Incidence proportions of brain metastases in patients diagnosed (1973 to 2001) in the Metropolitan Detroit Cancer Surveillance System. J Clin Oncol 2004;22(14):2865–72.

49. Hu DN, Yu GP, McCormick SA, et al. Population-based incidence of uveal melanoma in various races and ethnic groups. Am J Ophthalmol 2005; 140(4):612–7.

50. Kivelä T, Eskelin S, Kujala E. Metastatic uveal melanoma. Int Ophthalmol Clin 2006;46(1):133–49.

51. Schuster R, Bechrakis NE, Stroux A, et al. Circulating tumor cells as prognostic factor for distant metastases and survival in patients with primary uveal melanoma. Clin Cancer Res 2007;13(4): 1171–8.

52. Servois V, Mariani P, Malhaire C, et al. Preoperative staging of liver metastases from uveal melanoma by magnetic resonance imaging (MRI) and fluorodeoxyglucose-positron emission tomography (FDG-PET). Eur J Surg Oncol 2010;36(2):189–94.

53. Patel P, Finger PT. Whole-body 18F FDG positron emission tomography/computed tomography evaluation of patients with uveal metastasis. Am J Ophthalmol 2012;153(4):661–8.

54. Mervic L. Time course and pattern of metastasis of cutaneous melanoma differ between men and women. PLoS One 2012;7(3):e32955.

55. Soelberg KK, Bonnema SJ, Brix T, et al. Risk of malignancy in thyroid incidentalomas detected by 18F-fluorodeoxyglucose positron emission tomography. A systematic review. Thyroid 2012. [Epub ahead of print].

56. Kung B, Aftab S, Wood M, et al. Malignant melanoma metastatic to the thyroid gland: a case report and review of the literature. Ear Nose Throat J 2009;88(1):E7.

57. Haerle SK, Soyka MB, Fischer DR, et al. The value of 18F-FDG-PET/CT imaging for sinonasal malignant melanoma. Eur Arch Otorhinolaryngol 2011; 269(1):127–33. Available at: http://www.springer link.com.prospero.mc.utmck.edu:2048/content/r56 0m4w3641t1r43/fulltext.pdf.

58. Cone LA, Brochert A, Schulz K, et al. PET positive generalized lymphadenopathy and splenomegaly following interferon-alfa-2b adjuvant therapy for melanoma. Clin Nucl Med 2007;32(10):793.

59. Heusner T, Gölitz P, Hamami M, et al. "One-stop-shop" staging: should we prefer FDG-PET/CT or MRI for the detection of bone metastases? Eur J Radiol 2011;78(3):430–5.

60. "One-stop-shop" staging: should we prefer FDG-PET/CT or MRI for the detection of bone metastases? 2012;1–1.

61. Mayerhoefer ME, Prosch H, Herold CJ, et al. Assessment of pulmonary melanoma metastases with 18F-FDG PET/CT: which PET-negative patients require additional tests for definitive staging? Eur Radiol 2012;22(11):2451–7.

62. Cheng G, Newberg A. Metastatic melanoma causing complete atrioventricular block-the role of FDG PET/CT in diagnosis. Clin Imaging 2011; 35(4):312–4.

63. Karlen AI, Clark JJ, Wong LL. Two cases of partial hepatectomy for malignant melanoma. Hawaii J Med Public Health 2012;71(4):92–6.

64. Quarles UH, Zoon P, van Waes P, et al. Solitary splenic metastasis in a patient with a malignant melanoma diagnosed with F-18-FDG PET scanning. Clin Nucl Med 2005;30(8):582.

65. Meehan CP, Fuqua JL, Reiner AS, et al. Prognostic significance of adrenal gland morphology at CT in patients with three common malignancies. Br J Radiol 2012;85(1014):807–12.

66. Ozcan Kara P, Kara T, Kara Gedik G, et al. The role of fluorodeoxyglucose-positron emission tomography/computed tomography in differentiating between benign and malignant adrenal lesions. Nucl Med Commun 2010;32(2):106–12. Available at: http://graphics.tx.ovid.com.prospero.mc.utmck. edu:2048/ovftpdfs/FPDDNCFBAALFLG00/fs046/ov ft/live/gv023/00006231/00006231-201102000-00004. pdf.

67. Ozcan Kara P, Kara T, Kara Gedik G, et al. The role of fluorodeoxyglucose-positron emission tomography/computed tomography in differentiating between benign and malignant adrenal lesions. Nucl Med Commun 2011;32(2):106–12.

68. Vaz PS, Usurelu S, Monteiro A, et al. Small bowel metastatic of malignant melanoma: a rare cause of lower gastrointestinal bleeding. Acta Med Port 2011;24(1):179–82.

69. Patti R, Cacciatori M, Guercio G, et al. Intestinal melanoma: a broad spectrum of clinical presentation. Int J Surg Case Rep 2012;3(8):395–8.

70. Oudoux A, Rousseau T, Bridji B, et al. Interest of F-18 fluorodeoxyglucose positron emission tomography in the evaluation of vaginal malignant melanoma. Gynecol Oncol 2004;95(3):765–8. Available at: http://ac.els-cdn.com/S0090825804007024/1-s2.0-S0090825804007024-main.pdf?_tid=0a1b07fea10 cd5c14ec65e7f780a94cd&acdnat=1337983842_ 0594937df503e12badec82a7639b6e94.

Role of Positron Emission Tomography/Computed Tomography (PET/CT) in Head and Neck Cancer

Edward J. Escott, MD

KEYWORDS

- Head and neck cancer • PET/CT • Staging • Prognosis • FDG

KEY POINTS

- Positron emission tomography/computed tomography (PET/CT) is indicated for the staging of head and neck cancer.
- PET/CT may have a role in prognosis and in tailoring treatment.
- PET/CT can aid in detecting an unknown primary tumor in the head and neck.
- Optimally, a diagnostic quality CT scan is performed as part of a PET/CT. To obtain the full diagnostic value of a PET/CT, both the PET and CT components must be carefully evaluated.
- Incidental focal hypermetabolic thyroid lesions have a reasonably high likelihood of malignancy and require further evaluation.

INTRODUCTION

The term head and neck cancer generally encompasses malignant neoplasms of soft tissue origin of the oral cavity, lips, nasal cavity, paranasal sinuses, pharynx, larynx, and salivary glands, as well as sarcomas arising in this region.[1] The skin is sometimes included as well. About 95% or more are squamous cell carcinomas (or variants) arising from the mucosa or adenocarcinomas from the associated secretory glands.[1] Head and neck cancer also has a high propensity for developing distant metastases and second primary malignancies, with incidence ranging from 6.1% to 16.3%.[2] Distant metastases most frequently involve bone in nasopharyngeal carcinoma and the lung in other head and neck neoplasms.[2] Imaging plays a key role in the detection, staging, follow-up and treatment decisions for head and neck cancer. Not long ago this was accomplished with a thorough physical examination and supplemental CT scans, generally of the neck and chest. Magnetic resonance (MR) is also used for primary lesion evaluation, particularly for neoplasms of the oral cavity, salivary glands, and nasopharynx, and it can also be useful to evaluate for the invasion of local structures, as well as for the detection of adenopathy. More recently, PET, and then PET/CT, scanning has become a very useful tool in all aspects of head and neck cancer. This method can be used in the initial diagnosis to detect a primary tumor; in pretreatment staging, restaging, and in treatment follow-up; and for surveillance.[3] Although PET/CT can provide useful information, there are also several pitfalls and limitations associated with imaging of head and neck cancer. This article addresses all these issues and discusses some of the potential uses for PET/CT such as in prognosis and guiding therapy. This article also introduces radiopharmaceuticals other than [^{18}F]-2-fluoro-2-deoxy-D-glucose (F18-FDG) and their potential uses.

Department of Radiology, Division of Neuroradiology, University of Kentucky Medical Center, 800 Rose Street, Room HX-319A, Lexington, KY 40536-0293, USA
E-mail address: edward.escott@uky.edu

Radiol Clin N Am 51 (2013) 881–893
http://dx.doi.org/10.1016/j.rcl.2013.05.002
0033-8389/13/$ – see front matter © 2013 Elsevier Inc. All rights reserved.

ANATOMY AND IMAGING TECHNIQUES

The neck contains relatively complex anatomy in a fairly small space. Patients can present with a neck mass, in which case the goal of imaging is not only to define the mass but also to look for a possible primary head and neck neoplasm, in addition to any (additional) adenopathy. Imaging in the head and neck can be challenging because small mucosal lesions may be difficult to detect, and lesions in certain areas, such as the tongue or salivary glands, can be difficult to define, particularly on CT. CT and MR criteria for determining whether lymph nodes contain metastases have been published, but are imperfect, particularly because micrometastases cannot be detected.[4] There is considerable importance in identifying nodal metastases, as the treatment and prognosis of a patient with no nodal disease is significantly different from that of a patient with even a single metastatic lymph node.[5]

The traditional modalities used to image the neck and to stage disease are CT, MR, and ultrasonography. These modalities all have their advantages and limitations. For example, although morphologic features can help in identifying metastatic cervical lymph nodes, size is one of the major criteria used to determine whether lymph nodes are benign or malignant on CT and MR. The size criteria have been arrived at to provide a certain sensitivity and specificity, and inherent in this is that some malignant nodes will fall below the established criteria. PET/CT can be particularly helpful by demonstrating increased metabolic activity in these smaller lymph nodes. Likewise, in the postoperative or postradiation neck, the detection of recurrence or metastases at an early stage can be challenging on CT and MR because of architectural distortion and radiation-related soft tissue changes. PET/CT has the ability to better demonstrate metastases or recurrences in these morphologically altered regions (**Fig. 1**).[6]

PET/CT imaging in the head and neck is most commonly performed using one radiopharmaceutical, F18-FDG. FDG is a glucose analog that is transported into the cell but is not metabolized, and it therefore accumulates. It has been seen that there is increased utilization of glucose via glycolysis in cancer cells (as per the Warburg effect).[7] The uptake of FDG generally reflects glucose metabolism and is dependent on multiple factors, including at the cellular, tissue, and organ level, such as the amount of GLUT1 receptors, blood flow, tissue perfusion, hypoxia, and the amount of viable and inflammatory cells.[7] There will be resultant FDG uptake in cells exhibiting increased glucose metabolism. Therefore, FDG will accumulate in many tumor cells, but it can also accumulate in normal tissues and in nonmalignant processes.

The techniques and technical considerations for PET/CT have been outlined elsewhere and vary somewhat from institution to institution.[8,9] In brief, the patient receives similar screening and preparation for a contrast-enhanced CT scan of the neck, chest, abdomen, and pelvis as would normally be performed as per institutional protocol; this is

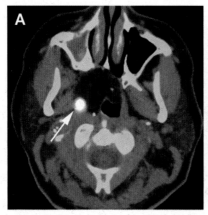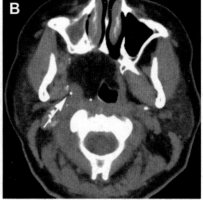

Fig. 1. PET/CT of a woman with prior resection of a right soft palate adenocarcinoma, as well as a maxillectomy, suprahyoid neck dissection, and radial forearm free flap reconstruction. (*A*) Fused PET/CT scan of the neck demonstrates increased uptake in nodular tissue (*arrow*) along the deep margin of the free flap, likely representing tumor recurrence. (*B*) The noncontrast CT scan component of the PET/CT demonstrates this nodular tissue (*arrow*); however, without the PET it would be difficult to definitively call this tumor rather than postoperative changes. As the patient was found to have sinonasal recurrent tumor as well as additional locoregional and distant metastases, this nodule is also presumably tumor recurrence. This case demonstrates why PET/CT can be very useful in patients who have significant postoperative or postradiation architectural alteration.

assuming that a "diagnostic" CT scan is to be obtained with both oral and intravenous (IV) contrast. If no contrast is to be administered, then no preparation would be needed. For the PET portion of the study, the patient must fast for 4 hours before the examination, but can drink water; in patients with diabetes, blood glucose level should be less than 200 mg/dL and the patient should be at a comfortable temperature to prevent shivering. An uptake phase of at least 60 minutes should be used, and the patient should be kept at a comfortable temperature and refrain from moving, speaking, or swallowing as much as possible, to minimize muscular and laryngeal uptake.[8,9]

ROLES OF PET

PET/CT has a variety of uses in head and neck cancer. Fletcher and colleagues,[3] in their "Recommendations on the Use of 18F-FDG PET in Oncology," which was based on an expert panel and reviews of the literature, recommend the use of PET for detection of an unknown primary neoplasm, for initial staging, particularly for local staging, and for the detection of tumor recurrence. The investigators did not recommend the use of PET for the initial diagnostic workup and defining the extent of primary head and neck malignancies. However, their recommendations were published in 2008 and did not include studies using PET/CT. Fukui and colleagues,[6] in their review of the diagnostic uses and pitfalls of PET/CT, report that the most powerful application of PET/CT was the detection of residual or recurrent primary neoplasm with a high sensitivity (95%) but not as high a specificity (60%). These investigators also found PET/CT useful in detecting recurrence or metastases of non–iodine-avid thyroid cancer and medullary thyroid cancer; in the detection of recurrent skull base neoplasms, where prior resection and treatment can significantly alter the anatomy and make detection of tumor by conventional means difficult; and for tumor staging, directing biopsy, and in posttreatment tumor surveillance.

PET VERSUS PET/CT

Difficulties can arise with PET alone because of the multiple causes of nonmalignant increased FDG update that can occur in the head and neck. It is generally accepted that PET/CT is superior to PET alone. Although overlap between tumor and physiologic uptake may confound interpretation, PET/CT allows direct correlation of FDG uptake with anatomic structures to reduce false-positive results.[6] Branstetter and colleagues[10] evaluated 65 consecutive patients with or suspected of

having head and neck cancer and found that PET/CT was superior to PET or CT alone. These investigators found that in addition to greater sensitivity and specificity for PET/CT, there was also greater radiologist confidence with PET/CT. Likewise, Jeong and colleagues,[11] in their evaluation of integrated PET/CT in the evaluation of cervical lymph nodes, also found PET/CT superior to PET or CT alone. Lesion localization is improved when using PET/CT rather than when using PET or CT alone. Syed and colleagues[12] demonstrated strong interobserver agreement in lesion detection and anatomic localization when using combined PET/CT and weaker correlation when using PET alone.

The CT scan obtained for PET/CT can be used in 2 ways. A CT scan using a relatively low dose can be obtained for attenuation correction and localization of metabolic activity, or a CT scan can be performed by a technique similar to a diagnostic study, including the use of iodinated and oral contrast. Imaging of the head and neck can be performed at a smaller field of view than for the body portion of the scan, with patients' arms down at their sides, to further improve the diagnostic quality of both the PET and the CT scan.[8] In order to obtain the most diagnostic value from a PET/CT, and to have a single report contain all relevant information for treatment planning, performing a diagnostic CT scan as a separate scan with a smaller field of view for the head and neck is preferable. If a diagnostic scan is not obtained as part of the PET/CT scan, then it is often obtained separately to provide the necessary anatomic information and additional morphologic information. It is critical that interpretation of a diagnostic CT scan accompany a PET/CT scan because there can be important diagnostic features such as a cystic or necrotic lymph node that does not demonstrate significant metabolic activity or small pulmonary nodules that might not be evident on the PET portion of the study (Fig. 2). In addition, important clinical information such as the accurate delineation of the tumor margins and invasion of local structures or the detection of extracapsular spread may be very difficult to detect on a nonoptimized CT scan.

IMAGING FINDINGS
Prognosis

PET/CT may have a role in prognosis and potentially in guiding therapy. Pretreatment SUV_{mean} has been suggested to be a useful prognostic parameter for patients who would be undergoing radiation therapy. Higgins and colleagues[13] found that only SUV_{mean} of the tumor had a statistically

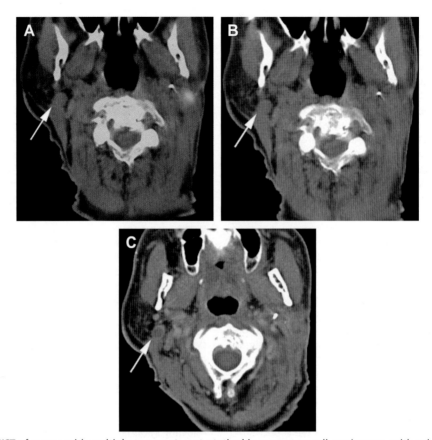

Fig. 2. PET/CT of a man with multiple recurrent, metastatic skin squamous cell carcinomas, with prior resection including partial left parotidectomy, and radiation therapy. An infiltrative metastasis was diagnosed in the left parotid gland and parotid bed. PET/CT was carried out to evaluate for additional disease. (*A*) Fused PET/CT scan demonstrates a rounded lymph node with mildly increased uptake along the deep margin of the right parotid tail (*arrow*). Note that there is significantly greater uptake seen in the left parotid region metastasis. (*B*) The noncontrast CT component of the PET/CT scan. The node (*arrow*) appears homogeneous, rounded, and borderline large. This lymph node was not interpreted as having a high likelihood of being a metastasis. (*C*) A "diagnostic" contrast-enhanced neck CT scan performed 2 days earlier. It can now clearly be seen that this lymph node has a cystic or necrotic central portion (*arrow*) and thus is likely a metastasis. Subsequent biopsy and surgery confirmed metastasis. This case demonstrates 2 important points. The first is that cystic or necrotic lymph nodes may have little to no increased uptake on the PET scan and the second is that it is crucial to correlate with and carefully evaluate a diagnostic CT scan when interpreting PET/CT.

significant correlation with disease-free survival (DFS). The investigators found that patients with pretreatment tumor SUV_{mean} that exceeded the median value (7) of the cohort demonstrated inferior 2-year DFS relative to patients with SUV_{mean} less than or equal to the median value of the cohort. It was found that there was a trend toward decreased DFS with increasing SUV_{max} of the primary tumor; however, this did not reach statistical significance. There was also no correlation between the SUV_{max} or SUV_{mean} of metastatic lymph nodes and the measured DFS parameters. The investigators focused on pretreatment FDG PET parameters with the goal of identifying a measurement that could help to identify a high-risk

group of patients that might respond poorly to conventional therapy. The investigators note that a potential pitfall of SUV_{mean} is the lesser degree of reproducibility relative to SUV_{max}. Traditionally, SUV_{max} has been the most common estimate of metabolic activity in clinical practice because it is thought to be the most reproducible.[13]

In a meta-analysis by Xie and colleagues[14] to evaluate the prognostic value of SUV from F18-FDG PET and PET/CT in patients with head and neck cancer, it was concluded that when evaluating patients before treatment as well as for treatment response, SUV (measurement method unspecified) correlated with overall survival, DFS, and local control in both groups. Torizuka and colleagues[15] evaluated the prognostic value of SUV in patients with head and neck cancer (multiple locations of primary tumors, all T stages). The investigators used a measurement that seems to be equivalent to SUV_{max} and found an inverse relationship between SUV and outcome parameters including local control and DFS. Furthermore, they found that SUV was associated as a continuous variable; in other words, the higher the value, the worse the prognosis. The investigators suggest that a more aggressive treatment approach should be considered for tumors with high FDG uptake.

Schinagl and colleagues[16] evaluated whether PET/CT could be predictive of outcome in patients with head and neck cancer who would be treated only with chemoradiation. The investigators evaluated multiple methods of determining the margins of the lesion on PET/CT including visual assessment and application of isocontours at different values or thresholds, and they also evaluated correlations based on different SUV measurements, such as SUV_{max}, SUV_{mean}, and an integrated SUV. While some of the volume measurements were found to be predictive of certain outcome parameters in some primary tumor sites, no correlation was found between SUV_{mean} and SUV_{max} and outcome. The investigators also reviewed the literature and reported mixed results, with about half the studies reviewed showing correlation and others showing no correlation between SUV and outcome. Therefore, although certainly some studies point to a value of PET/CT in predicting outcome or identifying tumors that might benefit from more aggressive therapy, it would seem that still more research needs to be done.

SUV: Value

An absolute SUV to differentiate benign and malignant disease in the head and neck has not been well defined. A variety of methods of using SUV in the head and neck have been reported. For example, Stoeckli and colleagues[17] (and others) judged nodes as metastatic if the uptake was clearly higher than that in the background tissue. In a meta-analysis by Kyzas and colleagues[18] evaluating the performance of PET/CT in metastatic lymph node detection, in 19 studies 18F-FDG PET positivity was stated to have been assessed in a qualitative manner, whereas in 8 studies it was stated to have been assessed by quantitative methods using standardized uptake values. The investigators found that the design of the study and the type of assessment of 18F-FDG PET positivity did not statistically significantly influence the reported diagnostic accuracy of the test. Fleming and colleagues[19] state that for the purpose of their study, an SUV level greater than 2.5 was considered consistent with abnormal, hypermetabolic activity in primary, regional, and distant disease. The investigators state that the currently accepted SUV level for a positive PET/CT scan is 2.5. Their reference for this statement is the article by Patz and colleagues[20] published in *Radiology* in 1993, which referred specifically to the PET evaluation of focal pulmonary abnormalities seen on chest radiographs and did not evaluate lymph nodes either in the chest or in the neck and did not evaluate anatomic sites other than the chest, so there is not clear evidence that this SUV value can be extrapolated to sites outside the lungs. In fact, Jeong and colleagues[11] in their study evaluating PET/CT in cervical nodal evaluation state with reference to SUV values used for cervical nodes (3.5) other than the jugulodigastric node (4.0) that "... we adopted the values (pSUV = 3.5 and 4.0) of our previous study for non-small cell lung cancer because there has been no strict cut off point for the SUV in the literature to differentiate benign from malignant tissues in both the primary site and the cervical lymph nodes in head and neck cancer". Hafidh and colleagues[21] in their evaluation of the impact of the addition of PET to the staging of head and neck cancers also evaluated the SUV values. The researchers found that using a cutoff of 2.9 and 3.2, the sensitivities were 100% and 97% and specificities were 20% and 40%, respectively. However, for an SUV cutoff of 5, sensitivity was 66.7% and specificity was 100%. The investigators used a cutoff of less than 3 for benignity and greater than 5 for malignancy, and 3 to 5 was considered indeterminate. This was one of the few studies that attempted to define SUV cutoff values in the head and neck. Another pitfall of using strict SUV criteria is that small lymph nodes may have an SUV value below an accepted threshold, but yet may subjectively have greater-than-expected metabolic activity for their size, thus making them concerning for harboring metastases. This again stresses the importance of careful correlation with the CT component of the PET/CT. Considering the evidence, subjective evaluation of increased metabolic activity and careful correlation with the CT scan likely provides the best diagnostic approach.

Staging

Many studies have evaluated the utility of PET/CT for the local and distant staging of head and neck cancer. While not all studies reached the same conclusion, PET/CT is probably useful for the staging of head and neck cancer, as long as there is not N0 disease.

Staging: Locoregional Disease

Stoeckli and colleagues[17] compared imaging modalities for staging the neck in a prospective cohort of patients evaluated by CT, ultrasonography with fine-needle aspiration cytology, and PET/CT with the histologic evaluation of the neck dissection as the standard of reference. The researchers found a fairly high rate of understaging among all modalities. The percentage of correctly staged necks was also fairly low. When evaluating the modalities in differentiating N0 from N+ necks, sensitivity, specificity, positive predictive value (PPV) and negative predictive value (NPV) for PET/CT of 86.4%, 76.9%, 95.0% and 52.6%, respectively, was found. The investigators thought that the inclusion of the clinically N0 necks adversely affected the results for PET/CT, and they conclude that none of the modalities is reliable enough to replace elective neck treatment in cN0 necks. They also thought that PET/CT performs best in trials only including patients with cN+, whereas the inclusion of patients with cN0 considerably reduces the accuracy.

A meta-analysis by Kyzas and colleagues[18] assessed the diagnostic accuracy of 18F-FDG PET in detecting lymph node metastases in patients with Head and Neck Squamous Cell Carcinoma (HNSCC). A total of 10 studies (311 patients) of cN0 patients and 19 studies (798 patients) with mixed patient populations were considered for analysis. It was found that the sensitivity for PET/CT overall was 79% and the specificity was 86%. However, for clinically N0 patients, the sensitivity was 50% and specificity was 87%. It was concluded that 18F-FDG PET has good diagnostic performance in the overall pretreatment evaluation of patients with HNSCC but still does not detect the disease in half of the patients with metastasis and cN0. It was also concluded that there was no solid evidence to support the routine clinical application of 18F-FDG PET in the pretreatment evaluation of the lymph node status in patients with HNSCC, including patients with clinically negative neck. The investigators thought that in patients with clinically positive nodal disease who will be treated surgically, PET or any other diagnostic test does not change management. However, because the accurate staging of disease might affect the extent of surgery, and certainly would affect the treatment of patients treated with chemoradiation, PET/CT may still be a worthwhile pretreatment diagnostic test.

Yoon and colleagues[22] evaluated CT, MR, ultrasonography, and PET/CT and their combined use in the assessment of cervical nodal metastasis in squamous cell carcinoma of the head and neck.

Clinical tumor stage or clinical N stages are not mentioned. Patients were imaged with all 4 imaging modalities before neck dissection to evaluate the performance of each modality separately and combined. CT and MR performed identically in their study. PET/CT had a small overall advantage. The investigators found that the overall sensitivity, specificity, and accuracy were 77.0%, 99.4%, and 95.3% for CT and MR; 78.4%, 98.5%, and 94.8% for ultrasonography; and 81.1%, 98.2%, and 95.0% for PET/CT, respectively. The criteria used for PET/CT positivity was both visual (greater than background activity) and semiquantitative using an SUV_{max} greater than 2.5. The researchers did not use any CT characteristics of malignancy in their interpretation of the PET/CT. They note that the addition of MR or CT to PET/CT improves sensitivity, but not to a statistically significant degree, and that the improvement comes from the identification of small necrotic nodes.

Fleming and colleagues[19] evaluated the use of PET/CT in the initial evaluation of newly diagnosed patients with head and neck cancer (all stages) and found that in patients with bilateral neck dissections, PET/CT had a sensitivity, specificity, PPV, and NPV of 86.3%, 94.1%, 89.7%, and 84.2%, respectively. PET/CT detected a possible synchronous primary neoplasm in 8.1% of patients (although 3 of 10 were false-positive results because of reactive lymph nodes and inflammatory changes) and distant metastases in 15.4%. The researchers conclude that PET/CT altered management in 30.9% of patients because of upstaging, diagnosing distant and unresectable disease, and working up second primary malignancies. They also concluded that although PET/CT is sensitive in detecting occult cervical nodal metastases, it does not yet have the ability to replace neck dissection as the diagnostic standard of care. Fletcher and colleagues,[3] in their review of studies and recommendations for the use of PET in head and neck cancer, concluded that PET should routinely be added to CT or MR imaging to improve nodal or distant-disease staging of head and neck cancer.

From these studies, it can be concluded that PET/CT is useful in the staging of locoregional disease, although it has limited utility in the N0 neck. However, one may want to consider PET/CT in the N0 neck, particularly if there are equivocal nodes seen on neck CT or MR, as the confirmation of a nodal metastasis may be helpful. It should be noted that a negative study in an N0 patient does not exclude nodal metastasis, however. Careful evaluation of the CT component of the study can help increase sensitivity by allowing the detection of cystic or necrotic lymph nodes that do not have significantly increased metabolic activity.

Staging: Distant Metastases

PET/CT also has a role in detecting distant metastases or a second primary tumor (**Fig. 3**). Xu and colleagues[23] performed a meta-analysis to evaluate whole-body PET and PET/CT for initial M staging of head and neck cancer and to determine whether integrating PET with CT could improve the diagnostic accuracy of PET alone. A total of 12 studies met their inclusion criteria and included 7 PET/CT studies and 8 PET studies consisting of a nearly equivalent number of patients. About 14.4% of patients had distant metastases or a second primary tumor. The pooled sensitivity for PET was 84.8%, and for PET/CT it was 87.5%. Pooled specificity was 95.2% and 95.0%. Based on likelihood ratios, the researchers concluded that a positive PET or PET/CT has a high probability of diagnosing a distant metastasis or second primary tumor; however, a negative PET or PET/CT scan result could not be used alone to exclude a distant metastasis or a second primary cancer. The investigators' overall conclusion is that current evidence suggests that whole-body PET/CT and PET have good diagnostic performance in M staging of head and neck cancer and that PET/CT tends to have higher accuracy than PET.

In another meta-analysis by Xu and colleagues[2] the role of 18FDG PET/CT in detecting distant metastases and second primary cancers in patients with head and neck cancer at staging was evaluated. A total of 12 articles again met their inclusion criteria. There was considerable overlap between the studies used in the 2 meta-analyses, but 3 studies were unique to this one, their references 27–29, and 3 studies included in the other were excluded. The investigators included 8 initial staging studies and 5 restaging studies (1 study evaluated both staging and restaging). Within these studies, 174 of 1276 eligible patients had distant metastases or second primary malignancies. When evaluating only posttreatment (restaging) patients, 81 of 452 had "distant failure" and/or second primary cancers. The pooled sensitivity for PET/CT for detecting distant metastases or a second primary was 88.8% and sensitivity was 95.1%, which are reasonably similar to the previous meta-analysis. The investigators found similar sensitivity and specificity for both the initial staging and restaging studies. It was concluded that current evidence suggests that 18FDG-PET/CT has good diagnostic performance in detecting distant metastases and second primary cancers of head and neck.

Residual or Recurrent Disease

Patients with unresectable disease have residual or recurrent disease following non-operative therapy, in 30% to 50% of cases.[24] Gupta and colleagues[24] performed a meta-analysis to evaluate the performance of PET or PET/CT in posttreatment response assessment and/or surveillance imaging of head and neck squamous cell carcinoma. A total of 2335 patients in 51 studies were included. The investigators carried out analyses based on the individual study data provided, for the site of the primary tumor, metastatic cervical nodes, and combined locoregional recurrence. They concluded that PET had an exceptionally high NPV and can be considered highly suggestive for the absence of viable disease. They also determined that scans performed 12 or more weeks after the completion of definitive therapy had a moderately higher diagnostic accuracy. The timing of posttreatment imaging has been investigated by several researchers. Andrade and colleagues[25] found that if patients were imaged after 8 weeks

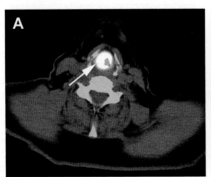
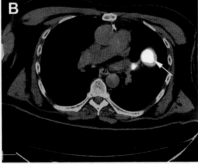

Fig. 3. PET/CT of a man who presented with T3N2B poorly differentiated squamous cell carcinoma of the supraglottic larynx. (*A*) Fused PET/CT demonstrates increased uptake in the supraglottic larynx, much greater on the right (*arrow*), corresponding to the patient's squamous cell carcinoma. There was also a large right level 2a lymph node (not shown) (*B*) Fused PET/CT through the chest also demonstrated a left lung mass with increased uptake (*arrow*). This was proved to be a second primary neoplasm, a non–small cell lung cancer. Note the adjacent left hilar metastatic lymph node. There were also additional mediastinal metastatic lymph nodes (not shown).

after radiation therapy, there was a substantially increased sensitivity and specificity for residual disease than if patients were scanned before this time. For some time after radiation therapy, there will be inflammatory changes that can result in false-positive or false-negative studies. PET/CT has greater diagnostic value after these reactive changes have subsided. Therefore, imaging should be performed no sooner than 8 to 12 weeks after treatment to increase sensitivity and specificity.

Unknown Primary Tumor

An unknown primary tumor is diagnosed when a patient presents with a neck metastasis but no primary tumor is found.[26] The workup generally consists of a full head and neck clinical examination, fiberoptic endoscopy and neck and chest CT and/or MR, and panendoscopy with blind biopsies and tonsillectomies.[19,26] PET/CT has been more recently added to the diagnostic workup. Although variable, the treatment of an unknown primary tumor can consist of up to bilateral neck dissections, tonsillectomies, and radiation therapy for all mucosal sites and both sides of the neck.[26] Detection of a primary tumor has implications for therapy in that targeted treatment of a known primary tumor can improve the chance of survival as well as lower the morbidity by better targeting the treatment options, including surgery, and decreasing the field of irradiation.[19,27] Pattani and colleagues[28] evaluated the utility of panendoscopy in patients with an unknown primary tumor after a negative PET/CT scan result. The investigators found that PET/CT detected an unknown primary tumor in 12 of 23 patients and that only 1 additional primary tumor was detected with panendoscopy. Fletcher and colleagues,[3] in their recommendations for the use of FDG PET in oncology, conclude that PET should be included in the workup of unknown primary tumors and will likely improve important health care outcomes. They stress that biopsy still needs to be performed whether the result of PET is positive or negative to evaluate for both false negatives and false positives. Fleming and colleagues,[19] in their evaluation of PET/CT in patients with previously untreated head and neck cancer, found that of the 22 patients in their series with unknown primary head and neck cancer, PET/CT correctly identified the primary site in 72.7% (16 of 22). Rudmik and colleagues[29] in their evaluation of the clinical utility of PET/CT in the evaluation of head and neck squamous cell carcinoma with an unknown primary tumor found that PET/CT increased the detection of a primary site from 25% to 55%

(5 vs 11 subjects). The researchers conclude that PET/CT performed before panendoscopy will increase the diagnostic yield in the unknown head and neck primary population, leading to more targeted, and less morbid, treatment. Overall, because of the change in management that results from the identification of an unknown primary tumor, it can be concluded that PET/CT is a useful adjunct to diagnosis in patients with an unknown primary tumor.

NON–SQUAMOUS CELL TUMORS
Thyroid

Thryoid cancer may be found incidentally with other cancers of the head and neck.[30] Incidental thyroid nodules are commonly encountered, with prevalence of 4% to 50% depending on demographics and diagnostic method, including autopsy.[30,31] Incidental focal thyroid lesions have been reported on PET in 1% to 4% of patients.[31] The risk of malignancy in these areas of focal uptake has been reported as 14% to 50%.[31] In a study by Kim and colleagues,[31] 159 patients with focal thyroid FDG-avid "incidentalomas" were evaluated during cancer evaluation. The incidence of a focal FDG thyroid incidentaloma was 1.23% with the risk of cancer being 23.3%. SUV_{max} (malignant: median 4.53, range 2.1–12.0; benign: median 3.08, range 1.6–35, $P = .0093$) but not the SUV_{mean} correlated with malignancy, but SUV_{max} had insufficient sensitivity and specificity. The investigators concluded that visual determination of degree of metabolic activity and size are potential predictors for malignancy. For visual grading, they used the liver as a reference, and lesions with greater intensity than liver had the highest likelihood of being malignant (26 of 50 nodules). Nam and colleagues[30] evaluated for the incidence of incidental hypermetabolic lesions in the thyroid gland in patients with nonthyroidal head and neck cancer. They found that 2.8% of 689 patients had incidental focal thyroid lesions on FDG-PET scans. Of these patients, 12 underwent further evaluation and 5 of these had thyroid malignancies, 4 had papillary carcinomas, and 1 had follicular carcinoma (42% malignant). The remaining lesions were follicular adenomas, Hürthle cell adenoma and nodular hyperplasia. These investigators found no significant difference in SUV_{max} between benign and malignant lesions. Eloya and colleagues[32] found incidental focal thyroid lesions on 4.8% of PET scans performed for nonthyroid cancers. They found 27.8% to be malignant tumors and suggested that most patients should undergo surgery because of the high risk of malignancy. Therefore, focal hypermetabolic thyroid lesions found on PET probably should be worked up further because of the relatively high risk of malignancy.

Generally, F18-FDG accumulation in normal thyroid tissue is usually low to absent.[33] Diffuse uptake of the thyroid gland usually represents benign conditions such as thyroiditis or Graves disease.[30] The most frequent cause of diffuse thyroid uptake is Hashimoto thyroiditis (chronic lymphocytic thyroiditis).[34] Chen and colleagues[34] evaluated 2594 PET/CT scans and found increased thyroid uptake in 3.8% of cases, with 1.8% being diffuse and 2.0% being focal. In the 21 patients with diffuse uptake for which they had results of thyroid functional assay and/or ultrasonography, all cases were diagnosed as chronic thyroiditis. Karantanis and colleagues[33] evaluated the clinical significance of diffusely increased uptake in the thyroid gland on PET/CT scans and found that 2.9% of 4732 patients had diffuse uptake (defined as visible on maximum intensity projection (MIP) images with liver windowed as light gray). In all patients in whom clinical information was available, the diffuse uptake corresponded to chronic lymphocytic thyroiditis. The SUV did not correlate with the degree of hypothyroidism or the titer of thyroid peroxidase antibodies.

With regard to thyroid cancer, most patients with the most common types (such as differentiated thyroid cancer [DTC]) are initially treated with thyroidectomy and I-131 ablation.[35] This treatment is then followed with measurement of thyroglobulin levels and cervical ultrasonography. If recurrence is suspected, additional imaging with whole-body I-131 (or I-123) scanning as well as CT and/or MR can be performed. However, not all disease recurrence is iodine avid, and in these cases, PET/CT has been found to be helpful.[35] The Society of Nuclear Medicine recommends that F-18 FDG PET should be routinely performed on patients previously treated for DTC when the findings of radioactive iodine whole-body scintigraphy are negative and the thyroglobulin (Tg) levels are more than 10 ng/mL.[36] Razfar evaluated 121 patients who were previously treated for thyroid cancer and suspected to have recurrence.[35] About 80.6% had negative whole-body I-131 scans. All patients underwent PET/CT, and there were positive findings in 75 patients, 71 of which represented true positives, for a sensitivity of 80.7%, specificity of 88.9%, PPV of 94.7%, and NPV of 65.3%. A total of 60 patients had positive findings on both PET and CT, 6 patients had positive CT findings only, and 5 patients had positive PET findings only, highlighting the importance of carefully evaluating the CT portion of a PET/CT scan. The investigators conclude

that PET/CT performed in patients with thyroid cancer having elevated thyroglobulin levels but non-I-131-avid tumors has high diagnostic accuracy for identifying local, regional, and distant metastases and can frequently guide clinical management. It has been demonstrated that F-18 FDG uptake represents less differentiated thyroid cancer cells or dedifferentiated cells and that PET-positive lesions are more likely to be resistant to 131I treatment.[36]

Some studies have suggested that PET is useful in patients with medullary thyroid carcinoma, particularly in those with elevated levels of calcitonin or other tumor markers and negative results of conventional imaging studies.[36] These same investigators in their review also state that PET is useful for evaluating disease extent and staging in anaplastic thyroid carcinoma and that the amount and degree of FDG uptake may also have additional prognostic significance.

Salivary Glands

For the evaluation, staging, and surveillance of salivary gland tumors, many studies suggest that PET has a role; however, it has been reported that some salivary gland tumors may not demonstrate increased metabolic activity and that some benign salivary gland neoplasms may demonstrate high FDG uptake.[37] A study by Razfar and colleagues[38] evaluated the role of PET/CT in the management of salivary gland malignancies. These investigators administered contrast on the CT portion of the study to obtain a "diagnostic" quality CT scan. They found that for salivary gland malignancies PET/CT had a sensitivity of 74.4%, specificity of 100%, PPV of 100%, and NPV of 61.5%. There was no significant difference in sensitivity between high-grade tumors and low-/intermediate-grade tumors. PET/CT altered or confirmed management in 26 patients (47.3%). It was found that 12 patients (21.8%) had distant metastasis at the time of initial PET/CT scan including 6 lung, 5 bone, 2 distant lymph node, and 1 liver metastases. Interestingly, all 12 of these patients had distant metastasis detected on the CT portion alone. Therefore, the researchers conclude that PET/CT is useful in the initial staging and for surgical and radiation therapy planning but has less added benefit in long-term surveillance and in detecting distant metastasis, where they thought CT with contrast is likely sufficient. Roh and colleagues[37] evaluated the clinical utility of PET in 34 patients with newly diagnosed salivary gland tumors who underwent both CT and PET before treatment and resection. These investigators found that PET had a greater sensitivity than CT for detecting primary tumors as well as metastases. PET only did not detect 3 primary tumors in this study, and this was thought to be due to 2 factors: (1) that salivary gland malignancies generally do not have as high an SUV as other head and neck malignancies such as squamous cell carcinoma and (2) therefore, these lesions are obscured by the normal metabolic activity of the salivary glands. The only metastatic lymph nodes that were not detected were smaller than 5 mm, and this was thought to be due to their small size. Interestingly, all the primary lesions that were not detected by PET were shown by contrast-enhanced CT (and all lesions not detected by CT were shown by PET), so this reinforces the point that both portions of a PET/CT study, or both a diagnostic CT and the PET scan, need to be very carefully evaluated. These investigators concluded that "the roles of 18F-FDG PET in initial staging and monitoring after treatment are significant, potentially affecting management for these patients. Histologic grade may be predicted by 18F-FDG uptake, providing useful preoperative information for surgical planning." However, the investigators did not find a relationship between SUV and survival. Uchida and colleagues[39] found 3 false negatives in their evaluation of PET and scintigraphy for the evaluation of parotid tumors. False-negative cases were found in 1 salivary duct carcinoma (SUV 2.01), 1 mucoepidermoid carcinoma (SUV 2.07), and 1 metastatic tumor of renal cell carcinoma (SUV 2.24). Tumor size of all false-negative cases was small (10 mm, 17 mm, and 20 mm, respectively). It seems that PET/CT may have more benefit for salivary tumors than was originally thought, particularly if both the PET and CT portions of the study are carefully evaluated.

PITFALLS

There are many sources of false-positive and false-negative findings in PET/CT of the head and neck, and these need to be well understood for accurate study interpretation (**Box 1**). In addition to malignancies, increased FDG uptake can be seen in inflammatory and infectious processes, including after radiation therapy.[3] Also, many benign lesions can also have increased metabolic activity such as thyroid adenomas, some salivary neoplasms, Graves disease, Paget disease, and fibrous dysplasia.[3,39] Normal structures such as muscle, brown fat, salivary glands, and lymphoid tissue, particularly the tissues of Waldeyer's ring, can have increased FDG uptake.[3,40] Asymmetric uptake can occur with vocal cord paralysis, resection of one or more salivary glands, and surgical or

---

Box 1
Potential pitfalls in PET/CT

Inflammation

Benign lesions

    Salivary (eg, Warthin tumor)

    Thyroiditis, thyroid adenomas

    Paget disease

    Fibrous dysplasia

Lymphoid tissue

    Waldeyer's ring

Brown fat

Salivary glands

Asymmetric uptake

    Vocal cord paralysis

    Unilateral salivary gland resection, inflammation, or atrophy

    Muscle

Intravenous or enteric contrast

Metallic implants

---

therapy-related changes, and there can be asymmetric muscle uptake.[40] There are also several PET/CT artifacts that do not occur on PET scanners including those due to metallic implants or other devices and dense IV or enteric contrast appearing as hypermetabolic areas. Careful correlation with the uncorrected images and CT images will allow correct interpretation. Many of the areas of increased FDG uptake that caused a diagnostic dilemma are now much less of a problem because of the common use of PET/CT, which allows precise localization of the uptake (such as within brown fat). The reader is directed to the excellent review of physiologic and artifactual uptake by Blodgett and colleagues[40] for a detailed review of this topic. In addition, malignant neoplasms with inherently low metabolic activity, such as some salivary neoplasms, and necrotic metastatic lymph nodes may also cause false-negative PET results.[6] Careful review of the CT images will help alleviate this pitfall.

FUTURE DIRECTIONS AND NEW TECHNIQUES

There are a few new compounds that may have promise for head and neck cancer evaluation and treatment planning including C11-acetate, C11-choline, F18-fluoromisonidazole (F18-FMISO), and 3'-deoxy-3'-18F-fluorothymidine (F18-FLT). These compounds overall may have the most use in targeting and modifying treatment, as well as assessing treatment efficacy. 1-C11-acetate (ACE) has been used to attempt to evaluate regions of tumor hypoxia. ACE is trapped in all tumor cells after conversion to C11-acetyl-CoA, but after oxidative metabolism, the $C11\text{-}CO_2$ created diffuses out of the cells. Therefore, it is retained in hypoxic cells. Tumor hypoxia has been said to be an important factor in determining treatment response.[41] Sun and colleagues[42] demonstrated that complete responders to radiation therapy had a higher oxidative metabolic rate than nonresponders (ie, nonresponders had greater tumor hypoxia) on initial scans. F18-FMISO also may have promise in detecting areas of tumor hypoxia. This compound diffuses into cells and becomes essentially trapped and bound to macromolecules under hypoxic conditions. However, imaging with this compound is faced with the disadvantage of decreased count statistics and increased image noise at the long delayed time points required for imaging. Combining delayed imaging with kinetic markers can increase the diagnostic yield.[43] Hendrickson and colleagues[44] evaluated whether using F18-FMISO could localize areas of tumor hypoxia for radiation dose escalation or dose boost to these regions and if this would have an effect on calculated estimated tumor control probability. They found that tumor control probability could be increased by 17% without an unacceptable increase in normal tissue complication probabilities. Rajendran and colleagues[45] used FMISO using a similar technique and evaluated the relationship of tumor hypoxia and the volume of hypoxic tumor to survival. They found an inverse relationship between length of survival and these variables. FMISO scanning has been used in clinical trials for chemotherapy agents targeting hypoxic cells.[46]

Another tumor characteristic that affects treatment outcome is accelerated tumor repopulation during therapy. F18-FLT uptake is enhanced during DNA synthesis and therefore provides a noninvasive way to image tumor cell proliferation.[47] Troost and colleagues[47] evaluated the feasibility of targeting Intensity-Modulated Radiation Therapy (IMRT) boost doses or dose escalation to areas of increased cellular proliferation based on FLT PET in oropharyngeal tumors. The investigators concluded that FLT is useful for early tumor response assessment and that FLT PET can define tumor subvolumes with high proliferative activity, and escalation of radiation dose within these regions is technically feasible. Menda and colleagues[48] investigated the kinetic behavior of F18-FLT before and early after the initiation of chemoradiation therapy in patients with squamous cell head and neck cancer. The researchers concluded that the initial F18-FLT uptake and

change early after treatment in squamous head and neck tumors can be adequately characterized with SUV obtained at 45 to 60 min, which demonstrates excellent correlation with influx parameters obtained from compartmental and Patlak analyses. C11-choline is a precursor for the biosynthesis of phosphatidylcholine and is incorporated into cells. This compound is potentially a useful tracer for detecting malignant tumors with elevated levels of phosphatidylcholine in the cell membrane. Ito and colleagues[49] evaluated whether a posttreatment F18-FDG PET or C11-choline PET scan obtained at 8 to 12 weeks after treatment was better at predicting tumor recurrence and also determined the best timing for the second follow-up scan. C11-choline turned out to be inferior to FDG for the detection of head and neck cancer, except at the skull base. This compound may have promise as a complementary study to FDG PET when patients present with tumors in this location.

SUMMARY

PET/CT has many uses in head and neck cancer, including the initial workup in cases of unknown primary tumors, for staging and restaging, and for tumor surveillance. These uses have been validated in the literature and are becoming standard practice. Additional uses for PET/CT are treatment planning and possibly helping to determine prognosis. Future uses may involve isotopes other than FDG and potential uses in further targeting and tailoring treatment.

REFERENCES

1. Johnson NW, Amarasinghe HK. Epidemiology and aetiology of head and neck cancers. In: Berner J, editor. Head and neck cancer: Multimodality management. New York: Springer Science+Business Media; 2011. p. 1–40.
2. Xu GZ, Guan DJ, He ZY. (18)FDG-PET/CT for detecting distant metastases and second primary cancers in patients with head and neck cancer. A meta-analysis. Oral Oncol 2011;47(7):560–5.
3. Fletcher JW, Djulbegovic B, Soares HP, et al. Recommendations on the use of 18F-FDG PET in oncology. J Nucl Med 2008;49:480–508.
4. Som PM. Detection of metastasis in cervical lymph nodes: CT and MR criteria and differential diagnosis. AJR Am J Roentgenol 1992;158(5):961–9.
5. Ozer E, Naiboğlu B, Meacham R, et al. The value of PET/CT to assess clinically negative necks. Eur Arch Otorhinolaryngol 2012;269(11):2411–4.
6. Fukui MB, Blodgett TM, Snyderman CH, et al. Combined PET-CT in the head and neck: part 2.

Diagnostic uses and pitfalls of oncologic imaging. Radiographics 2005;25(4):913–30.

7. Korn RL, Coates A, Milstine J. The role of glucose and FDG metabolism in the interpretation of PET studies. In: Lin E, Alavi A, editors. PET and PET/CT: a clinical guide. 2nd edition. New York: Thieme Medical Publishing; 2009. p. 22–9, Chapter 3.

8. Escott EJ. Positron emission tomography-computed tomography protocol considerations for head and neck cancer imaging. Semin Ultrasound CT MR 2008;29(4):263–70.

9. Wong TZ, Fras IM. PET/CT protocols and practical issues for the evaluation of patients with head and neck cancer. PET Clin 2007;2(4):413–21.

10. Branstetter BF 4th, Blodgett TM, Zimmer LA, et al. Head and neck malignancy: is PET/CT more accurate than PET or CT alone? Radiology 2005;235(2): 580–6.

11. Jeong HS, Baek CH, Son YI, et al. Use of integrated 18F-FDG PET/CT to improve the accuracy of initial cervical nodal evaluation in patients with head and neck squamous cell carcinoma. Head Neck 2007; 29(3):203–10.

12. Syed R, Bomanji JB, Nagabhushan N, et al. Impact of combined (18)F-FDG PET/CT in head and neck tumours. Br J Cancer 2005;92(6):1046–50.

13. Higgins KA, Hoang JK, Roach MC, et al. Analysis of pretreatment FDG-PET. Int J Radiat Oncol Biol Phys 2012;82(2):548–53.

14. Xie P, Li M, Zhao H, et al. 18F-FDG PET or PET-CT to evaluate prognosis for head and neck cancer: a meta-analysis. J Cancer Res Clin Oncol 2011; 137(7):1085–93.

15. Torizuka T, Tanizaki Y, Kanno T, et al. Prognostic value of 18F-FDG PET in patients with head and neck squamous cell cancer. AJR Am J Roentgenol 2009;192:W156–60.

16. Schinagl DA, Span PN, Oyen WJ, et al. Can FDG PET predict radiation treatment outcome in head and neck cancer? Results of a prospective study. Eur J Nucl Med Mol Imaging 2011;38(8):1449–58.

17. Stoeckli SJ, Haerle SK, Strobel K, et al. Initial staging of the neck in head and neck squamous cell carcinoma: a comparison of CT, PET/CT, and ultrasound-guided fine-needle aspiration cytology. Head Neck 2012;34(4):469–76.

18. Kyzas PA, Evangelou E, Denaxa-Kyza D, et al. 18F-fluorodeoxyglucose positron emission tomography to evaluate cervical node metastases in patients with head and neck squamous cell carcinoma: a meta-analysis. J Natl Cancer Inst 2008;100(10): 712–20.

19. Fleming AJ Jr, Smith SP Jr, Paul CM, et al. Impact of [18F]-2-fluorodeoxyglucose-positron emission tomography/computed tomography on previously untreated head and neck cancer patients. Laryngoscope 2007;117(7):1173–9.

20. Patz EF Jr, Lowe VJ, Hoffman JM, et al. Focal pulmonary abnormalities: evaluation with F-18 fluorodeoxyglucose PET scanning. Radiology 1993;188(2): 487–90.

21. Hafidh MA, Lacy PD, Hughes JP, et al. Evaluation of the impact of addition of PET to CT and MR scanning in the staging of patients with head and neck carcinomas. Eur Arch Otorhinolaryngol 2006; 263(9):853–9.

22. Yoon DY, Hwang HS, Chang SK, et al. CT, MR, US, 18F-FDG PET/CT, and their combined use for the assessment of cervical lymph node metastases in squamous cell carcinoma of the head and neck. Eur Radiol 2009;19(3):634–42.

23. Xu GZ, Zhu XD, Li MY. Accuracy of whole-body PET and PET-CT in initial M staging of head and neck cancer: a meta-analysis. Head Neck 2011;33:87–94.

24. Gupta T, Master Z, Kannan S, et al. Diagnostic performance of post-treatment FDG PET or FDG PET/CT imaging in head and neck cancer: a systematic review and meta-analysis. Eur J Nucl Med Mol Imaging 2011;38:2083–209.

25. Andrade RS, Heron DE, Degirmenci B, et al. Post-treatment assessment of response using FDG-PET/CT for patients treated with definitive radiation therapy for head and neck cancers. Int J Radiat Oncol Biol Phys 2006;65(5):1315–22.

26. Issing WJ, Taleban B, Tauber S. Diagnosis and management of carcinoma of unknown primary in the head and neck. Eur Arch Otorhinolaryngol 2003; 260(8):436–43.

27. Keller F, Psychogios G, Linke R, et al. Carcinoma of unknown primary in the head and neck: comparison between positron emission tomography (PET) and PET/CT. Head Neck 2011;33(11):1569–75.

28. Pattani KM, Goodier M, Lilien D, et al. Utility of panendoscopy for the detection of unknown primary head and neck cancer in patients with a negative PET/CT scan. Ear Nose Throat J 2011;90(8):E16–20.

29. Rudmik L, Lau HY, Matthews TW, et al. Clinical utility of PET/CT in the evaluation of head and neck squamous cell carcinoma with an unknown primary: a prospective clinical trial. Head Neck 2011;33(7): 935–40.

30. Nam SY, Roh JL, Kim JS, et al. Focal uptake of 18F-fluorodeoxyglucose by thyroid in patients with non-thyroidal head and neck cancers. Clin Endocrinol 2007;67:135–9.

31. Kim BH, Na MA, Kim IJ, et al. Risk stratification and prediction of cancer of focal thyroid fluorodeoxyglucose uptake during cancer evaluation. Ann Nucl Med 2010;24(10):721–8.

32. Eloya JA, Bretta EM, Fatterpekara GM, et al. The significance and management of incidental [18F]fluorodeoxyglucose–positron-emission tomography uptake in the thyroid gland in patients with cancer. AJNR Am J Neuroradiol 2009;30:1431–4.

33. Karantanis D, Bogsrud TV, Wiseman GA, et al. Clinical significance of diffusely increased 18F-FDG uptake in the thyroid gland. J Nucl Med 2007;48:896–901.

34. Chen W, Parsons M, Torigian D, et al. Evaluation of thyroid FDG uptake incidentally identified on FDG-PET/CT imaging. Nucl Med Commun 2009;30(3):240–4.

35. Razfar A, Branstetter BF 4th, Christopoulos A, et al. Clinical usefulness of positron emission tomography-computed tomography in recurrent thyroid carcinoma. Arch Otolaryngol Head Neck Surg 2010; 136(2):120–5.

36. Mosci C, Iagaru A. PET/CT imaging of thyroid cancer. Clin Nucl Med 2011;36(12):e180–5.

37. Roh JL, Ryu CH, Choi SH, et al. Clinical utility of 18F-FDG PET for patients with salivary gland malignancies. J Nucl Med 2007;48(2):240–6.

38. Razfar A, Heron DE, Branstetter BF 4th, et al. Positron emission tomography-computed tomography adds to the management of salivary gland malignancies. Laryngoscope 2010;120(4):734–8.

39. Uchida Y, Minoshima S, Kawata T, et al. Diagnostic value of FDG PET and salivary gland scintigraphy for parotid tumors. Clin Nucl Med 2005;30(3):170–6.

40. Blodgett TM, Fukui MB, Snyderman CH, et al. Combined PET-CT in the head and neck: part 1. Physiologic, altered physiologic, and artifactual FDG uptake. Radiographics 2005;25(4):897–912.

41. Hoogsteen IJ, Marres HA, Bussink J, et al. Tumor microenvironment in head and neck squamous cell carcinomas: predictive value and clinical relevance of hypoxic markers. A review. Head Neck 2007;29:591–604.

42. Sun A, Sörensen J, Karlsson M, et al. 1-[11C]-acetate PET imaging in head and neck cancer—a comparison with 18F-FDG-PET: implications for staging and radiotherapy planning. Eur J Nucl Med Mol Imaging 2007;34:651–65.

43. Wang W, Lee NY, Georgi JC, et al. Pharmacokinetic analysis of hypoxia (18)F-fluoromisonidazole dynamic PET in head and neck cancer. J Nucl Med 2010;51(1):37–45.

44. Hendrickson K, Phillips M, Smith W, et al. Hypoxia imaging with [F-18] FMISO-PET in head and neck cancer: potential for guiding intensity modulated radiation therapy in overcoming hypoxia-induced treatment resistance. Radiother Oncol 2011;101(3):369–75.

45. Rajendran JG, Schwartz DL, O'Sullivan J, et al. Tumor hypoxia imaging with [F-18] fluoromisonidazole positron emission tomography in head and neck cancer. Clin Cancer Res 2006;12(18):5435–41.

46. Rischin D, Peters L, Hicks R, et al. Phase I trial of concurrent tirapazamine, cisplatin, and radiotherapy in patients with advanced head and neck cancer. J Clin Oncol 2001;19(2):535–42.

47. Troost EG, Bussink J, Hoffmann AL, et al. 18F-FLT PET/CT for early response monitoring and dose escalation in oropharyngeal tumors. J Nucl Med 2010;51(6):866–74.

48. Menda Y, Boles Ponto LL, Dornfeld KJ, et al. Kinetic analysis of 3'-deoxy-3'-(18)F-fluorothymidine ((18)F-FLT) in head and neck cancer patients before and early after initiation of chemoradiation therapy. J Nucl Med 2009;50(7):1028–35.

49. Ito K, Yokoyama J, Kubota K, et al. 18F-FDG versus 11C-choline PET/CT for the imaging of advanced head and neck cancer after combined intra-arterial chemotherapy and radiotherapy: the time period during which PET/CT can reliably detect non-recurrence. Eur J Nucl Med Mol Imaging 2010;37(7):1318–27.

PET/CT in Gynecologic Malignancies

Jacqueline Brunetti, MD[a,b,*]

KEYWORDS

- FDG-PET • PET/CT • Ovarian cancer • Cervical cancer • Endometrial cancer

KEY POINTS

- Ovarian cancer and malignancies of the uterine cervix and corpus are the most commonly encountered gynecologic neoplasms in clinical practice.
- Fluorodeoxyglucose (FDG)-PET and PET/computed tomography (CT) are of little value in both diagnosis and early stage of gynecologic malignancy.
- FDG-PET and PET/CT provide accurate detection of metastatic disease in advanced malignancy and better delineation of recurrent disease compared with conventional imaging.

INTRODUCTION

The clinical usefulness of any imaging modality can be best determined by assessing the impact on decisions regarding diagnosis, disease treatment, and effect on patient outcome. This situation requires an understanding of the pathophysiology of the specific disease and the current accepted methods of diagnosis, initial staging, and restaging as well as treatment options. With current economic constraints on the availability of health care dollars, it is increasingly important for the imaging specialist to understand the specific disease state to recommend the imaging modality that gives the most accurate information at the least cost. For many malignancies, fluorodeoxyglucose (FDG)PET/computed tomography (CT) aids in optimized therapy decisions by providing the most precise information regarding local staging, identification of distant metastases, and possible synchronous neoplasm. For gynecologic malignancies (specifically, ovarian and endometrial cancers), treatment decisions are based on surgical staging of disease. Cervical cancer, on the other hand, is staged clinically. For each of these

malignancies, FDG-PET/CT can provide information that can improve therapy decision making when used in the appropriate clinical setting.

OVARIAN CANCER
Introduction

The American Cancer Society reports that approximately 22,000 women are diagnosed with ovarian cancer each year. Fifty percent of patients present with advanced (stage III or IV) disease. Ovarian cancer is a diverse group of malignancies that can occur in any age group, with highest incidence older than 65 years. Approximately 10% of ovarian cancers are related to specific genetic mutations. These mutations include mutations in tumor suppressor genes, BRCA 1 and BRCA 2, Lynch 2 syndrome (colorectal and extracolonic tumors), basal cell nevis syndrome, and multiple endocrine neoplasia type 1. Ninety percent of ovarian cancer is termed sporadic (ie, acquired).[1] A novel approach to classification of ovarian cancers groups the malignancies according to molecular and genetic features.[2] Type I tumors, approximately 25% of ovarian neoplasms,

Disclosures: None.
[a] Department of Radiology, Holy Name Medical Center, 718 Teaneck Road, Teaneck, NJ 07666, USA;
[b] NewYork-Presbyterian Hospital/Columbia University Medical Center, 177 Fort Washington Avenue, New York, NY 10032, USA
* Department of Radiology, Holy Name Medical Center, 718 Teaneck Road, Teaneck, NJ 07666.
E-mail address: brunetti@mail.holyname.org

typically are confined to the ovary at diagnosis and have an indolent course. This group includes low-grade serous, low-grade endometrioid, clear cell, and mucinous tumors. Type II tumors (75% of ovarian lesions), are high-grade serous and undifferentiated carcinomas and mixed meso-dermal tumors. Type II tumors typically present in advanced-stage and are responsible for 90% of ovarian cancer deaths. Best survival is achieved with early diagnosis and optimized tumor debulking.[3]

Diagnosis

Early diagnosis of ovarian cancer remains an enigma in clinical practice because of nonspecific symptomatology and lack of accurate screening methods. Consequently, two-thirds of ovarian cancers present at stage III or IV. Although epithelial cancer, which is responsible for 90% of ovarian malignancy, expresses a glycolytic phenotype that results in uptake of FDG, the sensitivity, specificity, and accuracy of FDG-PET and PET/CT in diagnosis vary significantly with lesion size and cellularity.[4] Although GLUT-1 overexpression, the basis of FDG uptake, is associated with reduced disease-free survival, the prognostic value of primary ovarian tumor standardized uptake value (SUV) has not been established.[5-7] Moreover, there is significant overlap in FDG uptake between benign and malignant lesions, as corpus luteum cysts, endometriomas, serous cystadenomas, and thecomas may show FDG uptake.[8] Normal physiologic uptake is also seen in the ovaries, particularly during the luteal phase (**Fig. 1**).

Consequently, incidental adnexal uptake on FDG-PET/CT should be interpreted with care, taking into account patient age, menstrual status, medications that may produce hormonal effect as well as the patient's primary tumor histology, specifically with respect to potential of adnexal metastatic disease. In the postmenopausal age group, adnexal deposition of FDG must be considered pathologic. Ovarian uptake of FDG should be evaluated with ultrasonography to differentiate benign from malignant disease.

FDG-PET and Initial Staging

The primary pattern of metastatic disease in ovarian cancer is serosal and is undetected by conventional imaging modalities until tumor bulk is sufficient to present as macroscopic foci greater than 0.5 mm (**Fig. 2**). Ovarian cancer is staged surgically, and tumor stage is based on histopathology of the primary lesion, the status of the uterus and contralateral ovary, pelvic, and retroperitoneal nodes, the omentum, and peritoneal surfaces (**Table 1**). Patient survival is directly related to the success of resection of all visible tumor, and unsuccessful debulking surgery (ie, residual tumor >1 cm) increases morbidity and

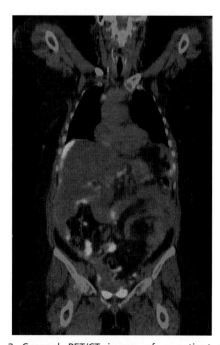

Fig. 2. Coronal PET/CT image of a patient with stage IV ovarian cancer shows typical plaquelike peritoneal metabolic uptake, indicating extensive serosal metastatic disease involving the liver and the pelvis. Nodal metastases are evident in the epigastrium and mediastinum.

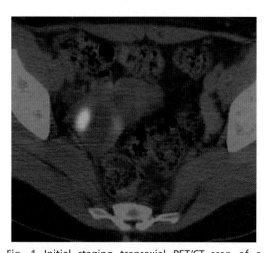

Fig. 1. Initial staging transaxial PET/CT scan of a 38-year-old woman shows focal FDG uptake in the wall of a right ovarian serous cystadenoma and low-level metabolic uptake in the left ovary, found to be histologically normal at surgery.

Table 1	
FIGO staging of ovarian cancer	
Stage	**Description**
I	Limited to ovaries
IA	1 ovary, capsule intact
IB	Both ovaries, capsules intact
IC	1 or both ovaries with capsule rupture, serosal tumor, ascites
II	1 or both ovaries with pelvic extension
IIA	Extension to uterus or tubes
IIB	Extension to other pelvic organs
IIC	Pelvic extension and malignant ascites
III	1 or both ovaries with microscopic peritoneal disease
IIIA	Microscopic peritoneal spread beyond pelvis
IIIB	Macroscopic peritoneal spread ≤ 2 cm
IIIC	Macroscopic peritoneal spread >2 cm or regional nodes
IV	Distant metastases (excluding peritoneal metastases)

Data from Benedet JL, Bender H, Jones H 3rd, et al. FIGO staging classifications and clinical practice guidelines in the management of gynecologic cancers. FIGO Committee on Gynecologic Oncology. Int J Gynaecol Obstet 2000;70(2):241.

cost without any gain in survival. Neoadjuvant chemotherapy is used to reduce tumor burden and optimize debulking. Although laparotomy remains the gold standard for staging, there are increasing data regarding the use of laparoscopy to not only predict the success of cytoreductive surgery but also for primary staging. Survival rates of early ovarian cancer staged laparoscopically are approximately 90% and similar to that reported with laparotomy.[9] Laparoscopy is beneficial in confirming extent of disease before primary cytoreductive surgery and thus avoiding futile debulking procedures.[10,11] PET/CT, used in combination with laparoscopy, can improve detection of metastatic foci within the abdomen and pelvis and therefore improve debulking outcomes.[12] PET/CT has been shown to be more accurate than CT and magnetic resonance (MR) imaging in identification of extra-abdominal metastatic lymphadenopathy adenopathy as well as detection of unexpected second primary malignancies (**Fig. 3**).[13,14] Detection of mediastinal metastatic lymphadenopathy on PET/CT in patients with advanced ovarian cancer is associated with higher mortality.[15] A preoperative PET/CT in patients with advanced ovarian cancer may alter therapy, direct surgery, and provide a baseline for subsequent treatment monitoring.

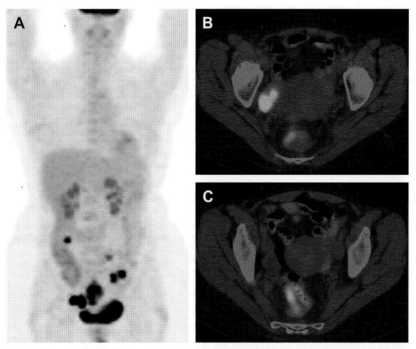

Fig. 3. Whole-body PET scan (*A*) of a 60-year-old woman with newly diagnosed ovarian cystadenocarcinoma with peritoneal metastases and coexisting sigmoid adenocarcinoma. Transaxial PET/CT (*B*) of the same patient shows intense metabolic activity within the right ovarian malignancy, low-level, normal physiologic uptake in the endometrium and left ovary and increased metabolic activity in the partially visualized rectosigmoid lesion. Transaxial PET/CT (*C*) shows hypermetabolic activity within the rectosigmoid adenocarcinoma and benign physiologic activity within the uterine endometrium.

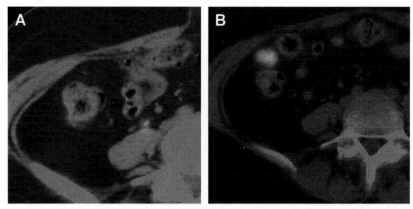

Fig. 4. Restaging transaxial PET/CT scan (*A*) of a 65-year-old woman with CA 125 level of 30.5 U/mL shows a 2.8-mm ametabolic mesenteric nodule in the right lower quadrant. A transaxial PET/CT scan (*B*) of the same patient, 11 months later, shows interval increase in size of the mesenteric nodule that is now 2.6 cm and shows metabolic uptake with SUV$_{max}$ 14.4. CA 125 level at the time of the second scan was 40.7 U/mL.

FDG-PET and Monitoring Therapy and Restaging

Physical examination and serial serum CA 125 determination are used for surveillance after primary therapy, with additional contrast-enhanced CT for investigation of symptoms or suspected recurrence. Detection of localized or disseminated recurrence dictates therapy choice. Although there is no confirmed survival benefit documented with early detection of metastatic disease, early intervention may delay onset of symptoms resulting from tumor burden, thereby improving quality of life for these patients.[16–18]

The established upper limit of normal for serum CA 125 is 35 U/mL and increasing levels after therapy highly correlate with changing tumor burden.[19] However, detecting residual or recurrent tumor solely by means of serum tumor marker fails to identify approximately 50% of patients with tumor, particularly those with tumor foci less than 2 cm (**Fig. 4**).[20–22]

PET/CT has been shown to be an effective imaging tool in patients with increased CA 125 level as well as in the setting of normal CA 125 level and clinical symptoms of recurrence. Detection of tumor recurrence has been shown to be better than conventional imaging, and accuracy and positive predictive value of FDG-PET/CT are reported to be greater than 90% (**Figs. 5–7**).[23–27] Most significant is the ability to detect tumor recurrence in the presence of normal CA 125 level. Review of uncorrected PET images aids in identification of subtle foci of uptake in metastases that might be overlooked (**Box 1, Fig. 8**).

CANCER OF THE UTERINE CERVIX
Introduction

Unlike ovarian cancer, cervical cancer is easily diagnosed in early and premalignant stage by Pap smear. The wide-scale adoption of cervical cancer screening with the Pap test has resulted in decreases in both incidence and mortality over the last 40 years. Risk factors for development of cervical malignancy include smoking, number of sexual partners, early age of first coitus, diethylstilbestrol exposure, compromised immune system,

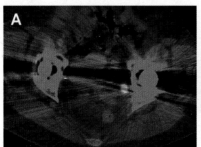
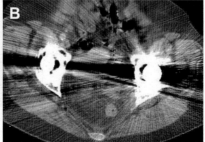

Fig. 5. Transaxial PET/CT (*A*) shows a focal metastasis in the left obturator region not visible on CT (*B*) because of scanning artifacts related to bilateral hip prostheses.

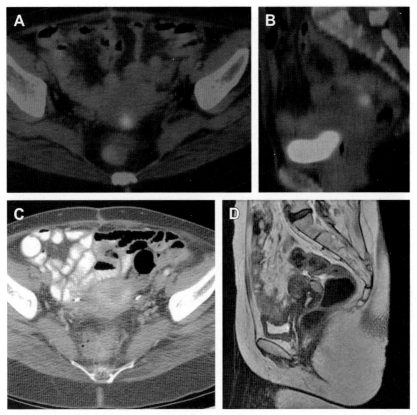

Fig. 6. Transaxial (*A*) and sagittal (*B*) restaging PET/CT images of a 45-year-old patient with ovarian cancer, status after oophorectomy with CA 125 level of 11.0 U/mL, showing focal increased metabolic activity on the posterior surface of the uterine fundus. Transaxial contrast-enhanced CT (*C*) shows subtle infiltrative soft tissue density posterior to the uterus, but identification of a focal fundal lesions is difficult. In a patient in this age group, the differential diagnosis includes both metastatic disease and uterine myoma. Sagittal T2 MR image (*D*) is definitive for a localized cystic serosal metastasis, confirmed as papillary serous adenocarcinoma at surgery.

long-term oral contraceptive use, and human papillomavirus (HPV).[28] Of the 100 recognized HPV viruses, HPV types 16 and 18 are oncogenic and responsible for approximately 75% of cervical cancers. The US Centers for Disease Control report that more than 10,000 new cases of HPV-associated cervical cancer are diagnosed in the United States each year. Although most HPV infections regress spontaneously in immunocompetent individuals, the high prevalence of HPV infection and the known oncogenic effects of the virus have led to development of vaccines that have been shown in phase III trials to have 100% efficacy in prevention of cervical dysplastic lesions

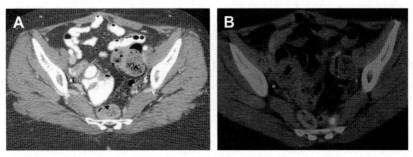

Fig. 7. Transaxial contrast-enhanced CT (*A*) and transaxial PET/CT (*B*) show a focal ovarian metastasis in the left presacral region. Although visible on the contrast-enhanced CT, it is easily overlooked, because it is similar in appearance to neighboring vessels.

that are precursors of invasive cervical cancer.[29] Vaccination has been recommended in females aged 9 to 26 years.

The histology of 95% of invasive cervical cancer is squamous cell with less than 5% being adenocarcinomas. Invasive cancer is preceded by dysplastic changes in the cervical squamous epithelium. If undetected in premalignant stage, cervical cancer invades the cervical stroma and spreads by direct invasion into the adjacent parametrium, uterine body, and vagina, then via lymphatics to pelvic, para-aortic, and supraclavicular nodes. Hematogenous dissemination typically occurs in more advanced disease. Treatment and survival are dictated by stage at diagnosis. The status of para-aortic lymph nodes directs therapy.

FDG-PET and Initial Staging

The Federation of Gynecology and Obstetrics (FIGO) staging of cancer of the uterine cervix is based on parameters of anatomic and compartmental spread (Table 2). Although recent advances in tumor imaging have influenced the staging of other malignancies, the FIGO staging system has remained essentially unchanged because of the unavailability of state-of-the-art imaging technology in developing nations, where there is a high incidence of cervical malignancy.

Carcinoma in situ and stage IA lesions are treated with resection, with expected 5-year survival of 93%. Locally invasive cancers can be managed with surgery, radiation, or a combination of surgery with preoperative adjuvant therapy and advanced disease with chemoradiation. The 5- year survival of patients with stage IV cancer is 16% (Fig. 9). The status of para-aortic lymph nodes and parametrial surgical margins dictates prognosis. The incidence of metastatic lymphadenopathy increases with FIGO stage. The presence of supraclavicular metastatic adenopathy is associated with extremely poor prognosis (Fig. 10).[30,31] Cervical cancer shows a glycolytic phenotype and imaging with FDG-PET/CT has been shown to be more accurate than conventional imaging with CT and MR imaging for detection of pelvic and para-aortic nodes.[32] Although published data show a high degree of accuracy for FDG-PET/CT in detection of metastatic lymphadenopathy, the sensitivity for detection of both pelvic and para-aortic lymph node metastases in early-stage cervical cancer is low, and, therefore, FDG-PET/CT cannot replace lymphadenectomy in the setting of early-stage disease (Table 3).[33–37]

The likelihood of a positive finding on FDG-PET/CT correlates with disease stage and tumor

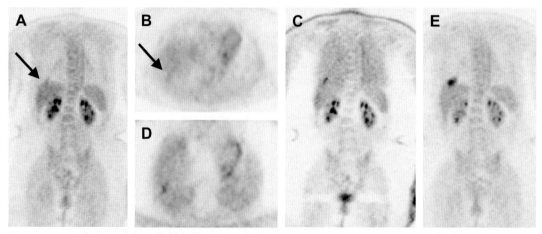

Fig. 8. Coronal (A) and transaxial (B) PET scans show a subtle focus of increased metabolic activity at the right lung base (arrow), which is best shown on the coronal image. On nonattenuation corrected coronal (C) and transaxial (D) images of the same patient, this region of focal uptake is accentuated. The CT image failed to show abnormality at this site. A coronal PET image of the same patient 9 months later (E) clearly shows focal metabolic activity, which on CT corresponded to a subdiaphragmatic hepatic serosal implant.

Table 2
FIGO staging of carcinoma of the uterine cervix

Stage	Description
0	Intraepithelial neoplasia, carcinoma in situ
I	Confined to cervix
IA1	Minimal microscopic stromal invasion
IA2	<5 mm depth invasion, <7 mm lateral spread
IB	>7 mm lateral spread
IIA	Invasion beyond cervix, upper 2/3rds vagina
IIB	Invasion of upper 2/3rds vagina and parametrial infiltration
III	Invasion to lateral pelvic sidewall, lower one-third vagina or hydronephrosis
IV	Invasion of urinary bladder mucosa, rectum or beyond pelvis

Data from Benedet JL, Bender H, Jones H 3rd, et al. FIGO staging classifications and clinical practice guidelines in the management of gynecologic cancers. FIGO Committee on Gynecologic Oncology. Int J Gynaecol Obstet 2000;70(2):223.

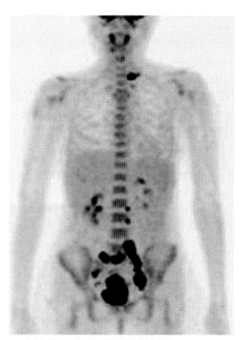

Fig. 10. Initial staging whole-body PET scan of a 36-year-old patient diagnosed with squamous cell cancer of the cervix shows intense metabolic activity within the cervical mass and metastatic adenopathy in pelvic, left para-aortic retroperitoneal, and left supraclavicular nodes.

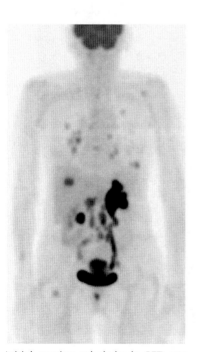

Fig. 9. Initial staging whole-body PET scan of an 86-year-old patient with stage IV cervical cancer showing pelvic, nodal, pulmonary, hepatic, and osseous metastases as well as left hydronephrosis caused by distal ureteral obstruction by the advanced cervical malignancy.

volume, and the sensitivity of FDG-PET/CT for detection of metastases in patients with advanced-stage disease increases to 95%.[38–40] In the setting of advanced cervical cancer, FDG-positive extrapelvic lymphadenopathy may alter therapy choice but does not alter the initial clinical stage. FDG-PET/CT is routinely used to optimize radiation therapy planning in advanced stage disease, and results of FDG-PET/CT modify treatment volumes in approximately 30% of patients; more precise definition of metastatic disease allows escalation of radiation dose, potentially improving local response (Fig. 11).

A pretreatment PET/CT provides prognostic information regarding survival that is not obtained by clinical staging. Overexpression of GLUT-1 transporters in various neoplasms typically correlates with degree of tumor aggressiveness and in cervical cancer correlates with quantitative SUV_{max} measurements but not FIGO stage or initial tumor grade.[41] A high SUV_{max} (>10) in the primary cervical neoplasm and pelvic nodes as well as FDG-positive para-aortic lymph nodes is associated with poor outcomes, with SUV of pelvic nodes being an independent prognostic factor for posttreatment persistent disease.[42–49] SUV_{max} is a useful biomarker in patients who have cervical

Table 3
FDG-PET/CT: detection of lymph node metastases in early-stage cervical cancer

Reference	Number of Patients	Stage	Sensitivity (%)	Specificity (%)	Positive Predictive Value (%)	Negative Predictive Value (%)
Chung et al,[35] 2009	34	IA2-IIB	36.4	98.8	85.7	88.9
Signorelli et al,[37] 2011	159	IB1-IIa	32.1	96.9	69.2	87
Ramirez et al,[33] 2011	60	IB2-IVa	36	96		
Leblanc et al,[34] 2011	125	IB2-IVA	33.3	94.2	53.8	87.5

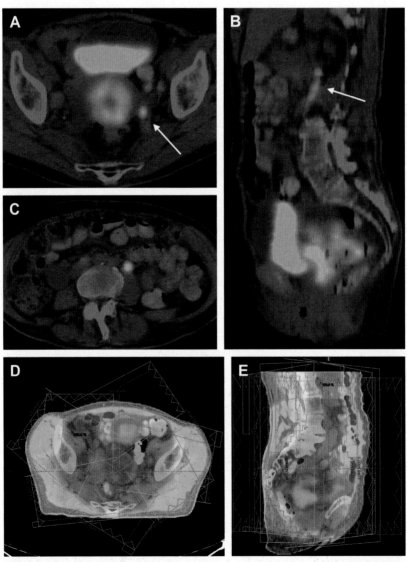

Fig. 11. PET/CT images of a 54-year-old patient with stage IV cervical cancer invading the urinary bladder and rectum with metastatic pelvic and retroperitoneal adenopathy. Transaxial PET/CT image (A) demonstrates intense activity within the cervical lesion and lower level activity within bilateral pelvic nodes. An obstructed ureter, not to be confused with pathologic adenopathy, is seen in the left hemipelvis (arrows) on fused axial (A, C) PET/CT images. Sagittal PET/CT image (B) demonstrated hypermetabolic activity within the bulk cervical mass inseparable from the bladder and rectum with a dilated ureter (arrow) in the retroperitoneum. Fused axial (D) and sagittal (E) PET/CT radiation planning demonstrate a palliative IMRT planning target volume that encompasses the pelvis and paraortic nodes.

cancer predicting treatment response, risk of pelvic recurrence, and disease-free survival and may influence initial treatment planning and surveillance.[50–53]

FDG-PET and Monitoring Therapy and Restaging

Relapse occurs within the first 2 years after therapy. Posttherapy surveillance protocols typically include physical examination, cervical and vaginal cytology, and chest radiograph obtained at recommended intervals for 5 years. The 2012 National Comprehensive Cancer Network (NCCN) guidelines for cervical cancer surveillance also include PET/CT for patients at high risk for local-regional failure.[54] Accurate detection of asymptomatic persistent or recurrent disease may allow early initiation of therapy that could affect both quality of life and survival outcomes. Sensitivity rates of 86% to 100% have been reported for detection of recurrent or persistent tumor with FDG-PET/CT.[55–57] Pattern of metabolic response after primary therapy for cervical cancer is predictive of disease-free interval and overall survival. Patients whose posttherapy PET/CT shows progressive disease have a significantly decreased overall survival (0%–18%) compared with those patients with complete metabolic response (86%–99%) (Box 2).[58–60]

ENDOMETRIAL CANCER
Introduction

The American Cancer Society estimated that more than 47,000 new cases of cancer of the uterine corpus would be diagnosed for 2012. This estimate represents approximately 4 times the number of newly diagnosed cervical cancers. Risk factors include abdominal obesity, multiparity, late menopause, smoking, unopposed estrogen therapy, tamoxifen, Lynch syndrome, and diabetes. Long-term unopposed estrogen therapy, no longer prescribed for treatment of menopause, was associated with a 2 to 10 times increased risk.[61]

Most patients are postmenopausal, but 20% to 25% present in the premenopausal age group. Two histologic subtypes of endometrial carcinoma are identified: type 1 estrogen-associated carcinoma accounts for approximately 75% to 80% of cases and is related to estrogen excess and is well differentiated and classified as endometrioid adenocarcinoma cell type; type 2 estrogen-independent cancers are aggressive, undifferentiated tumors of serous or clear cell type and typically develop in atrophic endometrium, as might occur in elderly women or after pelvic irradiation.[62,63]

Patients typically present with postmenopausal bleeding and combination of postmenopausal bleeding, and sonographic documentation of endometrial thickness greater than 3 mm is highly suggestive of malignancy and should warrant hysteroscopy and curettage.[64,65] The clinical onset of abnormal vaginal bleeding that occurs early in this disease results in 75% of patients being diagnosed at an early stage.

Endometrial cancer is staged surgically, including total abdominal hysterectomy, bilateral salpingo-oophorectomy, pelvic and para-aortic lymphadenectomy (Table 4). Treatment and prognosis are dictated by the surgical stage, as identified by tumor size, depth of myometrial invasion, lymphovascular invasion, lymph node status, and histologic subtype.

Box 2
FDG-PET/CT: cervical cancer

- Improved detection of metastatic disease in locally advanced cancers
  - Little value in early-stage disease
- Improved treatment planning
- Improved detection of recurrence
  - Asymptomatic patients
  - Unexplained increased tumor markers
- Possible prognostic value of SUV_{max} of pelvic nodal metastases

---

Table 4
FIGO staging: endometrial cancer

IA	Confined to uterus, <50% myometrial invasion
IB	Confined to uterus, >50% myometrial invasion
II	Cervical stromal invasion
IIIA	Invasion into serosa, adenexa
IIIB	Parametrial, vaginal invasion
IIIC1	+Pelvic nodes
IIIC2	+Para-aortic nodes
IVA	Bladder, bowel invasion
IVB	Distant metastasis

Data from Benedet JL, Bender H, Jones H 3rd, et al. FIGO staging classifications and clinical practice guidelines in the management of gynecologic cancers. FIGO Committee on Gynecologic Oncology. Int J Gynaecol Obstet 2000;70(2):230.

FDG-PET and Initial Staging

As with other gynecologic malignancies, the added value of FDG-PET in initial staging of early-stage endometrial cancer is limited. Endometrial cancer spreads by local extension, lymphatic, and hematogenous routes. Similar to cervical cancer, endometrial cancer shows an intensely positive glycolytic phenotype, and although specificity for detection of the nodal metastases is as high as 100%, the reported sensitivity of 57% to 63% is insufficient to replace lymphadenectomy.[66–69] Even patients with locally advanced disease benefit from surgical debulking and positive findings on FDG-PET before therapy does not deter surgical intervention. However, FDG-PET/CT imaging in selected patients with high-risk disease may identify distant metastases that obviate surgical staging. For those patients who are candidates for radiation therapy, either curative or palliative, FDG-PET/CT provides more accurate delineation of both the primary and metastatic lesions and potentially allows radiation dose escalation that can affect effectiveness in local tumor control.

Although FDG-PET does not significantly affect initial staging of patients with endometrial cancer, the quantitative measure of SUV_{max} of the primary

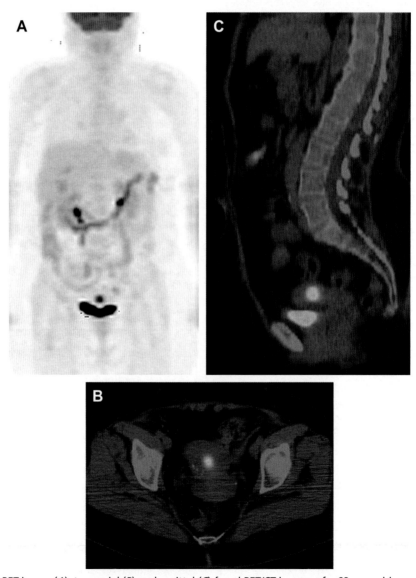

Fig. 12. MIP PET image (*A*), transaxial (*B*) and sagittal (*C*) fused PET/CT images of a 68-year-old woman with new diagnosis of endometrial adenocarcinoma show neoplastic hypermetabolic activity (SUV 9.5) localized to the endometrial cavity of the body of the uterus.

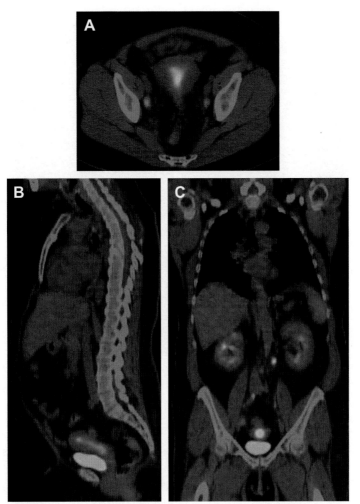

Fig. 13. Transaxial (*A*) and sagittal (*B*) initial and coronal (*C*) PET/CT images of a 72-year-old woman with endometrial cancer shows neoplastic hypermetabolic activity (SUV$_{max}$ 37) throughout the endometrial cavity to the level of the endocervical canal as well as within metastatic pelvic and retroperitoneal lymph nodes (SUV 7.1).

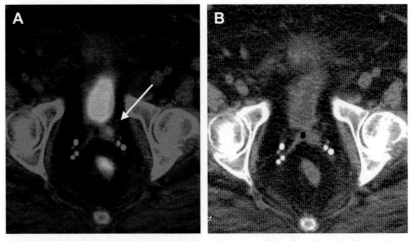

Fig. 14. Transaxial (*A*) fused PET/CT and noncontrast CT (*B*) images show focal metabolic activity within a recurrent tumor nodule (*arrow*) at the vaginal apex. Careful evaluation of subtle changes in the shape of the vaginal apex helps identify tumor recurrence at this site. Care should be taken to exclude refluxed radioactive urine within the vagina as a cause of increased metabolic activity at this site.

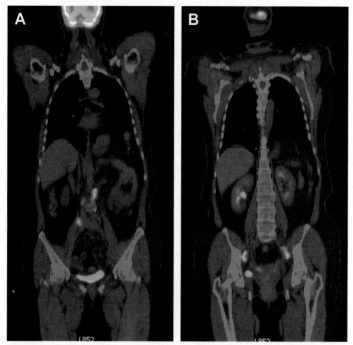

Fig. 15. Coronal (*A, B*) fused PET/CT images of a 72-year-old patient with recurrent endometrial adenocarcinoma demonstrates typical pelvic and retroperitoneal nodal metastatic pattern.

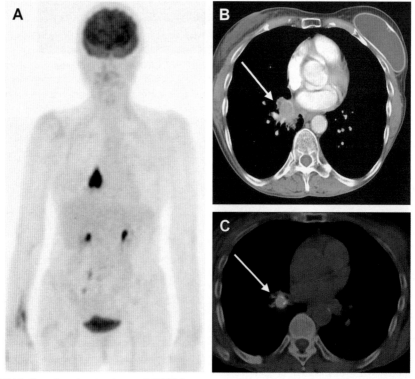

Fig. 16. PET/CT (*A, C*) and contrast-enhanced CT (*B*) images of a 76-year-old patient with previous history of breast cancer and tamoxifen-related endometrial cancer show a right lower lobe endobronchial metastasis (*arrow*).

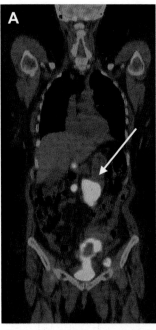
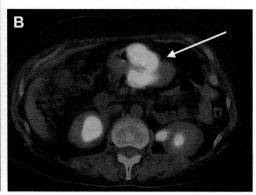

Fig. 17. Restaging coronal (*A*) and axial (*B*) fused PET/CT images of an 82-year-old patient with advanced metastatic endometrial cancer show an unusual metastasis to the gastric wall (*arrow*) as well as other nodal and pelvic sites of tumor recurrence.

uterine lesion correlates with tumor aggressiveness, and data suggest that SUV_{max} greater than 12 may be a useful biomarker to predict treatment failure (**Figs. 12** and **13**).[70–72]

FDG-PET Monitoring Therapy and Restaging

Most recurrences of endometrial cancer occur within the first 3 years after diagnosis. Tumor recurrences are most frequently found in the abdomen and pelvis, with approximately 20% involving the vagina (**Fig. 14**). It is not unusual to find distant metastatic lesions, either above the diaphragm or skeletal.[73] Routine surveillance includes periodic physical examinations, vaginal cytology, and CT or MR imaging as clinically indicated. Detection of tumor recurrence based on clinical and laboratory findings is suboptimal, because at least 20% of patients have asymptomatic metastatic disease.[74] High-grade tumor histology is associated with increased incidence of recurrence and reduced overall survival even when diagnosed at stage I.[73] Although FDG-PET/CT is not included in the NCCN guidelines for routine follow-up of endometrial cancer, the modality provides high sensitivity and accuracy in detection of both local recurrence and distant metastatic disease and potentially a better surveillance tool for high-risk patients (**Figs. 15–17, Table 5**).[75–80] Persistent posttreatment FDG

Table 5
FDG-PET: endometrial recurrence

Reference	Number of Patients	Sensitivity (%)	Specificity (%)	Positive Predicted Value (%)	Negative Predictive Value (%)	ACC
Belhocine et al,[75] 2002	34	96	78	89	91	90
Saga et al,[76] 2003	21	100	88.2			93.3
Sironi et al,[77] 2007	25	92.9	100	100	91.7	96
Kitajima et al,[78] 2008	30	93	93			93
Ryu et al,[79] 2010	127	100	88	59	100	
Sharma et al,[80] 2012	12	85.7	100			93.3

Abbreviation: ACC, accuracy.

> **Box 3**
> **FDG-PET/CT: endometrial cancer**
>
> - Not indicated early-stage disease
> - Cannot replace staging lymphadenectomy
> - High accuracy in detection of recurrent disease
> - Careful assessment of pelvic floor may aid in identification of local recurrence
> - High FDG avidity of metastases optimizes radiation therapy planning
> - Possible usefulness in treatment monitoring

uptake as measured by SUV_{max} is reported to be inversely proportional to patient survival and may be useful as a prognostic biomarker in the posttherapy setting (**Box 3**).[81]

REFERENCES

1. Copeland LJ. Epithelial ovarian cancer. In: DiSaia PJ, Creasman WT, editors. Clinical gynecologic oncology. 7th edition. Philadelphia: Mosby Elsevier; 2007. p. 313–67.
2. Kurman RJ, Shih IeM. The origin and pathogenesis of epithelial ovarian cancer–a proposed unifying theory. Am J Pathol 2010;34:433–43.
3. Mould T. An overview of current diagnosis and treatment in ovarian cancer. Int J Gynecol Cancer 2012;22:S2–4.
4. Cantuaria G, Magalhaes A, Penalver M, et al. Expression of GLUT-1 transporter in borderline and malignant epithelial tumors of the ovary. Gynecol Oncol 2000;79:33–7.
5. Semaan A, Munkarah AR, Arabi H, et al. Expression of GLUT-1 in epithelial ovarian carcinoma: correlation with tumor cell proliferation, angiogenesis, survival and ability to predict optimal cytoreduction. Gynecol Oncol 2011;121:181–6.
6. Cantuaria G, Fagotti A, Ferrandina G, et al. GLUT-1 expression in ovarian carcinoma: association with survival and response to chemotherapy. Cancer 2001;92:1144–50.
7. Risum S, Loft A, Hogdall C, et al. Standardized FDG uptake as a prognostic variable and as a predictor of incomplete cytoreduction in primary advanced ovarian cancer. Acta Oncol 2011;50:415–9.
8. Fenchel S, Grab D, Nuessle K, et al. Asymptomatic adnexal masses: correlation of FDG PET and histopathologic findings. Radiology 2002;223:780–8.
9. Ghezzi F, Cromi A, Sieto G, et al. Laparoscopy staging of early ovarian cancer our experience and review of the literature. Int J Gynecol Cancer 2009;19:S7–13.
10. Weber S, McCann CK, Boruta DM, et al. Laparoscopic surgical staging of early ovarian cancer. Rev Obstet Gynecol 2011;4:117–22.
11. Rutten MJ, Gaarenstroom KN, Van Gorp T, et al. Laparoscopy to predict the result of primary cytoreductive surgery in advanced ovarian cancer patients (LapOvCa-trial): a multicentre randomized controlled study. Cancer 2012;12:31–6.
12. De Iaco P, Musto A, Orazi L, et al. FDG PET/CT in advanced ovarian cancer staging: value and pitfalls in detecting lesions in different abdominal and pelvic quadrants compared with laparoscopy. Eur J Radiol 2010;80:e98–103.
13. Nam EJ, Yun MJ, Oh YT, et al. Diagnosis and staging of primary ovarian cancer: correlation between PET/CT, Doppler UD, and CT or MRI. Gynecol Oncol 2010;116:3389–94.
14. Yuan Y, Gu ZX, Tao XF, et al. Computer tomography, magnetic resonance imaging, and positron emission tomography or positron emission tomography/computer tomography for detection of metastatic lymph nodes in patient with ovarian cancer: a meta-analysis. Eur J Radiol 2012;81:1002–6.
15. Bats AS, Hugonnet F, Huchon C, et al. Prognostic significance of mediastinal 18F-FDG uptake in PET/CT in advanced ovarian cancer. Eur J Nucl Med Mol Imaging 2012;39:474–80.
16. Pignata S, Cannella L, Leopardo D, et al. Follow-up with CA125 after primary therapy of advanced ovarian cancer: in favor of continuing to prescribe CA125 during follow-up. Ann Oncol 2011; 22(Suppl 8):viii40–4.
17. Hall M, Rustin G. Recurrent ovarian cancer: when and how to treat. Curr Oncol Rep 2011;13:459–71.
18. Geurts SM, de Vegt F, van Altena AM, et al. Considering early detection of relapsed ovarian cancer: review of the literature. Int J Gynecol Cancer 2011;21:837–45.
19. Kumar P, Rehani MM, Kumar L, et al. Tumor marker CA-125 as an evaluator and response indicator in ovarian cancer: its quantitative correlation with tumor volume. Med Sci Monit 2005;11:CR84–9.
20. Patsner B, Orr JW Jr, Mann WJ Jr, et al. Does serum CA-125 level prior to second-look laparotomy for invasive ovarian carcinoma predict size of residual disease? Gynecol Oncol 1990;38:373–6.
21. Podczaski E, Whitney C, Manetta A, et al. Use of CA 125 to monitor patients with ovarian epithelial carcinomas. Gynecol Oncol 1989;33:193–7.
22. Meier W, Stieber P, Eiermann W, et al. Serum levels of CA 125 and histological findings at second-look laparotomy in ovarian carcinoma. Gynecol Oncol 1989;35:44–6.
23. Pan HS, Lee SL, Huang LK, et al. Combined positron emission tomography and tumor markers for detecting ovarian cancer. Arch Gynecol Obstet 2011;283:335–41.

24. Peng NJ, Liou W, Liu RS, et al. Early detection of recurrent ovarian cancer in patients with low-level increases in serum CA-125 levels by 2-[F-18]fluoro-2-deoxy-D-glucose-positron emission tomography/computed tomography. Cancer Biother Radiopharm 2011;26:175–81.

25. Bhosale P, Peungjesada S, Wei W, et al. Clinical utility of positron emission tomography/computed tomography in the evaluation of suspected recurrent ovarian cancer in the setting of normal CA-125 levels. Int J Gynecol Cancer 2010;20: 936–44.

26. Palomar A, Nanni C, Castelucci P, et al. Value of FDG PET/CT in patients with treated ovarian cancer and raised CA125 serum levels. Mol Imaging Biol 2012;14:123–9.

27. Sari O, Kaya B, Kara PO, et al. The role of FDG-PET/CT in ovarian cancer patients with high tumor markers or suspicious lesions on contrast-enhanced CT in evaluation of recurrence and/or in determination of intraabdominal metastases. Rev Esp Med Nucl 2012;31:3–8.

28. Duarte-Franco E, Franco EL. Cancer of the uterine cervix. BMC Womens Health 2004;4(Suppl 1):S13.

29. Ibeanu OA. Molecular pathogenesis of cervical cancer. Cancer Biol Ther 2011;11:295–306.

30. Tran BN, Grigsby PW, Dehdashti F, et al. Occult supraclavicular lymph node metastasis identified by FDG-PET in patients with carcinoma of the uterine cervix. Gynecol Oncol 2003;90(3):572–6.

31. Qiu JT, Ho KC, Lai CH, et al. Supraclavicular lymph node metastases in cervical cancer. Eur J Gynaecol Oncol 2007;28(1):33–8.

32. Choi HJ, Ju W, Myung SK, et al. Diagnostic performance of computer tomography, magnetic resonance imaging, and positron emission tomography/computed tomography for detection of metastatic lymph nodes in patients with cervical cancer: meta-analysis. Cancer Sci 2010;101(6):1471–9.

33. Ramirez PT, Jhingran A, Macapinlac HA, et al. Laparoscopic extraperitoneal para-aortic lymphadenectomy in locally advanced cervical cancer: a prospective correlation with surgical findings with positron emission tomography/computed tomography findings. Cancer 2011;117(9):1928–34.

34. Leblanc E, Gauthier H, Querleu D, et al. Accuracy of 19-fluoro-2-deoxy-D-glucose positron emission tomography in the pretherapeutic detection of occult para-aortic node involvement in patients with locally advanced cervical carcinoma. Ann Surg Oncol 2011;18(8):2302–9.

35. Chung HH, Park NH, Kim JW, et al. Role of integrated PET-CT in pelvic lymph node staging of cervical cancer before hysterectomy. Gynecol Obstet Invest 2009;67(1):61–6.

36. Ferrandina G, Petrillo M, Restaino G, et al. Can radicality of surgery be safely modulated on the basis of MRI and PET/CT imaging in locally advanced cervical cancer patients administered preoperative treatment? Cancer 2012;118(2):392–403.

37. Signorelli M, Guerra L, Montanelli L, et al. Preoperative staging of cervical cancer: is 18-FDG-PET/CT really effective in patients with early stage disease? Gynecol Oncol 2011;123(2):236–40.

38. Yen TC, Ng KK, Ma SY, et al. Value of dual-phase 2-fluoro-2-deoxy-d-glucose positron emission tomography in cervical cancer. J Clin Oncol 2003; 21(19):3651–8.

39. Rose AG, Adler LP, Rodriguez M, et al. Positron emission tomography for evaluating para-aortic nodal metastases in locally advanced cervical cancer before surgical staging: a surgicopathologic study. J Clin Oncol 1999;17(1):41–5.

40. Wright JD, Dehdashti F, Herzog TJ, et al. Preoperative lymph node staging of early-stage cervical carcinoma by [18F]-fluoro-2-deoxy-D-glucose-positron emission tomography. Cancer 2005;104(11): 2484–91.

41. Tzu-Chen Y, Lai-Chu S, Chyong-Huey L, et al. 18F-FDG uptake in squamous cell carcinoma of the cervix is correlated with glucose transporter 1 expression. J Nucl Med 2004;45(1):22–9.

42. Unger JB, Lilien DL, Caldito G, et al. The prognostic value of pre-treatment 2-(18F)-fluoro-2-deoxy-D-glucose positron emission tomography scan in women with cervical cancer. Int J Gynecol Cancer 2007;17(5):1062–7.

43. Grigsby PW. The prognostic value of PET and PET/CT in cervical cancer. Cancer Imaging 2008; 8:146–55.

44. Chung HH, Nam BH, Kim JW, et al. Preoperative [18F]FDG PET/CT maximum standardized uptake value predicts recurrence of uterine cervical cancer. Eur J Nucl Med Mol Imaging 2010;37(8): 1467–73.

45. Chou HH, Chang HP, Lai CH, et al. (18)F-FDG PET in stage IB/IIB cervical adenocarcinoma/adenosquamous carcinoma. Eur J Nucl Med Mol Imaging 2010;37(4):728–35.

46. Kidd EA, Siegel BA, Dehdashti F, et al. Pelvic lymph node F-18 fluorodeoxyglucose uptake as a prognostic biomarker in newly diagnosed patients with locally advanced cervical cancer. Cancer 2010;116(6):1469–75.

47. Kang S, Park JY, Lim MC, et al. Pelvic lymph node status assessed by 18F-fluorodeoxyglucose positron emission tomography predicts low-risk group for distant recurrence in locally advanced cervical cancer: a prospective study. Int J Radiat Oncol Biol Phys 2011;70(3):788–93.

48. Pan L, Cheng J, Zhou M, et al. The SUVmax (maximum standardized uptake value for F-18 fluorodeoxyglucose) and serum squamous cell carcinoma antigen (SCC-ag) function as prognostic

biomarkers in patients with primary cervical cancer. J Cancer Res Clin Oncol 2012;138(2):239–46.

49. Kidd EA, El Naqa I, Siegel BA, et al. FDG-PET-based prognostic nomograms for locally advanced cervical cancer. Gynecol Oncol 2012; 127(1):136–40.

50. Dolezelova H, Slampa P, Ondrova B, et al. The impact of 18FDG in radiotherapy treatment planning and in prediction in patients with cervix carcinoma: results of pilot study. Neoplasma 2008; 55(5):437–41.

51. Esthappan J, Chaudhari S, Santanam L, et al. Prospective clinical trial of positron emission tomography/computed tomography image-guided intensity-modulated radiation therapy for cervical carcinoma with positive para-aortic lymph nodes. Int J Radiat Oncol Biol Phys 2008;72(4): 1134–9.

52. Mutic S, Malyapa RS, Grigsby PW, et al. PET-guided IMRT for cervical carcinoma with positive para-aortic lymph nodes–a dose-escalation treatment planning study. Int J Radiat Oncol Biol Phys 2003;55(1):28–35.

53. Caroli P, Fanti S. PET/CT and radiotherapy in gynecologic malignancy. Q J Nucl Med Mol Imaging 2010;54(5):533–42.

54. National Comprehensive Cancer Institute Guidelines. Version 2012 MS-7.

55. Havrilesky LJ, Wong TZ, Secord AA, et al. The role of PET scanning in detection of recurrent cervical cancer. Gynecol Oncol 2003;90(1):186–90.

56. Chung HH, Kim SK, Kim TH, et al. Clinical impact of FDG-PET imaging in post-therapy surveillance of uterine cervical cancer: from diagnosis to prognosis. Gynecol Oncol 2006;103(1):165–70.

57. Cetina L, Serrano A, Cantu-de-Leon D, et al. F18-FDG-PET/CT in the evaluation of patients with suspected recurrent or persistent locally advanced cervical cancer. Rev Invest Clin 2011; 63(3):227–35.

58. Grigsby PW, Siegel BA, Dehdashti F, et al. Posttherapy surveillance of cervical cancer by FDG-PET. Int J Radiat Oncol Biol Phys 2003;55(4):907–13.

59. Siva S, Herschtal A, Thomas JM, et al. Impact of post-therapy emission tomography on prognostic stratification and surveillance after chemoradiation for cervical cancer. Cancer 2011;117(17):3981–8.

60. Hoon CH, Kim JW, Kang KW, et al. Predictive role of post-treatment [(18)F]FDG PET/CT in patients with uterine cervical cancer. Eur J Radiol 2012; 81(8):e817–22.

61. Cramer DW. The epidemiology of endometrial and ovarian cancer. Hematol Oncol Clin North Am 2012;26(1):1–12.

62. Liu FS. Molecular carcinogenesis of endometrial cancer. Taiwan J Obstet Gynecol 2007;46(1): 26–32.

63. Lax SF, Kurman RJ. A dualistic model for endometrial carcinogenesis based on immunohistochemical molecular genetic analysis. Verh Dtsch Ges Pathol 1997;81:228–32.

64. Timmermans A, Opmeer BC, Khan KS, et al. Endometrial thickness measurement for detecting endometrial cancer in women with postmenopausal bleeding: a systematic review and meta-analysis. Obstet Gynecol 2010;116(1):160–7.

65. van Hanegem N, Breijer MC, Khan KS, et al. Diagnostic evaluation of the endometrium in postmenopausal bleeding: an evidence-based approach. Maturitas 2011;68(2):155–64.

66. Chang MC, Chen JH, Liang JA, et al. 18F-FDG PET or PET-CT for detection of metastatic lymph nodes in patients with endometrial cancer: a systematic review and meta-analysis. Eur J Radiol 2012; 81(11):3511–7.

67. Kitajima K, Suzuki K, Senda M, et al. Preoperative nodal staging of uterine cancer: is contrast-enhanced PET/CT more accurate than non-enhanced PET/CT or enhanced CT alone? Ann Nucl Med 2011;25(7):511–9.

68. Suga T, Nakamoto Y, Saga T, et al. Clinical value of FDG-PET for preoperative evaluation of endometrial cancer. Ann Nucl Med 2011; 25(4):269–75.

69. Picchio M, Mangilli G, Samanes Gajate AM, et al. High-grade endometrial cancer: value of [(18)F] FDG PET/CT in preoperative staging. Nucl Med Commun 2010;31(6):506–12.

70. Kitajima K, Kita M, Suzuki K, et al. Prognostic significance of SUVmax (maximum standardized uptake value) measured by [(18)F] FDG PET/CT in endometrial cancer. Eur J Nucl Med Mol Imaging 2012;39(5):840–5.

71. Nakamura K, Hongo A, Kodama J, et al. The measurement of SUVmax of the primary tumor is predictive of prognosis for patients with endometrial cancer. Gynecol Oncol 2011;123(1):82–7.

72. Lee HJ, Ahn BC, Hong CM, et al. Preoperative risk stratification using (18)F-FDG PET/CT in women with endometrial cancer. Nuklearmedizin 2011; 50(5):204–13.

73. Esselen KM, Boruta DM, del Carmen M, et al. Defining prognostic variables in recurrent endometriod endometrial cancer: a 15-year single-institution review. Int J Gynecol Cancer 2011; 21(6):1078–83.

74. Berchuck A, Anspach C, Evans AC, et al. Postsurgical surveillance of patients with FIGO stage I/II endometrial adenocarcinoma. Gynecol Oncol 1995;59(1):20–4.

75. Belhocine T, De Barsy C, Husyinx R, et al. Usefulness of ^{18}F-FDG PET in the post-therapy surveillance of endometrial carcinoma. Eur J Nucl Med 2002;29:1132–9.

76. Saga T, Higashi T, Ishimori T, et al. Clinical value of FDG-PET in the follow up of post-operative patients with endometrial cancer. Ann Nucl Med 2003;17(3): 197–203.

77. Sironi S, Picchio M, Landoni C, et al. Post-therapy surveillance of patients with uterine cancer: value of integrated FDG PET/CT in the detection of recurrence. Eur J Nucl Med Mol Imaging 2007;34(4): 472–9.

78. Kitajima K, Murakami K, Yamasaki E, et al. Performance of FDG-PET/CT in the diagnosis of recurrent endometrial cancer. Ann Nucl Med 2008;22(2): 103–9.

79. Ryu SY, Kim K, Kim Y, et al. Detection of recurrence by ^{18}F-FDG PET in patients with endometrial cancer showing no evidence of disease. J Korean Med Sci 2010;25(7):1029–33.

80. Sharma P, Kumar R, Singh H, et al. Role of FDG PET-CT in detecting recurrence in patients with uterine sarcoma: comparison with conventional imaging. Nucl Med Commun 2012;33(2):185–90.

81. Chung HH, Kim JW, Kang KW, et al. Post-treatment [18F] FDG maximum uptake value as a prognostic marker of recurrence in endometrial carcinoma. Eur J Nucl Med Mol Imaging 2011; 38(1):74–80.

Positron Emission Tomography in Radiation Treatment Planning
The Potential of Metabolic Imaging

Junzo Chino, MD[a],*, Shiva Das, PhD[a],
Terence Wong, MD, PhD[b]

KEYWORDS

- Radiation therapy • Positron emission tomography • Adaptive planning • Metabolic imaging
- Functional imaging

KEY POINTS

- Positron emission tomography (PET) has proved to be an indispensable tool in the staging of many malignancies, as well as in discriminating responses to therapy.
- Technologic advances in radiation therapy planning and delivery have made highly conformal and accurate treatments a reality.
- Integration of PET into radiation treatment planning is a method of accurate target definition at the initiation of treatment, but also is during potentially adaptive treatment that depends on response.
- Future research should be focused on determining the potential benefits of such adaptations in a prospective manner, as well as exploring new tracers that may improve existing results.

INTRODUCTION

Radiation therapy and diagnostic radiology have always enjoyed a close relationship, and both have evolved from a common specialty. Advances in diagnostic imaging have resulted in parallel changes in the planning of radiation therapy. The development of cross-sectional imaging with computed tomography led to the transition from 2-dimensional treatment planning based on plain films to volumetric 3-dimensional therapy planning, and has become the standard method of radiation therapy planning. Similarly, magnetic resonance (MR) imaging is gradually being more commonly used in integrated treatment planning in the brain, head and neck, and pelvis, owing to the superior tissue contrast afforded.

Until recently, radiation treatment planning has been based on anatomically defined targets. This paradigm has several limitations; tumor margins are often not well defined on computed tomography (CT) or MR images. Active tumor may extend beyond the anatomically defined boundaries. In other cases, the tumor may be surrounded by or contain regions of edema, necrosis, or fibrosis, which may increase the apparent target treatment volume, and therefore increase the potential for adverse effects. The advent of functional and metabolic imaging techniques, such as positron emission tomography (PET), allows for novel information to be combined with the anatomic definition provided by CT or MR imaging.

Disclosures: The authors have no relevant conflicts of interest to disclose.
[a] Department of Radiation Oncology, Duke University Medical Center, DUMC 3085, Durham, NC 27710, USA;
[b] Department of Radiology, Duke University Medical Center, DUMC 3949, Durham, NC 27710, USA
* Corresponding author.
E-mail address: junzo.chino@duke.edu

In parallel, radiation-therapy treatment planning and delivery has benefited from new technology and techniques. Intensity-modulated radiation therapy techniques have been developed to allow higher doses to be delivered in a highly conformal manner. Image-guided techniques allow for these treatments to be delivered accurately on a daily basis, and are able to appropriately control for target motion within the body, whether it be due to respiration or distension/emptying of hollow organs.

Given the convergence of the improved ability to image active tumor and the delivery of radiation to very specific targets, the implications for a tighter integration of PET imaging with radiation treatment planning are apparent. This fusion has the potential to improve the therapeutic ratio in 2 ways: (1) PET imaging may identify targets that would benefit from dose escalation, improving the control achieved with radiation; and (2) PET may conversely identify regions that may not require a full dose, allowing for de-escalation and sparing of nontarget normal tissue. This article summarizes developments in radiation therapy technology and the application of various PET tracers in diseases treated by radiation therapy, and looks to future possibilities of combining these modalities.

RADIATION THERAPY TECHNOLOGY

The treatment of cancers with external beam radiation therapy has evolved over time, largely because of rapid improvements in technology. Earlier external-beam treatment machines used a radioactive Cobalt-60 source mounted within the gantry head. The gantry was capable of rotating around a patient positioned supine/prone on a couch, delivering radiation to the tumor from multiple directions. Subsequently, linear accelerators were developed specifically for radiation therapy. Unlike radioactive sources, which had the potential to accidentally deliver radiation even when the machine was not turned on, linear accelerators work by accelerating electrons to collide with a fixed metal target, in turn producing megavoltage-energy photons used to treat the tumor. The beam aperture through which the photons stream out are typically shaped by heavy jaws that collimate the beam to a rectangular shape of a size somewhat larger than the tumor being irradiated. To reduce the incidental irradiation of normal organs surrounding the tumor, additional blocking is used to conform the radiation shape to only treat the tumor and some uniform surrounding margin. This additional blocking is achieved in modern-day machines by a system of parallel metal "leaves" (multileaf collimator) oriented such that each leaf is capable of protruding into the rectangular jaw aperture to cast a narrow blocking shadow on the radiation beam. Positioning the leaves to protrude to various lengths creates a customized blocking pattern that excludes tissue outside of some margin surrounding the tumor (**Fig. 1**).

Modern-day treatments with external-beam linear accelerators equipped with multileaf collimators may be classified as either conformal radiation therapy (CRT) or intensity-modulated radiation therapy (IMRT). CRT uses beams with customized blocking patterns, as previously described, to irradiate a target volume within the patient. The target volume comprises a clinical target volume (gross tumor volume plus microscopic extension) and margin to account for setup uncertainties and tumor motion, generated by the treating radiation oncologist. Megavoltage-beam doses fall off almost exponentially as a function of depth after entering the patient's body. For deep-seated tumors, this implies that normal structures on the entrance side of the beam will receive a far higher dose than the tumor. To reduce normal structure doses to a tolerable level, multiple beams from various entrance directions around the patient are used. Because each of these beams is aimed at the tumor, their combined dosage will be received by the tumor, whereas only a fraction of the dose will be received by normal structures. For example, if one is to assume that 7 beams are used to treat a tumor, approximately one-seventh of the dose should be delivered to normal structures in the path of any one beam. In reality, however, the beam widths necessary to irradiate the target are large enough such that the entrances and exits of beams will overlap even at some distance away from the tumor. This overlapping implies that, in some situations, CRT may not be capable of reducing normal structure doses below the levels required for acceptable toxicity.

IMRT is capable of reducing normal structure doses to a level significantly below that from CRT. As with CRT, IMRT irradiates the target from multiple directions. Unlike CRT, the field aperture for each IMRT beam does not provide a uniform intensity across the opening. In other words, for any one beam the photon intensity is higher in some portions of the aperture and lower in others. This arrangement is analogous to a shower head delivering the same flow of water through each of its nozzle openings (CRT) versus water flow rates that differ between the nozzle openings (IMRT). This effect is physically achieved by dynamically moving the multileaf collimator

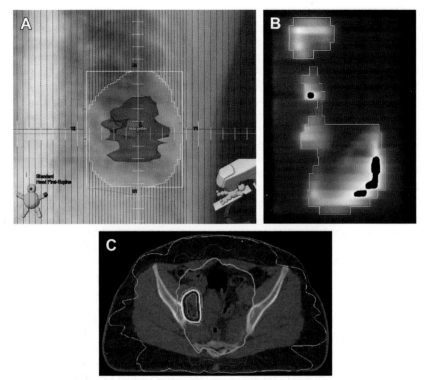

Fig. 1. Modern radiation treatment. (*A*) A "beam's eye view" of a single field from a 3-dimensional conformal treatment of an inoperable early-stage lung cancer. The leaves of the multileaf collimator (MLC) are shown in blue, conforming to the red-contoured target with margin for beam penumbra. (*B*) Photon fluence from a single beam in an 11-beam intensity-modulated plan. These maps are generated via algorithmic optimization based on volumes and constraints provided by the radiation oncologist, and are achieved by moving individual leaves of the MLC while the beam is on. The pure black reflects regions where the dose was at the upper limit of the quality-assurance film used for this image. (*C*) A conformal isodose distribution for a patient with node-positive cervical cancer, tightly conforming to the lymph node basins at risk, avoiding normal tissue. Note that in this case a higher dose is being given to a lymph node that was identified by diagnostic PET (the *orange isodose line* is 45 Gy; the *yellow isodose line* is 60 Gy).

leaves across the aperture while the beam is on. The idea behind varying the intensity is as follows. The beam apertures in CRT irradiate the target and any critical organs within the aperture view. Some portions of the aperture see only the target, whereas others see the target overlapped with critical organs. It would seem to make sense, then, to deliver a higher dose through the portion of the aperture that only sees the target, relative to the portion that sees the target overlapping with critical organs. For any one beam, this also means that the beam has not delivered the requisite amount of dose to some regions of the target. This dose deficit is compensated by other beams that are able to deliver relatively higher doses to the underdosed target regions. The interaction between beams is complex, because dose deficits from each beam (as a consequence of reducing critical structure doses within its aperture) must be compensated by an increased dose from other

beams. The net effect is that IMRT is usually capable of delivering a dose pattern that uniformly irradiates the target while sculpting and redistributing the dose outside the target to reduce irradiation of critical organs.

A direct consequence of this more conformal method of treatment planning and delivery is that volumes must be more precisely defined than what was acceptable in CRT plans. Radiation oncologists have had to rethink what is absolutely required to be within the irradiated volume, and what can be safely spared. Therefore, much attention recently has been focused on which are the appropriate volumes, and how they are generated via segmentation or contouring.

SEGMENTATION (CONTOURING)

An important use of ^{18}F-labeled fluorodeoxyglucose (FDG) PET imaging in radiotherapy is accurate segmentation of the PET-avid region so that it can be included in the target. The consequence of not including some portion of the PET-avid region is to underdose that region, potentially leading to lowered tumor control and the risk of recurrence. Segmenting the PET-avid region is not an easy task, because the region could look very different depending on the window level used to visualize the image (**Fig. 2**).

Other factors also confound a "clean" identification of the PET-avid region. PET detectors have some inherent resolution, on the order of several millimeters, implying that the boundaries of the high-uptake region will appear blurred on the image. If the high-uptake region is very small this blurring effect can also diminish the overall intensity, making it more difficult to distinguish from the background. In addition to the blurring effect, image noise is also always present. Motion of the tumor, as in lung or liver, can also blur tumor boundaries. Uptake intensity in tumors near the bladder will also be deliberately diminished owing to a "void" effect created by the presence of high intensity in the bladder (**Fig. 3**). The time point at which the image is acquired after injection can also influence the appearance of the high-uptake region relative to background.

Manual segmentation of the PET-avid region in radiotherapy is very dependent on individual practices. Typically the CT acquired at the time of PET (CT-PET imaging) is used as a guide. Modern radiotherapy planning systems are capable of superimposing the PET image on the CT, or MR imaging via image fusion, to aid in using the strengths of all modalities (**Fig. 4**). The radiation oncologist then adjusts the PET window level and manually outlines the PET-avid region while simultaneously visualizing the CT image. The PET window-level adjustment is subjective and, hence, can be highly variable between institutions and even between radiation oncologists in a single institution. Some radiation oncologists use guidelines previously provided from phantom experiments or patient imaging. Phantom experiments have suggested setting the lower window level to 42% of the maximum intensity in the PET-avid region and using this threshold for segmentation.[1] Earlier PET studies in patients with lung cancer[2] have suggested setting the threshold for malignancy using a standardized uptake value (SUV) of 2.5 (SUV is the measured activity within the region normalized to the injected activity and body weight). However, these threshold levels have not been universally applicable or reliable, and it is known that benign processes such as post-therapy inflammation, granulomatous disease, and infection can also have SUVs greater than this threshold.

As a consequence of the subjective nature of manual segmentation, automatic segmentation methods have been developed with the aim of arriving at the ground truth. These methods are typically developed in phantom experiments where several inserts (usually spherical) filled with FDG to concentrations seen in human tumors are placed within a large container filled with some background concentration. These experiments are typically performed with the ratios of insert to background concentrations varied over ranges seen in human scans. Because the insert volumes (ie, the ground truth) are known, automatic segmentation methods can be developed and tested on them. A popular class of methods uses threshold intensities,[1,3–5] whereby any intensity higher than a certain threshold is deemed to be the true metabolic volume. Erdi and colleagues[1] developed a formalism whereby the threshold depended on the signal-to-background ratio and tumor volume. In fact, the 42% threshold intensity mentioned earlier was their recommendation for

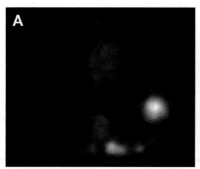
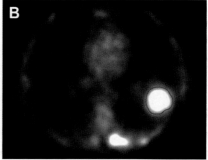

Fig. 2. The effect of windowing on PET-generated contours. (*A, B*) Two target contours (*red border*) generated from the same FDG PET images of an early-stage lung cancer to be treated with stereotactic body radiotherapy (SBRT). One can see subtle but significant changes in the contour size and shape, which become clinically significant when extremely conformal and precise techniques are used.

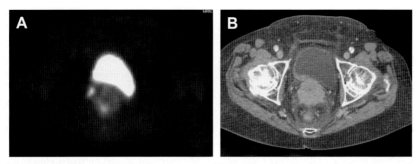

Fig. 3. (*A*) Axial section of the FDG PET of a woman with locally advanced cervical cancer at the level of the bladder. Note that owing to the high concentration of FDG in the normal urine, the full extent of disease may be underestimated on PET imaging alone; as the CT image correlates at the same level (*B*), clear invasion into the posterior wall of the bladder is demonstrated.

volumes greater than 4 mL. Subsequently, Jentzen and colleagues[5] refined this approach with a scheme that iteratively changed the threshold to more accurately arrive at the true volume. Yet another method advocates using a threshold of 15% of the mean tumor intensity over the background intensity.[3] Another class of methods uses the gradient (slope) of the intensity fall-off at the

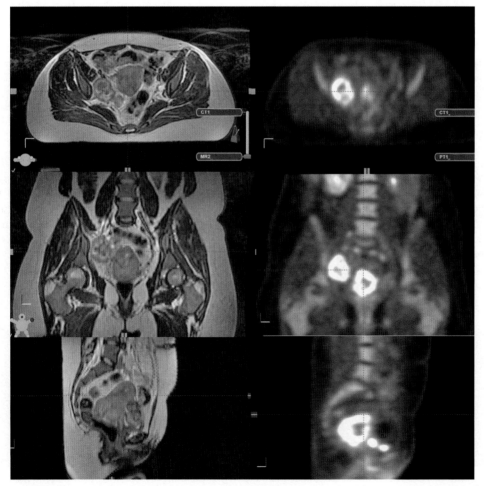

Fig. 4. Fused FDG PET and MR imaging. These merged image sets were obtained for optimal treatment planning for a patient with node-positive cervical cancer. The PET images demonstrate clearly the regions of highest metabolic activity while MR imaging provides superior soft-tissue contrast.

edge of the tumor to determine the tumor boundary.[6,7] The idea here is that the true tumor boundary will correspond to a rapid drop in intensity. Yet another method starts with the maximum-intensity pixel in the tumor and iteratively adds on pixels to expand outwards to the tumor boundary.[8] The important point to note with all of these methods is that they have only largely been tested and validated in phantoms, and have not been extensively validated in animals or humans. The general feeling is that there is still not a universally accepted automatic segmentation method.

USE OF FDG PET IN TREATMENT PLANNING

FDG PET is typically used in radiotherapy planning to guide the segmentation of the high-uptake portion of the tumor and nodes, as previously described (**Figs. 5** and **6**). These segmented volumes are then included as part of the larger target region. The radiotherapy prescription usually takes

the larger target region to some primary dose and then boosts the gross tumor volume (including high-uptake regions) to a higher dose. The primary and boost doses are typically planned for spatially homogeneous delivery to their respective target regions.

Of late there has been increasing clinical interest in delivering a nonhomogeneous dose to the target based on FDG PET uptake, with the aim of improving local control.[9,10] The idea is to take avid regions to still higher doses while maintaining critical-organ doses below acceptable dose limits. This approach, whereby high-uptake regions are either uniformly taken to a higher dose or have a more tailored pattern with higher doses to higher voxel intensities, has been shown to be technically feasible in the past.[11–14] However, PET volumes can change during the course of treatment as a consequence of radiation,[15] implying that a plan generated on the PET image before radiotherapy may be less relevant during radiotherapy (see

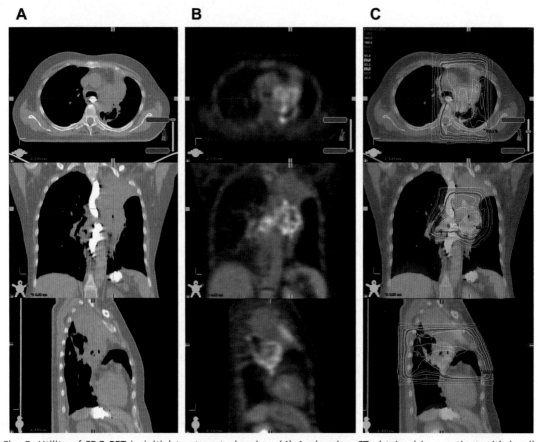

A   **B**   **C**

Fig. 5. Utility of FDG PET in initial treatment planning. (*A*) A planning CT obtained in a patient with locally advanced non–small cell lung cancer (NSCLC). There is a significant degree of lung collapse associated with the tumor, although the exact borders are unclear. (*B*) A fused planning FDG PET, demonstrating a clear delineation of the metabolically active tumor. (*C*) The treatment plan for the patient, sparing all nontarget lung.

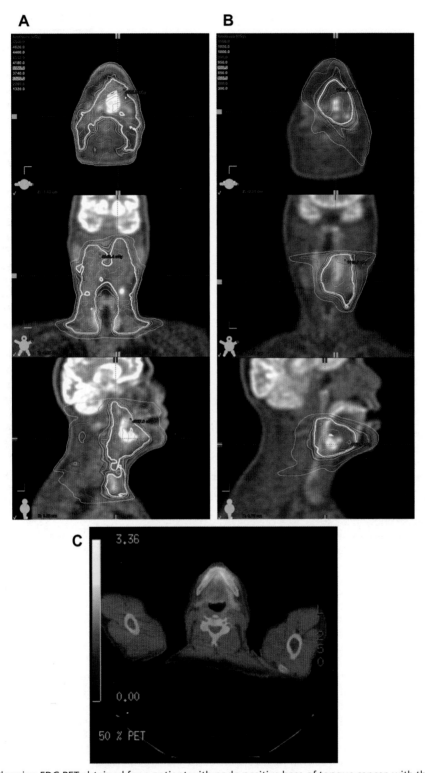

Fig. 6. (*A*) Planning FDG PET obtained for a patient with node-positive base of tongue cancer, with the optimized plan showing good coverage of the primary tumor in the base of tongue as well as elective coverage of the neck. (*B*) A repeat FDG PET after 2 weeks of concurrent chemoradiotherapy. The boost plan was developed based on these images, as opposed to the initial PET-positive volumes, as part of a clinical trial at the Duke Cancer Center. (*C*) Diagnostic PET obtained 3 months after completion of treatment, showing a complete resolution of PET abnormality.

Fig. 5). A study of patients with non–small cell lung cancer (NSCLC) reveals that although the volumes themselves may become smaller, areas of low and high PET uptake overlap reasonably well on serial images acquired at various time points during the course of radiotherapy.[16] This finding supports the premise that a plan generated with the initial PET image may remain relevant throughout the course of therapy. Two recent clinical studies have instituted the approach of tailoring the dose to high-uptake regions such that the dose at each voxel is in proportion to the voxel activity. One is an ongoing phase 2 trial for Stage 2 to 3 NSCLC,[10] and the other is a phase 1 trial for determining maximum tolerated dose in squamous cell carcinoma of the head and neck.[17] With growing interest in this approach, more of these studies are likely to be initiated in the near future.

RESPONSE TO THERAPY

PET is widely used to assess response to radiotherapy with or without chemotherapy. Response assessment has generally used imaging at 1 or more of the time points pretherapy, intratherapy, and/or post-therapy.

Pretherapy or Post-Therapy

In squamous cell carcinoma of the head and neck,[18] preradiotherapy mean tumor SUV higher than the median was associated with worse 2-year disease-free survival. Also in squamous cell carcinoma of the head and neck,[19] post-chemoradiotherapy imaging versus pathologic/clinical response showed a low positive predictive value and a high negative predictive value for the primary tumor, but high positive and negative predictive values for nodes.

Pretherapy and Post-Therapy

This category assesses metabolic response by comparing post-therapy image uptake with pre-therapy uptake. In patients with anal squamous cell carcinoma,[20] both the 2-year and 5-year survivals were significantly higher for complete metabolic responders compared with partial metabolic responders or nonresponders. Patients with locally advanced rectal adenocarcinoma[21] were graded for regression at surgery after radiotherapy, to determine how well the assessment correlated with metabolic response (preradiotherapy vs postradiotherapy before surgery). Reductions in both maximum and mean SUV were significantly different between responders and nonresponders. A cutoff of 24.5% in the mean SUV reduction gave a sensitivity, specificity, accuracy, positive predictive value, and negative predictive value of 80%, 72%, 76%, 70%, and 82%, respectively. By contrast,[22] also for locally advanced rectal cancer, the change in SUV was not found to be predictive of regression grading at surgery. In locally advanced squamous cell carcinoma of the head and neck,[23] PET response assessed via visual examination was significantly different for 2-year survival between complete responders and nonresponders, whereas response assessment with clinical examination and CT were not significantly different.

Pretherapy and Intratherapy

This category assesses metabolic response by comparing PET imaging pretherapy with imaging during therapy. In advanced NSCLC,[24] imaging at 40 Gy into the radiotherapy course showed fairly high sensitivity, specificity, and accuracy for determining tumor response using the metrics of maximum SUV, mean SUV, and metabolic tumor volume. In patients with stage 1 to 3 small cell lung cancer,[25] the change in metabolic tumor volume after the first cycle of chemotherapy (before radiotherapy) was correlated with survival. Tumor regression grading in locally advanced rectal cancer[26] was predicted by the change in maximum SUV between the pre-chemoradiotherapy image and the image at 15 days into radiotherapy. A reduction in maximum SUV of 43% resulted in a sensitivity of 77% and specificity of 93%. This category of assessment is most useful in being able to change the course of therapy based on the response. Poorly responding patients could thus be moved to a more aggressive chemoradiotherapy regimen. Nonresponders might be best served by no further chemoradiotherapy, thereby at least reducing the likelihood of chemoradiotherapy-induced complications (Fig. 7). There are several cautionary notes, however, when using this category. If the intratherapy image is acquired too late into radiotherapy, radiotherapy-induced inflammatory response could actually result in an increased SUV.[27] Consistency in the imaging parameters is important for not underestimating or overestimating the metabolic response.[28,29] For example, intratherapy imaging at a different time point after injection, compared with pretherapy imaging, will capture a different SUV dynamic and skew the change in SUV metrics. Patients' fasting parameters and serum glucose before imaging should be consistent, as far as possible. It is also imperative that PET scanning parameters (uptake time, acquisition parameters, and reconstruction parameters) be consistent between the 2 sets of images. In general, this means that the pretherapy

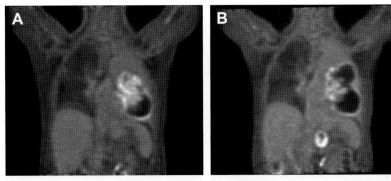

Fig. 7. (A) Initial planning PET for a patient with NSCLC. A conformal IMRT plan was developed, which was performed for 4 weeks. (B) Intratreatment planning PET demonstrating only modest response of the primary, unfortunately also showing new metastatic disease in the adrenal gland. For this reason, radiation was ceased. The patient was not a good candidate for systemic chemotherapy, and so went into hospice care.

and intratherapy PET/CT scans should be performed on the same scanner. If pretherapy scans are obtained on a different PET/CT scanner (even if the vendor is the same), correlation with the intratherapy scan is likely to be invalid. Unfortunately, this may necessitate repeating the baseline PET/CT scan for treatment planning purposes.

ADAPTIVE RADIOTHERAPY

An assumption underpinning the majority of fractionated radiotherapy planning and delivery is that the target volumes change little throughout the course of treatment, and that a full course might be designed based entirely on initial imaging. This most assuredly is not the case for many situations, and replanning based on CT imaging has been explored in multiple clinical scenarios, demonstrating improved coverage of targets with increased sparing of normal tissue.[30]

A pilot study from Belgium examined the effect of replanning 10 patients with head and neck cancer 4 times throughout treatment, using PET/CT data for each iteration.[31] This study demonstrated a 7% reduction in the dose received to the spinal cord with the adaptive plan, as well as a 10% reduction in dose to the oral cavity and improved sparing of the parotid glands. The investigators also observed significant variability in the response to treatment; those patients with the largest decrease in gross tumor volume (GTV) also had the largest benefit to adaptive planning. An National Cancer Institute study of 10 patients with head and neck cancer with a CT-based adaptive plan at 3 weeks intratreatment showed significant reductions in maximum dose to spinal cord, brainstem, larynx, and parotid glands.[32]

A series of 13 patients with NSCLC were replanned with an intratreatment CT at weeks 3

and 5 of radiation therapy.[33] A single adaptive plan resulted in a decrease in the mean lung dose by 5%, and with 2 adaptive plans the dose was reduced by 8%. The investigators were also able to increase the dose to the GTV from 67 Gy with the conventional plan to 74 Gy with adaptive treatment, while keeping the dose to lung constant.

Although PET-based adaptive planning is in its infancy, there is significant opportunity to adjust fields for those with an excellent response early in treatment, potentially reducing the dose to normal tissues; conversely, those with a less than optimal response might be considered for treatment intensification, either by a higher radiotherapy dose or by addition of chemotherapeutic agents (**Fig. 8**).

OTHER PET TRACERS FOR TREATMENT PLANNING

Glucose metabolism, as reflected on FDG PET scans, is a general indicator of malignant activity; however, there are limitations to this as a sole metric for treatment planning. Active malignancies tend to have high glucose metabolism, and glucose metabolism decreases in response to therapy. However, a major limitation of FDG PET is that inflammatory processes may result in high FDG accumulation, indistinguishable from malignancy. Reactive lymph nodes thus may have FDG uptake similar to that of metastatic adenopathy. Furthermore, radiation therapy itself frequently results in an inflammatory response associated with macrophage infiltration, which is in turn metabolically active on FDG PET imaging. Finally, evaluation of primary and metastatic brain tumors is difficult with FDG PET, owing to high

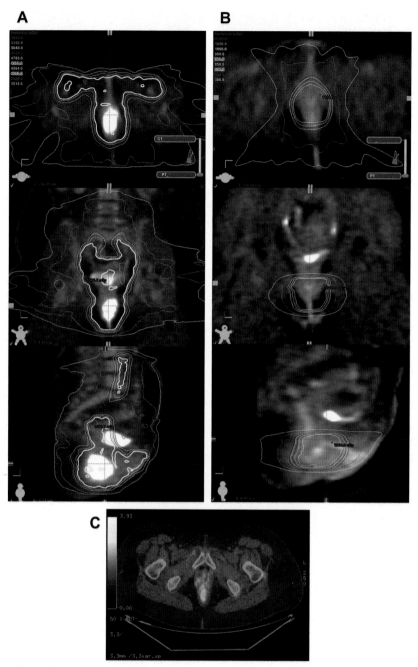

Fig. 8. (*A*) Planning FDG PET obtained in a woman with a posteriorly located vulvar cancer, extending into the rectovaginal septum. A large initial field was designed to cover all areas of PET-positive disease as well as elective nodal basins at risk. (*B*) Adaptive PET planning scan after 4 weeks of treatment as part of a clinical trial. Near complete response is noted, and the boost fields are replanned to the new anatomy, significantly reducing the dose to the normal rectum and anal canal. (*C*) Posttreatment diagnostic PET, 3 months after completion of therapy, with a metabolic complete response.

background physiologic activity in the cerebral cortex.

Although FDG has been proved to be a useful PET tracer for radiation therapy planning, other tracers are being investigated that may (1) allow radiotherapy targeting of other important physiologic parameters, or (2) address limitations of FDG imaging. The main non–FDG PET tracers that are currently being investigated for radiation therapy planning are markers for cell proliferation and hypoxia. PET tracers labeled with ^{18}F have advantages over others, because the infrastructure for ^{18}F production and national distribution of ^{18}F radiotracers is available because of the commercial production of FDG. The most promising tracers are reviewed here.

^{18}F-Fluorothymidine

^{18}F-fluorothymidine (FLT) is a surrogate tracer for cellular proliferation. FLT is phosphorylated by thymidine kinase in metabolically active cells, where it is trapped intracellularly, but not incorporated into DNA.[34] FLT has relatively high physiologic uptake in the liver and bone marrow, reducing sensitivity for evaluating tumors in these organs.

There have been several pilot studies investigating potential applications for FLT PET/CT in treatment planning. Troost and colleagues[35] performed a study using FLT PET/CT in 10 patients with oropharyngeal tumors, and concluded that radiotherapy dose-escalation planning was feasible using the GTV determined by serial FLT PET/CT scans. Han and colleagues[36] compared treatment planning for esophageal cancer using FDG PET and FLT PET; their findings suggested that lung and cardiac dose was reduced using FLT-based treatment planning. Patel and colleagues[37] compared FDG PET/CT and FLT PET/CT for treatment planning of rectal cancer, and found that the GTV was similar for both tracers. FLT PET has potential advantages over FDG PET for defining therapy targets in brain tumors, because it does not have the high cortical uptake that is intrinsic to FDG.[38]

FLT PET is less susceptible to false-positive activity from inflammatory changes following radiation therapy in esophageal cancer.[39] However, as with FDG, reactive lymph nodes may have FLT uptake that is indistinguishable from active tumor.[40,41]

Hypoxia Tracers

Hypoxia is a major factor in radioresistance, so that imaging hypoxic cells could potentially have great value in treatment planning; for example, enabling delivery of a higher radiation dose to the most resistant cell population.[42] Hypoxia tracers generally enter the target cells where they are reduced and trapped under hypoxic conditions. Under normoxic conditions, the compound is not reduced and is free to exit the cell. Several redox PET tracers have been investigated for the imaging of hypoxic cells, including ^{18}F-labeled fluoromisonidazole (FMISO), fluoroazomycinarabinofuranoside (FAZA), EF5, fluoroerythronitroimidazole, fluoroetanidazole, and ^{64}Cu-, ^{60}Cu-, or ^{62}Cu-labeled diacetyl-bis(N^4-methylthiosemicarbazone) (ATSM).[43] Considerations for incorporating hypoxia imaging into radiation treatment planning have been recently summarized by Thorwarth and Alber.[44]

It has been long established that hypoxia is a significant negative prognostic factor for patients with head and neck cancer, and currently this represents the major use of hypoxia imaging in radiotherapy planning.[45] Several preliminary studies have demonstrated the feasibility of improving tumor control using IMRT treatment plans based on FMISO PET or FAZA PET scans designed to selectively deliver a higher dose to hypoxic tumor regions in patients with head and neck cancer.[46–49] However, there are some potential difficulties in using these hypoxia tracers. Lin and colleagues[50] studied the repeatability of FMISO PET scans in a small study of 7 patients, and found that the pattern of hypoxia changed over 3 days in 4 of the patients. This finding suggests that tumor hypoxia may be a dynamic process with acute and chronic components, which may complicate PET-based treatment planning. In addition, the target-to-background activity of hypoxia tracers is substantially less than is typically seen in FDG PET scans.

SUMMARY

In the past decade, PET has proved to be an indispensable tool in the staging of many malignancies as well as in discriminating responses to therapy. In parallel, technologic advances in radiation therapy planning and delivery have made highly conformal and accurate treatments a reality. Integration of PET into radiation treatment planning is thus a natural evolution of both technologies, as a method of accurate target definition both at the initiation of treatment and during potentially adaptive treatment that is dependent on response. Future research should be focused on determining the potential benefits of such adaptations in a prospective manner, and exploring new tracers that can improve on existing results.

REFERENCES

1. Erdi YE, Mawlawi O, Larson SM, et al. Segmentation of lung lesion volume by adaptive positron emission tomography image thresholding. Cancer 1997;80:2505–9.
2. Patz EF, Lowe VJ, Hoffman JM, et al. Persistent or recurrent bronchogenic carcinoma—detection

with PET and 2-F-18-2-deoxy-D-glucose. Radiology 1994;191:379–82.

3. Nestle U, Kremp S, Schaefer-Schuler A, et al. Comparison of different methods for delineation of F-18-FDG PET-positive tissue for target volume definition in radiotherapy of patients with non-small cell lung cancer. J Nucl Med 2005;46: 1342–8.

4. Black QC, Grills IS, Kestin LL, et al. Defining a radiotherapy target with positron emission tomography. Int J Radiat Oncol Biol Phys 2004;60: 1272–82.

5. Jentzen W, Freudenberg L, Eising EG, et al. Segmentation of PET volumes by iterative image thresholding. J Nucl Med 2007;48:108–14.

6. Werner-Wasik M, Nelson AD, Choi W, et al. What is the best way to contour lung tumors on PET scans? Multiobserver validation of a gradient-based method using a NSCLC digital PET phantom. Int J Radiat Oncol Biol Phys 2012;82:1164–71.

7. Geets X, Lee JA, Bol A, et al. A gradient-based method for segmenting FDG-PET images: methodology and validation. Eur J Nucl Med Mol Imaging 2007;34:1427–38.

8. Li H, Thorstad WL, Biehl KJ, et al. A novel PET tumor delineation method based on adaptive region-growing and dual-front active contours. Med Phys 2008;35:3711–21.

9. Bentzen SM, Gregoire V. Molecular imaging-based dose painting: a novel paradigm for radiation therapy prescription. Semin Radiat Oncol 2011; 21:101–10.

10. Aerts H, Lambin P, De Ruysscher D. FDG for dose painting: a rational choice. Radiother Oncol 2010; 97:163–4.

11. Meijer G, Steenhuijsen J, Bal M, et al. Dose painting by contours versus dose painting by numbers for stage II/III lung cancer: Practical implications of using a broad or sharp brush. Radiother Oncol 2011;100:396–401.

12. Vanderstraeten B, Duthoy W, De Gersem W, et al. F-18 fluoro-deoxy-glucose positron emission tomography (F-18 FDG-PET) voxel intensity-based intensity-modulated radiation therapy (IMRT) for head and neck cancer. Radiother Oncol 2006;79: 249–58.

13. Das SK, Miften MM, Zhou S, et al. Feasibility of optimizing the dose distribution in lung tumors using fluorine-18-fluorodeoxyglucose positron emission tomography and single photon emission computed tomography guided dose prescriptions. Med Phys 2004;31:1452–61.

14. Alber M, Paulsen F, Eschmann SM, et al. On biologically conformal boost dose optimization. Phys Med Biol 2003;48:N31–5.

15. Geets X, Tomsej M, Lee JA, et al. Adaptive biological image-guided IMRT with anatomic and functional imaging in pharyngo-laryngeal tumors: impact on target volume delineation and dose distribution using helical tomotherapy. Radiother Oncol 2007;85:105–15.

16. Aerts H, Bosmans G, van Baardwijk AA, et al. Stability of F-18-deoxyglucose uptake locations within tumor during radiotherapy for NSCLC: a prospective study. Int J Radiat Oncol Biol Phys 2008; 71:1402–7.

17. Madani I, Duprez F, Boterberg T, et al. Maximum tolerated dose in a phase I trial on adaptive dose painting by numbers for head and neck cancer. Radiother Oncol 2011;101:351–5.

18. Higgins KA, Hoang JK, Roach MC, et al. Analysis of pretreatment FDG-PET SUV parameters in head-and-neck cancer: tumor SUV(mean) has superior prognostic value. Int J Radiat Oncol Biol Phys 2012;82:548–53.

19. Gupta T, Jain S, Agarwal JP, et al. Diagnostic performance of response assessment FDG-PET/CT in patients with head and neck squamous cell carcinoma treated with high-precision definitive (chemo)radiation. Radiother Oncol 2010;97:194–9.

20. Day FL, Link E, Ngan S, et al. FDG-PET metabolic response predicts outcomes in anal cancer managed with chemoradiotherapy. Br J Cancer 2011;105:498–504.

21. Everaert H, Hoorens A, Vanhove C, et al. Prediction of response to neoadjuvant radiotherapy in patients with locally advanced rectal cancer by means of sequential ^{18}FDG-PET. Int J Radiat Oncol Biol Phys 2011;80:91–6.

22. Martoni AA, Di Fabio F, Pinto C, et al. Prospective study on the FDG-PET/CT predictive and prognostic values in patients treated with neoadjuvant chemoradiation therapy and radical surgery for locally advanced rectal cancer. Ann Oncol 2011; 22:650–6.

23. Passero VA, Branstetter BF, Shuai Y, et al. Response assessment by combined PET-CT scan versus CT scan alone using RECIST in patients with locally advanced head and neck cancer treated with chemoradiotherapy. Ann Oncol 2010; 21:2278–83.

24. Huang W, Zhou T, Ma L, et al. Standard uptake value and metabolic tumor volume of (18)F-FDG PET/CT predict short-term outcome early in the course of chemoradiotherapy in advanced non-small cell lung cancer. Eur J Nucl Med Mol Imaging 2011;38:1628–35.

25. van Loon J, Offermann C, Ollers M, et al. Early CT and FDG-metabolic tumour volume changes show a significant correlation with survival in stage I-III small cell lung cancer: a hypothesis generating study. Radiother Oncol 2011;99:172–5.

26. Janssen MH, Ollers MC, Riedl RG, et al. Accurate prediction of pathological rectal tumor response

after two weeks of preoperative radiochemotherapy using (18)F-fluorodeoxyglucose-positron emission tomography-computed tomography imaging. Int J Radiat Oncol Biol Phys 2010;77:392–9.

27. Wiegman EM, Pruim J, Ubbels JF, et al. (18)F-FDG PET during stereotactic body radiotherapy for stage I lung tumours cannot predict outcome: a pilot study. Eur J Nucl Med Mol Imaging 2011;38:1059–63.

28. Boellaard R. Standards for PET image acquisition and quantitative data analysis. J Nucl Med 2009;50:11S–20S.

29. Boellaard R, Oyen WJ, Hoekstra CJ, et al. The Netherlands protocol for standardisation and quantification of FDG whole body PET studies in multi-centre trials. Eur J Nucl Med Mol Imaging 2008;35:2320–33.

30. Wu QJ, Li T, Wu Q, et al. Adaptive radiation therapy: technical components and clinical applications. Cancer J 2011;17:182–9.

31. Castadot P, Geets X, Lee JA, et al. Adaptive functional image-guided IMRT in pharyngo-laryngeal squamous cell carcinoma: is the gain in dose distribution worth the effort? Radiother Oncol 2011;101(3):343–50.

32. Simone CB 2nd, Ly D, Dan TD, et al. Comparison of intensity-modulated radiotherapy, adaptive radiotherapy, proton radiotherapy, and adaptive proton radiotherapy for treatment of locally advanced head and neck cancer. Radiother Oncol 2011;101(3):376–82.

33. Guckenberger M, Wilbert J, Richter A, et al. Potential of adaptive radiotherapy to escalate the radiation dose in combined radiochemotherapy for locally advanced non-small cell lung cancer. Int J Radiat Oncol Biol Phys 2011;79:901–8.

34. Shields AF. PET imaging with 18F-FLT and thymidine analogs: promise and pitfalls. J Nucl Med 2003;44:1432–4.

35. Troost EG, Bussink J, Hoffmann AL, et al. ^{18}F-FLT PET/CT for early response monitoring and dose escalation in oropharyngeal tumors. J Nucl Med 2010;51:866–74.

36. Han D, Yu J, Yu Y, et al. Comparison of (18)F-fluorothymidine and (18)F-fluorodeoxyglucose PET/CT in delineating gross tumor volume by optimal threshold in patients with squamous cell carcinoma of thoracic esophagus. Int J Radiat Oncol Biol Phys 2010;76:1235–41.

37. Patel DA, Chang ST, Goodman KA, et al. Impact of integrated PET/CT on variability of target volume delineation in rectal cancer. Technol Cancer Res Treat 2007;6:31–6.

38. Grosu AL, Weber WA. PET for radiation treatment planning of brain tumours. Radiother Oncol 2010;96:325–7.

39. Yue J, Chen L, Cabrera AR, et al. Measuring tumor cell proliferation with ^{18}F-FLT PET during radiotherapy of esophageal squamous cell carcinoma: a pilot clinical study. J Nucl Med 2010;51:528–34.

40. van Waarde A, Elsinga PH. Proliferation markers for the differential diagnosis of tumor and inflammation. Curr Pharm Des 2008;14:3326–39.

41. Troost EG, Vogel WV, Merkx MA, et al. ^{18}F-FLT PET does not discriminate between reactive and metastatic lymph nodes in primary head and neck cancer patients. J Nucl Med 2007;48:726–35.

42. Rajendran JG, Hendrickson KR, Spence AM, et al. Hypoxia imaging-directed radiation treatment planning. Eur J Nucl Med Mol Imaging 2006;33(Suppl 1):44–53.

43. Hoigebazar L, Jeong JM. Hypoxia imaging agents labeled with positron emitters. Recent Results Cancer Res 2012;194:285–99.

44. Thorwarth D, Alber M. Implementation of hypoxia imaging into treatment planning and delivery. Radiother Oncol 2010;97:172–5.

45. Brizel DM, Sibley GS, Prosnitz LR, et al. Tumor hypoxia adversely affects the prognosis of carcinoma of the head and neck. Int J Radiat Oncol Biol Phys 1997;38:285–9.

46. Hendrickson K, Phillips M, Smith W, et al. Hypoxia imaging with [F-18] FMISO-PET in head and neck cancer: potential for guiding intensity modulated radiation therapy in overcoming hypoxia-induced treatment resistance. Radiother Oncol 2011;101:369–75.

47. Choi W, Lee SW, Park SH, et al. Planning study for available dose of hypoxic tumor volume using fluorine-18-labeled fluoromisonidazole positron emission tomography for treatment of the head and neck cancer. Radiother Oncol 2010;97:176–82.

48. Lee NY, Mechalakos JG, Nehmeh S, et al. Fluorine-18-labeled fluoromisonidazole positron emission and computed tomography-guided intensity-modulated radiotherapy for head and neck cancer: a feasibility study. Int J Radiat Oncol Biol Phys 2008;70:2–13.

49. Grosu AL, Souvatzoglou M, Roper B, et al. Hypoxia imaging with FAZA-PET and theoretical considerations with regard to dose painting for individualization of radiotherapy in patients with head and neck cancer. Int J Radiat Oncol Biol Phys 2007;69:541–51.

50. Lin Z, Mechalakos J, Nehmeh S, et al. The influence of changes in tumor hypoxia on dose-painting treatment plans based on ^{18}F-FMISO positron emission tomography. Int J Radiat Oncol Biol Phys 2008;70:1219–28.

Role of Positron Emission Tomography/Computed Tomography in Dementia

Sidney R. Hinds II, MD[a],*, Derek J. Stocker, MD[a],
Yong C. Bradley, MD[b]

KEYWORDS

- Positron emission tomography • Dementia • Amyloid • Tau • PiB • Florbetapir

KEY POINTS

- Numerous positron emission tomography (PET) radiotracers for imaging dementia are being evaluated for efficacy, whereas only a few are clinically available for patient care.
- As the era of molecular imaging proceeds, target-specific imaging for the relevant disease will become more important.
- Further research into the cause and significance of the specific visualized pathologic hallmarks of the dementia disorders will be crucial for directing diagnosis, treatment, and possibly cure.
- At present, an arsenal of PET imaging agents is proving to be an effective tool in the clinical diagnosis of dementia.

INTRODUCTION

Dementia, with a worldwide prevalence of approximately 24 million, covers the broad category of traumatic, metabolic, or neurodegenerative processes that lead to a loss of overall function.[1] Alzheimer disease (AD) is the most common recognized cause of dementia, followed by dementia with Lewy bodies (DLB) and vascular dementia (VaD). A diagnosis of dementia has profound implications for those affected and their loved ones, as well as a significant impact on available health care resources. The United States spends more than $172 billion on the health care costs of AD alone. Although there are no current cures for the neurodegenerative causes of dementia, effective management depends on the most accurate diagnosis of the cause. Positron emission tomography (PET) with its molecular imaging approach is expertly situated to provide increased diagnostic efficacy that can support accurate diagnosis, thus improving disease outcome and morbidity. In an

effort to provide a target-specific PET neuroimaging agent for the evaluation of dementias, the US Food and Drug Administration (FDA) recently approved the amyloid imaging radiotracer (E)-4-(2-(6-(2-(2-(2-(^{18}F-fluoroethoxy)ethoxy)ethoxy) pyridin-3-yl)vinyl)-N-methyl benzenamine, also known as ^{18}F-florbetapir or ^{18}F-AV-45.[2,3] The National Institute of Neurologic and Communicative Disorders and Stroke and Alzheimer's Disease and Related Disorders Association (NINCDS-ADRDA) revises and refines the diagnostic criteria for dementias.[4,5] The goal of establishing clinical dementia criteria is to improve the clinical reliability of a diagnosis of dementia and thus improve the treatment of patients who are diagnosed. Despite guidelines, pathologic findings on autopsy have shown that frontotemporal lobar dementia (FTLD) and AD are clinically misdiagnosed based on clinical criteria alone. Varma and colleagues[6] reported that 77% (20 patients) who were diagnosed with AD had autopsy findings consistent with FTLD. Among the many causes of dementia, clinical

[a] Walter Reed National Military Medical Center, Bethesda, MD 20814, USA; [b] University of Tennessee Medical Center, 1924 Alcoa Highway, Knoxville, TN 37920, USA
* Corresponding author.
E-mail address: sidney.r.hinds.mil@mail.mil

Radiol Clin N Am 51 (2013) 927–934
http://dx.doi.org/10.1016/j.rcl.2013.06.002
0033-8389/13/$ – see front matter © 2013 Elsevier Inc. All rights reserved.

symptoms may overlap, confounding an accurate analysis. The goal of neuroimaging is to aid in the accurate and early diagnosis and therefore provide treatment that is appropriate for the dementia type.

NEUROIMAGING

Anatomic imaging may underdiagnose the various types of dementia, especially when used early in the disease. However, computed tomography (CT) and magnetic resonance (MR) can also have a role in the evaluation of structural abnormalities that may mimic dementia or of other dementia causes, such as space-occupying lesions and stroke. CT does not possess the resolution of MR imaging. Volumetric/morphometric analysis with MR has proved that MR is able to identify areas of neuronal loss, especially in the hippocampus. Walhovd and colleagues[7] used morphometric MR imaging, [^{18}F]-2-fluoro-2-deoxy-D-glucose (FDG) PET, and cerebrospinal fluid (CSF) biomarker methodology and found that the MR volumetric analysis was sensitive to the diagnosis of AD versus normal controls. FDG-PET adds similar information, but FDG-PET and MR imaging, when coupled with CSF biomarkers (tau/Aβ42), increased the differentiation. MR with a morphometric analysis and FDG-PET were superior to CSF biomarkers in clinical prognosis. Nuclear medicine and molecular imaging (particularly PET) offer disorder-specific radiotracers to address the disparate neurologic processes causing dementia. Diffusion tensor imaging (DTI) is another MR technique that may be useful, and not only in differentiating between the various dementias. Based on the anisotropic water diffusion pattern of water within white matter (WM), DTI can image WM bundles to detect fiber loss. WM diminishing fiber loss then represents an indirect measure of neuronal loss.[8]

The ideal PET radiotracer would yield a superior target/background ratio; image the region, function, or disorder of interest; and be readily available for use by a large number of institutions. Numerous agents have been used in attempts to image the pathophysiology of the dementing disorders: ^{15}O-H$_2$0 cerebral (blood flow) perfusion, ^{18}F-FDG (metabolism), ^{11}C/^{18}F amyloid, dopamine, acetylcholine, and ^{11}C microglia ligands. Cyclotrons are not as abundant as PET imaging systems or commercial PET radiotracer distributions centers; therefore short-lived radioligands are less suitable for widespread use of the dementia radiotracers.

AD

Alois Alzheimer described the clinical and pathologic findings of the disease that would bear his name in 1907, but it was not until recently that the development of the amyloid cascade has dominated.[9] The pathogenesis of the phenotype still eludes the medical profession. AD is the most common cause of dementia and may be sporadic or associated with genetic factors (specifically mutation in the amyloid precursor protein, and ε4 allele of apolipoprotein E [APOE4]). The main features of neuronal degeneration in AD are neuronal loss leading to cerebral atrophy especially in the temporal lobe, parietal lobe, posterior cingulate gyrus, and hippocampus. Extracellular amyloid deposition with amyloid-containing neuritic plaques and intracellular neurofibrillary tangles containing tau (microtubule-associated protein) are a pathologic finding in AD.[10] Amyloid accumulation begins early in the disease process, but tau appears earlier, especially in the hippocampus and entorhinal cortex. Tau deposition correlates with the level of cognitive dysfunction, whereas amyloid does not reliably predict disease severity.[11]

FDG is a radioligand that represents the cerebral metabolic rate of glucose (CMR$_{glc}$). With the widespread usage of PET, the commercially available FDG has been the mainstay for clinical imaging. Neurons preferentially use glucose as their source of energy and thus this radiotracer is well suited to evaluate alterations in neuronal/cerebral metabolism. Qualitative visual as well as semiquantitative and quantitative methods have been used to evaluate relative changes in cerebral glucose metabolism.[12–14]

It is widely accepted that the sensitivity and specificity for molecular imaging dementia using FDG are both high. The region and magnitude of FDG hypometabolism directly correlates with the decline in cognitive function once the diagnosis is established.

N-methyl-^{11}C-2-(-4′-methylaminophenyl)-6-hydroxy-benzothiazole (11C-6-OH-BTA-1; also called Pittsburgh compound B [^{11}C-PiB]) heralded the AD target-specific radiotracer. Although not the first amyloid radiotracer to attempt to image Aβ, this radiotracer revealed that a disorder-specific agent may increase the specificity for AD. Klunk and colleagues[15] conducted the first in vivo human trials of ^{11}C-PiB in 2004, revealing the usefulness of this radiotracer in capturing Aβ density. PiB is a benzothiazole chosen because the dye thioflavin-T is able to penetrate the blood-brain barrier and bind to amyloid. It reveals preferential activity, which is consistent with postmortem amyloid deposits, within the frontal, temporal, and parietal cortices. Early in its evaluation, ^{11}C-PiB activity was inversely correlated with FDG activity in patients with AD.[15] Aβ accumulates early and progresses in the AD process. However, it also accumulates in normal aging, healthy adults without cognitive dysfunction, and mild cognitive impairment (MCI). The clinical picture is clouded further because Aβ is also present in other dementias such as DLB. It was apparent early in the evaluation of PET amyloid ligands that the amount or intensity of the identified amyloid deposition did not correlate with the clinical severity of the dementia.[16] In addition, ^{11}C-PiB does not expose the AD-associated disorder in the hippocampus or entorhinal cortex, which is predominantly neurofibrillary tangles. Quantitative analysis and qualitative analysis with ^{11}C-PiB are similar and reportedly have accuracies of 95% and 90%.[13] However, the implementation of cyclotron-produced ^{11}C-PiB caused a race to develop and prove ^{18}F-based PET Aβ radiotracers. Furthermore, ^{18}F has a more favorable half-life of 110 minutes, compared with 20 minutes for [11]C.

As noted earlier, the FDA recently approved ^{18}F florbetapir injections for the evaluation of neurocognitive decline and for AD.[2,3] This action will allow PET centers access to an [18]F Aβ agent. The current indications for use are to estimate brain Aβ density in MCI in patients being evaluated for AD or other cognitive decline. It is not approved for predicting development of AD or monitoring response to AD drugs.[2,3] Wong and colleagues[17] performed the first human trial of ^{18}F-florbetapir and noted similar ^{11}C-PiB patterns of uptake in patients with AD and normal control patients. Activity was greatest in the frontal, temporal, and precuneus lobes in patients with AD. AD-patterned activity was noted in 2 of the control patients, confirming the ^{11}C-PiB findings that cognitively normal individuals may also have Aβ deposition.

Fleischer and colleagues[18] evaluated APOE4 healthy and AD participants and noted that carriers of the APOE4 (healthy normal, MCI, or AD) had increased amyloid activity within the frontal, parietal, and temporal cortices as well as the precuneus and posterior cingulate. This study suggests that APOE4 carriers may hasten AD by up to 20 years. Negative ^{18}F-florbetapir studies occurred in 16% of patients with AD, but none was a carrier of APOE4. This study suggests non-APOE4 carrier AD patients without amyloid activity on imaging represent pathological variants. Low ^{11}C-PiB was noted in patients with the early-onset familial AD Arctic APP mutation who had hypometabolism on FDG-PET.[19] Newberg and colleagues[20] evaluated the observer's ability to differentiate normal participants from participants with clinically diagnosed AD using ^{18}F-florbetapir and FDG. The sensitivity and specificity were 95% and 95% for ^{18}F-florbetapir and 89% and 86% for FDG. Clark and colleagues[21] conducted

a multicenter, prospective cohort trial with ^{18}F-florbetapir to determine the observer's ability to identify Aβ plaques compared with postmortem autopsy results. The sensitivity and specificity were 92% and 100% respectively.

1,1-Dicyano-2-[6-(dimethylamino)naphthalen-2-yl]propene (DDNP), also called ^{18}F-FDDNP, is a radiotracer that has an affinity for amyloid but also binds to tau-containing neurofibrillary tangles.[22] This radioligand may prove more useful in differentiating frontotemporal lobar dementia versus AD, and imaging Parkinson disease, Parkinson disease dementia, or possible chronic traumatic encephalopathy (CTE). ^{18}F-Florbetaben (^{18}F-BAY94-9172) imaging has been used effectively to characterize the Aβ in patients with clinically confirmed AD.[23–25]

Although amyloid ligand imaging accurately documents the density of plaques and aids in the diagnostic assuredness of AD, amyloid-modifying drugs are not meeting with success as therapeutic agents. This failure suggests that amyloid deposition may not be the cause of neuronal demise (**Fig. 1**).[26,27]

FRONTOTEMPORAL LOBAR DEMENTIA

Frontotemporal lobar dementia (FLTD) is categorized as one of the tauopathies, a heterogeneous family of related disorders whose main pathologic feature is the accumulation of intracellular tau.[28,29] FTLD reflects several distinct phenotypes of dementia that present with neuronal loss in the frontal and temporal lobes: frontal or behavioral variant, primary progressive aphasia, semantic dementia, and frontotemporal dementia with motor neuron disease.[10,30] Overlap between FLTD and AD may occur, but the clinical characteristics of FLTD can support a differential diagnosis. FDG in the evaluation is particularly helpful in identifying neuronal loss in the classic frontal lobe and temporal lobes.[31] Aβ deposition is not a pathologic feature of FTLD and therefore imaging with 1 amyloid radioligand has proved to be helpful in differentiating FTLD from AD. Rabinovici and colleagues[32] reported similar qualitative and quantitative sensitivities and specificities for both FDG and ^{11}C-PiB in differentiating between AD (n = 62) and FTLD (n = 45). Histopathology was available for 12 patients. FDG had an accuracy of 87%, whereas the accuracy of PiB was 87% in predicting AD versus FTLD. No FDA-approved drug exists for FTLD. Although acetylcholinesterase (ACh) inhibitors are used to modify AD, FTLD patients have preserved the metabolic functions of acetylcholine. Some reports suggest that ACh inhibitors have effects on frontal lobe function and may be detrimental in

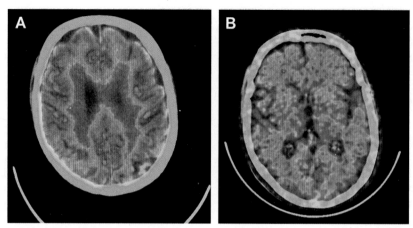

Fig. 1. (A) FDG-PET/CT shows mild to moderately decreased metabolic uptake of the parietal lobes suspicious for Alzheimer disease. (B) ^{18}F-florbetapir reveals cortical uptakes in the frontal and occipital lobes consistent with Alzheimer disease.

FTLD, especially those involved with disinhibition or compulsion.[33] Therefore differentiation between FTLD and AD is clinically relevant and not simply academic. In a pilot study, Chow and colleagues[34] used FDG-PET to evaluate metabolism in the semantic dementia form of FTLD after a 6-month trial of the N-methyl-D-aspartic acid (NMDA) receptor antagonist memantine. Although no clinical improvement was noted in the study patients, a small normalization of cortical metabolism was noted (Fig. 2).

DLB

DLB is the second most common neurodegenerative cause of dementia and is defined by dementia and 2 of the following: fluctuating cognition, visual hallucinations, or movement disorder. On histopathology, alpha-synuclein–containing neuronal inclusions called Lewy bodies and neurites are found predominantly in the substantia nigra, brainstem nuclei, and limbic system.[10,35] In addition, neurofibrillary tangles and amyloid plaques are also seen in DLB. The movement disorder typically associated with DLB consists of extrapyramidal movement consistent with parkinsonism, but the dementia precedes or presents in conjunction with parkinsonism.[10,35,36] Sensitivity to antipsychotic drugs is a well-known component of this disorder and is why distinguishing DLB from other forms of dementia is crucial in the proper medical management of the demented. Also, antiparkinsonism drugs may exacerbate the visual hallucinations and delusion that are prominent in DLB. FDG-PET imaging studies have hypometabolism with the occipital lobes compared with the hypometabolism of the temporal, parietal, and frontal lobes and hippocampus that is seen in AD.

Sensitivity and specificity of FDG in distinguishing DLB from AD has been reported to be 90% and 80% respectively.[37] ^{11}C-PiB has been able to differentiate DLB among normal controls, Parkinson disease dementia (PDD) with MCI, and PDD, and may help to explain the disparate temporal relationship of dementia and parkinsonian movement in PDD and DLB (Fig. 3).[38,39]

PDD

Idiopathic parkinsonism (PD) has a classic presentation of resting tremor, bradykinesia, and cogwheel rigidity. The reported prevalence of patients progressing from PD to PDD varies from approximately 4% to 90%.[28] The chief pathologic abnormalities are the presence of Lewy bodies within the cortices and neuronal degeneration of subcortical cells, especially of dopaminergic neurons in the nigrostriatal region.[40] Using previously known study findings of decreased glucose metabolism within the posterior cingulate, Bohnen and colleagues[40] followed patients with PD without a diagnosis of PDD and imaged them with FDG. When the patients progressed to clinical diagnoses of PDD, decreased glucose metabolism was found in the primary visual cortex, posterior cingulate, and variably within the cortices using statistical parametric analyses.

Patients with PD experience visual hallucinations in the course of the disease process, but hallucinations are late features of PD and the onset is a distinguishing feature compared with DLB.[36] Aβ deposition does not occur as part of PD and therefore Aβ PET imaging does not reveal positive studies. In addition, if the radiotracer is visualized it does not usually reach the significance seen in AD.[38,41]

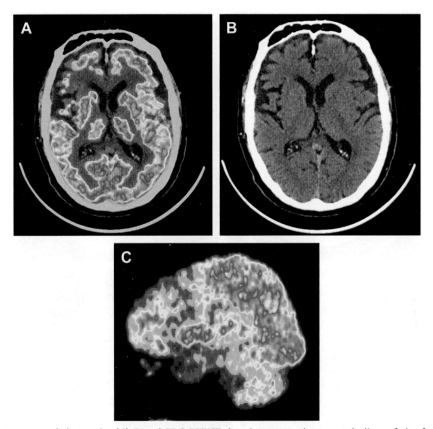

Fig. 2. Frontotemporal dementia. (*A*) Fused FDG-PET/CT showing severe hypometabolism of the frontal lobes, with right greater than left. (*B*) CT showing moderate cortical loss in the frontal lobes. (*C*) Maximal intensity projection reveals the extensive hypometabolism of the frontal and temporal lobes.

VAD

VaD is the third leading cause of dementia. The direct relationship with cerebrovascular disease such as strokes is associated with cognitive deficits and dementia. Hachinski and colleagues[42] dubbed the cognitive decline secondary to several infarcts, multi-infarct dementia. Characteristic patterns of gray matter and WM changes on MR are routinely visualized. Diffusion-weighted MR imaging is particularly useful in evaluating areas of vascular damage. No pathognomonic lesion exists for this dementia type; therefore symptoms are related to involved brain parenchyma. However, they may not fully explain the clinical manifestation. Risk factors include genetic and molecular causes of vascular damage in addition to any factor that contributes to atherosclerosis. The challenge in any imaging modality is to distinguish among the dementia, which usually begins in later decades, and coexisting intracerebral atherosclerotic changes.[43] MR evaluations of patients with dementia are revealing microhemorrhages, which are of unknown significance in the causality of dementia. One of the most common causes of

intracranial bleeds is cerebral amyloid angiopathy (CAA)/CAA-related hemorrhage (CAAH). The link between AD and CAA is still unclear, but it has been reported that up to 30% of patients with CAAH have characteristics of AD. Ly and colleagues[44] performed a prospective study on patients with probable CAAH and confirmed the increased diffuse ^{11}C-PiB cortical activity.

MCI

As emphasized earlier, correctly discriminating among the causes of dementia leads to correct treatment of the affected patient. Patients with MCI, especially amnestic MCI, are most at risk of developing AD. The rate of progression is approximately 10% to 15% per year.[45] In a multicenter longitudinal study, Mosconi and colleagues[12] reported an accuracy of 98% in distinguishing MCI from normal functioning using FDG. Okello and colleagues[45] evaluated MCI to AD converters and noted that 15 of 31 patients with MCI converted to AD. Fourteen of the 15 had ^{11}C-PiB–positive baseline imaging. Accumulation of Aβ precedes the onset of MCI. The accumulation of

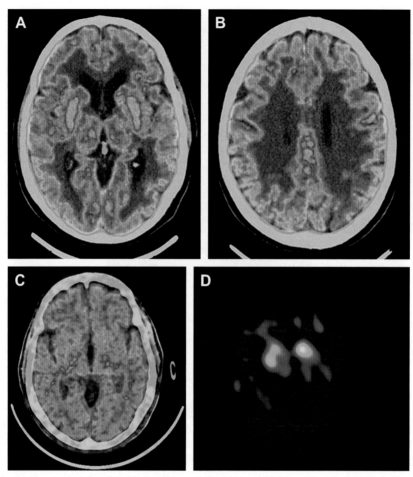

Fig. 3. Lewy body disease. (*A, B*) FDG-PET/CT shows moderate to severe hypometabolism in the occipital and parietal lobes bilaterally. Posterior cingulate gyri are also decreased. (*C*) F-18 florbetapir image reveals diffuse cortical uptake in both the frontal and occipital lobes. (*D*) I Dapscan reveals bilaterally decreased in the basal ganglia consistent with Lewy body disease.

Aβ continues, eventually plateaus, and the radioligand activity does not correlate with the progress of cognitive symptoms. This finding is supported by the imaging results of patients with MCI who proceed to a diagnosis of AD. These patients revealed a similar pattern on amyloid imaging to patients with AD, but did not reveal an appreciable level of increased activity once the clinical diagnosis of AD was made. It seems that clinical symptoms follow neuronal degeneration rather than amyloid deposition.

CENTERS FOR MEDICARE AND MEDICAID SERVICES

At present the only reimbursement for the evaluation of dementia is in the differentiation between AD and frontotemporal lobar dementias. Only FDG-PET is approved for PET imaging, and only when specific prerequisites exist. In addition, FDG-PET imaging may be covered if parts of US Centers for Medicare and Medicaid Services (CMS)–approved clinical trials involving the neurodegenerative diseases that are known to cause dementia are included. Medicare Evidence Development & Coverage Advisory Committee (MED-CAC) met in January 2013 and gave a low to intermediate confidence rating for ^{18}F-florbetapir. CMS will meet in July 2013 to determine whether ^{18}F-florbetapir will be reimbursed.[46,47]

SUMMARY

Numerous PET radiotracers for imaging dementia are being evaluated for efficacy, whereas only a few are clinically available for patient care. As the era of molecular imaging proceeds, target-specific imaging for the relevant disease process will become more important. Further research into the causes and significance of the specific visualized pathologic hallmarks of the dementia disorders will be crucial for directing diagnosis, treatment, and possibly cure. At present, an arsenal of PET imaging agents is proving to be an effective tool in the clinical diagnosis of dementia.

REFERENCES

1. Reitz C, Brayne C, Mayeux R. Epidemiology of Alzheimer disease. Nat Rev Neurol 2011;7(3):137–52.

2. FDA approves 18F-florbetapir PET agent. J Nucl Med 2012;53(6):15N.

3. Yang L, Rieves D, Ganley C. Brain amyloid imaging–FDA approval of florbetapir F18 injection. N Engl J Med 2012;367(10):885–7.

4. Knopman DS, DeKosky ST, Cummings JL, et al. Practice parameter: diagnosis of dementia (an evidence-based review). Report of the Quality Standards Subcommittee of the American Academy of Neurology. Neurology 2001;56(9):1143–53.

5. Petersen RC, Stevens JC, Ganguli M, et al. Practice parameter: early detection of dementia: mild cognitive impairment (an evidence-based review). Report of the Quality Standards Subcommittee of the American Academy of Neurology. Neurology 2001;56(9):1133–42.

6. Varma AR, Snowden JS, Lloyd JJ, et al. Evaluation of the NINCDS-ADRDA criteria in the differentiation of Alzheimer's disease and frontotemporal dementia. J Neurol Neurosurg Psychiatry 1999;66(2):184–8.

7. Walhovd KB, Fjell AM, Brewer J, et al. Combining MR imaging, positron-emission tomography, and CSF biomarkers in the diagnosis and prognosis of Alzheimer disease. AJNR Am J Neuroradiol 2010;31(2):347–54.

8. Oishi K, Mielke MM, Albert M, et al. DTI analyses and clinical applications in Alzheimer's disease. J Alzheimers Dis 2011;26(Suppl 3):287–96.

9. Cipriani G, Dolciotti C, Picchi L, et al. Alzheimer and his disease: a brief history. Neurol Sci 2010;32(2):275–9.

10. Daroff RB, Bradley WG. Bradley's neurology in clinical practice. 6th edition. Philadelphia: Elsevier/Saunders; 2012.

11. Harrington CR. The molecular pathology of Alzheimer's disease. Neuroimaging Clin N Am 2012;22(1):11–22, vii.

12. Mosconi L, Tsui WH, Herholz K, et al. Multicenter standardized 18F-FDG PET diagnosis of mild cognitive impairment, Alzheimer's disease, and other dementias. J Nucl Med 2008;49(3):390–8.

13. Ng S, Villemagne VL, Berlangieri S, et al. Visual assessment versus quantitative assessment of 11C-PIB PET and 18F-FDG PET for detection of Alzheimer's disease. J Nucl Med 2007;48(4):547–52.

14. Lopresti BJ, Klunk WE, Mathis CA, et al. Simplified quantification of Pittsburgh compound B amyloid imaging PET studies: a comparative analysis. J Nucl Med 2005;46(12):1959–72.

15. Klunk WE, Engler H, Nordberg A, et al. Imaging brain amyloid in Alzheimer's disease with Pittsburgh compound-B. Ann Neurol 2004;55(3):306–19.

16. Wolk DA, Price JC, Madeira C, et al. Amyloid imaging in dementias with atypical presentation. Alzheimers Dement 2012;8(5):389–98.

17. Wong DF, Rosenberg PB, Zhou Y, et al. In vivo imaging of amyloid deposition in Alzheimer disease using the radioligand 18F-AV-45 (flobetapir F 18). J Nucl Med 2010;51(6):913–20.

18. Fleisher AS, Chen K, Liu X, et al. Apolipoprotein E epsilon4 and age effects on florbetapir positron emission tomography in healthy aging and Alzheimer disease. Neurobiol Aging 2013;34(1):1–12.

19. Scholl M, Wall A, Thordardottir S, et al. Low PiB PET retention in presence of pathologic CSF biomarkers in Arctic APP mutation carriers. Neurology 2012;79(3):229–36.

20. Newberg AB, Arnold SE, Wintering N, et al. Initial clinical comparison of 18F-florbetapir and 18F-FDG PET in patients with Alzheimer disease and controls. J Nucl Med 2012;53(6):902–7.

21. Clark CM, Pontecorvo MJ, Beach TG, et al. Cerebral PET with florbetapir compared with neuropathology at autopsy for detection of neuritic amyloid-beta plaques: a prospective cohort study. Lancet Neurol 2012;11(8):669–78.

22. Shin J, Kepe V, Barrio JR, et al. The merits of FDDNP-PET imaging in Alzheimer's disease. J Alzheimers Dis 2011;26(Suppl 3):135–45.

23. Rowe CC, Ackerman U, Browne W, et al. Imaging of amyloid beta in Alzheimer's disease with 18F-BAY94-9172, a novel PET tracer: proof of mechanism. Lancet Neurol 2008;7(2):129–35.

24. Villemagne VL, Mulligan RS, Pejoska S, et al. Comparison of 11C-PiB and 18F-florbetaben for Abeta imaging in ageing and Alzheimer's disease. Eur J Nucl Med Mol Imaging 2012;39(6):983–9.

25. Villemagne VL, Ong K, Mulligan RS, et al. Amyloid imaging with (18)F-florbetaben in Alzheimer disease and other dementias. J Nucl Med 2011;52(8):1210–7.

26. Niedowicz DM, Nelson PT, Murphy MP. Alzheimer's disease: pathological mechanisms and recent insights. Curr Neuropharmacol 2012;9(4):674–84.

27. Lee VM. Amyloid binding ligands as Alzheimer's disease therapies. Neurobiol Aging 2002;23(6):1039–42.

28. Kadir A, Nordberg A. Target-specific PET probes for neurodegenerative disorders related to dementia. J Nucl Med 2010;51(9):1418–30.

29. Goedert M, Hasegawa M. The tauopathies: toward an experimental animal model. Am J Pathol 1999;154(1):1–6.

30. Neary D, Snowden JS, Gustafson L, et al. Frontotemporal lobar degeneration: a consensus on clinical diagnostic criteria. Neurology 1998;51(6):1546–54.

31. Jeong Y, Cho SS, Park JM, et al. 18F-FDG PET findings in frontotemporal dementia: an SPM analysis of 29 patients. J Nucl Med 2005;46(2):233–9.

32. Rabinovici GD, Rosen HJ, Alkalay A, et al. Amyloid vs FDG-PET in the differential diagnosis of AD and FTLD. Neurology 2011;77(23):2034–42.

33. Mendez MF, Shapira JS, McMurtray A, et al. Preliminary findings: behavioral worsening on donepezil in patients with frontotemporal dementia. Am J Geriatr Psychiatry 2007;15(1):84–7.

34. Chow TW, Fam D, Graff-Guerrero A, et al. Fluorodeoxyglucose positron emission tomography in semantic dementia after 6 months of memantine: an open-label pilot study. Int J Geriatr Psychiatry 2013;28(3):319–25.

35. Macijauskiene J, Lesauskaite V. Dementia with Lewy bodies: the principles of diagnostics, treatment, and management. Medicina (Kaunas) 2012;48(1):1–8.

36. McKeith IG, Dickson DW, Lowe J, et al. Diagnosis and management of dementia with Lewy bodies: third report of the DLB Consortium. Neurology 2005;65(12):1863–72.

37. Minoshima S, Foster NL, Sima AA, et al. Alzheimer's disease versus dementia with Lewy bodies: cerebral metabolic distinction with autopsy confirmation. Ann Neurol 2001;50(3):358–65.

38. Gomperts SN, Locascio JJ, Marquie M, et al. Brain amyloid and cognition in Lewy body diseases. Mov Disord 2012;27(8):965–73.

39. Gomperts SN, Rentz DM, Moran E, et al. Imaging amyloid deposition in Lewy body diseases. Neurology 2008;71(12):903–10.

40. Bohnen NI, Koeppe RA, Minoshima S, et al. Cerebral glucose metabolic features of Parkinson disease and incident dementia: longitudinal study. J Nucl Med 2011;52(6):848–55.

41. Petrou M, Bohnen NI, Muller ML, et al. Abeta-amyloid deposition in patients with Parkinson disease at risk for development of dementia. Neurology 2012;79(11):1161–7.

42. Hachinski VC, Lassen NA, Marshall J. Multi-infarct dementia. A cause of mental deterioration in the elderly. Lancet 1974;2(7874):207–10.

43. Korczyn AD, Vakhapova V, Grinberg LT. Vascular dementia. J Neurol Sci 2012;322(1–2):2–10.

44. Ly JV. 11C-PIB binding is increased in patients with cerebral amyloid angiopathy-related hemorrhage. Neurology 2010;74(6):487–93.

45. Okello A, Koivunen J, Edison P, et al. Conversion of amyloid positive and negative MCI to AD over 3 years: an 11C-PIB PET study. Neurology 2009; 73(10):754–60.

46. MEDCAC Meeting 1/30/2013-Beta amyloid positron emission tomography (PET) in dementia and neurodegenerative disease. 2012. Available at: http://www.cms.gov/medicare-coverage-database/details/medcac-meeting-details.aspx?MEDCACId=66&TimeFrame=90&DocType=All&bc=AQAAIAAAAAAA&. Accessed September 16, 2012.

47. Medicare national coverage determinations manual chapter 1, part 4 (sections 200-310.1) coverage determinations (Rev.08/03/12). 2012 [PET coverage determinations]. Available at: http://www.cms.gov/Regulations-and-Guidance/Guidance/Manuals/Downloads/ncd103c1_Part4.pdf. Accessed September 16, 2012.

Index

Note: Page numbers of article titles are in **boldface** type.

Radiol Clin N Am 51 (2013) 935–940
http://dx.doi.org/10.1016/S0033-8389(13)00138-3
0033-8389/13/$ – see front matter © 2013 Elsevier Inc. All rights reserved.

radiologic.theclinics.com

Moving?

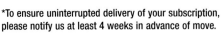

Make sure your subscription moves with you!

To notify us of your new address, find your **Clinics Account Number** (located on your mailing label above your name), and contact customer service at:

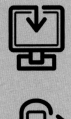

Email: journalscustomerservice-usa@elsevier.com

800-654-2452 (subscribers in the U.S. & Canada)
314-447-8871 (subscribers outside of the U.S. & Canada)

Fax number: 314-447-8029

Elsevier Health Sciences Division
Subscription Customer Service
3251 Riverport Lane
Maryland Heights, MO 63043

*To ensure uninterrupted delivery of your subscription, please notify us at least 4 weeks in advance of move.